THE

Administrative
DENTAL ASSISTANT

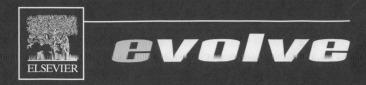

ELSEVIER

evolve

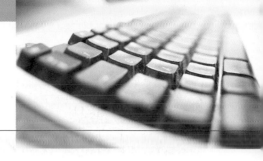

THE
Administrative
DENTAL ASSISTANT

LINDA J. GAYLOR, RDA

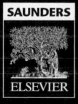

SAUNDERS

ELSEVIER

SECOND EDITION

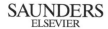

11830 Westline Industrial Drive
St. Louis, Missouri 63146

THE ADMINISTRATIVE DENTAL ASSISTANT,
SECOND EDITION

ISBN-13: 978-1-4160-2566-5
ISBN-10: 1-4160-2566-9

ISBN-13: 978-1-4160-2566-5
ISBN-10: 1-4160-2566-9

Publishing Director: Linda Duncan
Senior Editor: John Dolan
Developmental Editor: John Dedeke
Editorial Assistant: Marcia Bunda
Publishing Services Manager: Pat Joiner
Senior Project Manager: Karen M. Rehwinkel
Design Direction: Julia Dummitt
Cover Designer: Julia Dummitt

Printed in Canada

Last digit is the print number: 9 8 7 6 5 4 3 2 1

The second edition of The Administrative Dental Assistant
*is dedicated to Vivian Muensterman,
my mentor and friend.*

*As a teacher, the student was always first.
Her caring heart, enthusiastic teaching style,
and amazing personality inspired countless students
to achieve more than they ever thought possible.*

*As a mentor, Vivian inspired new and old teachers
with her creativity, passion, love,
and dedication to the noblest of all professions, teaching.*

REVIEWERS

Roberto Albano, CDA, RDH, Med
Professor
Dental Radiology and Dental Assisting
Center for Business and Technology
Springfield Technical Community College
Springfield, Massachusetts

Robin M. Caplan, CDA, QDT, DRT
Owings Mills, Maryland

Scott Chavez, RDA
Director
Dental Assisting Program
Bryman College
Los Angeles, California

Tracy McLaughlin, MPA
Dental Instructor
IntelliTec Medical Institute
Colorado Springs, Colorado

Janet Wilburn, CDA
Director
Dental Assisting Program
Phoenix College
Phoenix, Arizona

Tracy Wilson
Dental Assisting Instructor
IntelliTec Medical Institute
Colorado Springs, Colorado

ABOUT THE AUTHOR

Linda Gaylor holds a Bachelor of Science degree in Public Administration, with a minor in Organizational Management, and a Master of Education degree from the University of La Verne. She currently holds RDA licensure from California and the DANB CDPMA. Organization membership includes the American Dental Assistants Association and Health Occupations Students of America. Ms. Gaylor worked extensively in private practice as an administrative assistant, office manager, and registered dental assistant for more than 20 years. She also developed and participated in a consulting firm specializing in dental and medical business office organization and insurance processing. Ms.

Gaylor's career also includes 15 years of classroom and clinical instruction teaching registered dental assisting, dental assisting, and administrative dental assisting.

Currently Ms. Gaylor is employed by the California Department of Education (CDE) as a health science and medical technology education program consultant. Duties at the CDE include serving as State Advisor for HOSA, assisting in statewide health science and medical technology program coordination, and acting as lead consultant for the development and adoption of the California Career and Technical Education Model Curriculum Standards and Framework (standards adopted May 2005).

PREFACE

In today's dental practices, organizing and operating an efficient dental business presents many challenges. A well-qualified administrative dental assistant will understand basic business concepts, understand all facets of the dental practice, and be a loyal and active member of the dental healthcare team. The purpose of this book is to provide a comprehensive textbook that illustrates the functions of the dental business office and to provide information on how to organize tasks, complete procedures, develop effective communication skills, and acquire a professional outlook toward dentistry.

The second edition of *The Administrative Dental Assistant* continues to provide the basic skill and knowledge necessary to work in a progressive dental practice. Added to this edition are the introduction and application of regulations enacted by the Health Insurance Portability and Accountability Act of 1996 (HIPAA) and real-world computer application (activities in the workbook). As we move away from the traditional paper-based dental practice into a computer-based environment, it will be necessary to become proficient in basic essential skills, such as problem solving, critical thinking, teamwork, and leadership, to adapt to the new and emerging technology. Although the technology is changing, the basic procedures and routines remain the same. For an administrative assistant to move beyond a data entry technician it will be necessary to become skilled in communications, basic bookkeeping, appointment control, and records management, as well as fundamental dental procedures and terminology. With a solid foundation, the administrative dental assistant will be able to quickly adapt to the rapidly changing role of technology in the field of dental practice management.

Specifically in this second edition the reader will find the following:
- Application of HIPAA regulations
- Basic dental anatomy, charting, terminology, and common dental procedures
- Communication skills that take into consideration the entire dental healthcare team, patient relations, record management, and risk management
- Controlled record management
- Effective scheduling, insurance processing, recall systems, and inventory control, with suggested steps for developing a routine
- A basic foundation in bookkeeping accounts receivable and payable in which theories can be applied to a manual system and transferred to a computerized system
- A needs assessment for a computerized system and application of current technology; introduction to Dentrix, a leading dental practice software system
- Employment skills necessary to obtain a position as an administrative dental assistant and assistance in cultivating skills necessary to remain employed

The Administrative Dental Assistant package includes a textbook, interactive CD-ROM, workbook (practical application of a variety of tasks, both manual and computerized), and an instructor's manual. The book and accompanying ancillaries include many features that encourage learning and cultivate comprehension. Critical Thinking Questions challenge the student to reach beyond basic learning, to research subjects, and to express an opinion based on knowledge obtained in the textbook, additional resources, and interactive discussions.

THE TEXTBOOK

The following features are included in the textbook to help the student learn facts, apply procedures, synthesize concepts, and evaluate outcomes:
- Outlines at the beginning of each chapter can be used as a study guide.
- Key terms and concepts identify terminology and concepts that are highlighted in the chapter.
- Objectives clearly state what the student needs to know and be able to do.
- HIPAA boxes identify where regulations need to be applied.

- "Remember" icons alert the student to important information.
- "Food for Thought" boxes emphasize relevant principles.
- Boxed information is used to highlight key points, organize information, and give examples for easy reference.
- Examples show what or what not to say or do as an administrative dental assistant.
- "Anatomy of" illustrations show the function of forms and procedures used by the administrative dental assistant through labeling of key features.
- Illustrations and figures offer visual support in the explanation of information and procedures.
- Step-by-step procedures show the student, simply and logically, how to perform business office tasks correctly and completely.
- Key points at the end of each chapter summarize the chapter and can be used as a study tool.
- Critical Thinking Questions challenge the student to evaluate information, perform problem-solving tasks, research and support answers, and complete tasks.
- Web Watch identifies locations for additional information on relevant topics. Although websites change, these sites should offer resources and links to other sites.
- The Glossary at the end of the text defines terms and concepts as they apply to the text.

THE COMPANION CD-ROM

The features of the interactive software included in this textbook are designed to guide the student through simulated tasks typical to a dental business office. Students can begin exploring elements of the CD from the beginning. Each "day of the week" in the program increases the difficulty and introduces new concepts. Concepts are directly related to material in the textbook. Later days of the week will require students to independently apply information and concepts that they have learned in the textbook. Students may find the exercises to have more significance after completing Chapters 3 through 15.

The interactive program simulates a "Day in the Life of an Administrative Dental Assistant" and challenges students to complete tasks as they would occur in the work place. Students organize functions, prioritize tasks, solve problems, and complete daily tasks typical of an administrative dental assistant.

- With the use of a mouse and a simulated computer screen, students will select a variety of tasks that are typical in practice management software: enter and update patient data, post payment and treatment procedures using codes, submit insurance e-claims for payment, evaluate reports, and schedule appointments.
- Patients arrive for appointments and the student must complete related tasks (update patient information and complete the checkout process). The mail arrives on a daily basis and must be processed. The telephone rings and the student must take care of the caller.
- Popups ask the student questions about a particular subject relevant to the task at hand. Prompts inform students if they have answered the question correctly or incorrectly and give a rationale (students are able to go back and view the correct response if they have answered incorrectly).

THE WORKBOOK

New to the workbook is the inclusion of a fully functional copy of DENTRIX, a leading dental practice management software program. The student will be able to manage a dental practice, create patient files, and perform common tasks required in a computerized dental practice.

The design of the workbook helps students apply information they have learned in a fun and stimulating way. The activities are project based and simulate a real-world application. Each activity is integrated and provides the student with guided and independent practice. At the conclusion of the project the student will have completed a variety of routine daily functions of a dental business office.

- Objectives are stated at the beginning of the chapter and identify what the student will accomplish.
- Exercises include listing and defining terms, multiple choice questions, short answers, puzzles and, when applicable, completing relevant forms and computer application.
- Activities are designed to be completed sequentially, simulating real-world conditions and application.

Dentrix practice management software activities include guided practice through structured tutorials and independent practice with real-world routines and application.

THE INSTRUCTOR'S RESOURCE MANUAL

Features of the instructor's resource manual include answers to exercises and a section on additional activities that can be applied to the lesson. The instructor's resource manual also includes the following:

- Questions, Critical Thinking Questions, and Activities identified by objective
- Answers to exercises and puzzles in the student workbook
- Test Bank and Test Bank Answer Key with answers and rationales
- Additional classroom activities

TEXTBOOK ADAPTATION

The textbook and ancillaries have been carefully designed to provide the skills and knowledge necessary for the efficient operation of a dental business office and can be adapted and adopted for the following:

- A one-semester course for the administrative dental assistant
- To fulfill the business component of a dental assisting course
- As a resource for those dental assistants who want to upgrade their skills
- As a resource for review before an examination
- As a resource for an on-the-job trained administrative dental assistant
- As a basic course with real-world application for dental hygiene and dental students

LINDA J. GAYLOR

ACKNOWLEDGMENTS

A project such as this does not happen in a vacuum. It is the result of countless hours of hard work by all those involved. First and foremost is the support of my family and friends. Their understanding and encouragement is the motivation that kept me going. A special thank you to my sons, Phil and Rob; daughters-in-law, Diane and Deanna; and my grandchildren, Kyra, Justin, and Stephen, who served as models throughout the text. Thanks also to Margie Shamblin, Baldy View Regional Occupational Program, Registered Dental Assisting Program, for providing valued resources and opening their clinic for photo sessions.

I extend a special thank you to William Domb, DMD, for his contributions to dentistry and to dental assisting education, and for his photographic talents. Dr. Domb shared his talent, time, staff, and office during the production of several photographs used throughout this text. In addition, over the years he has served on numerous committees and panels, contributing professional expertise and sharing his love of dentistry.

I acknowledge the contribution of the entire publishing team at Elsevier: John Dolan, John Dedeke, Marcia Bunda, Karen Rehwinkel, and Julia Dummitt.

Thank you to the entire group of professionals, family, and friends that have made the dream of *The Administrative Dental Assistant* a reality.

CONTENTS

THE

Administrative
DENTAL ASSISTANT

OUTLINE

KEY TERMS AND CONCEPTS

Administrative Dental Assistant
Administrative Simplification
American Dental Assistants Association
Appointment Clerk
Board of Dental Examiners
Bookkeeper
Business Manager
Certified Dental Assistant
Certified Dental Practice Management Assistant
Chairside Dental Assistant
Circulating (Roving) Assistant
Code on Dental Procedures and Nomenclature
Current Dental Terminology
Data Processor
Dental Assisting National Board, Inc.
Dental Auxiliary
Dental Healthcare Team

Dental Hygienist
Dental Practice Act
Dental Public Health
Doctor of Dental Surgery
Doctor of Medical Dentistry
Electronic Protected Health Information
Endodontics
Ethics
Expanded (Extended) Function Assistant
Health Insurance Portability and Accountability Act of 1996
HOSA
Insurance Clerk
Legal Standards
Licensure
National Provider Identifier Standard
Occupational Safety and Health Administration (OSHA)

Office Manager
Oral and Maxillofacial Pathology
Oral and Maxillofacial Radiology
Oral and Maxillofacial Surgery
Orthodontics and Dentofacial Orthopedics
Pediatric Dentistry
Periodontics
Privacy Officer
Prosthodontics
Protected Health Information
Receptionist
Records Manager
Registration
Standards for Privacy of Individually Identifiable Health Information
Standards for Security of Individually Identifiable Health Information
Transactions and Code Sets

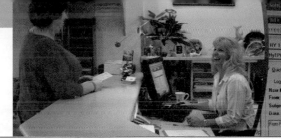
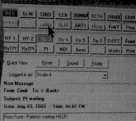

CHAPTER 1

Orientation to the Dental Profession

LEARNING OBJECTIVES

The student will:

1. List the different traits of an administrative dental assistant.
2. Describe the many roles of the administrative dental assistant, office manager, business manager, receptionist, insurance clerk, records manager, data processor, bookkeeper, and appointment clerk.
3. Name the various members of the dental healthcare team and discuss the roles they play in the delivery of dental care.
4. Identify the rules and function of the Health Insurance Portability and Accountability Act of 1996, Administrative Simplification, as it applies to the dental healthcare system.
5. Examine the American Dental Association's *Principles of Ethics and Code of Professional Conduct* and demonstrate an understanding of their content by explaining, discussing, and applying the principles.

INTRODUCTION

The dental profession in the 21st century will be a complex healthcare delivery system. The profession will use the latest technology and will demand caring, well-trained, multiskilled dental auxiliaries. The dental assistant will require knowledge of all phases of the dental practice and of the daily business operations. Those who excel and become vital members of the dental healthcare team will have mastered multiple skills, will be flexible, and will work well in a team environment.

The primary objective of dentistry is to provide quality care for all patients. This care is given without regard to social standing, insurance coverage, ethnic background, or ability to pay. A dentist can provide quality care for all patients only if the total picture of dentistry is taken into consideration.

Dentistry is a service of providing dental care to improve and maintain dental health. Dental professionals of the 21st century will need to consider the business side of dentistry in the total treatment of their patients. Without a well-developed business understanding, the dental healthcare team will not be able to satisfy the needs of their patients. Patients want and will demand that they be treated by qualified professionals, who provide quality care while treating them as individuals. Patients will expect to be treated with respect for themselves and their time, they will expect that the dental healthcare team members will be skillful in the performance of their duties, and they will expect the dental healthcare team to work in harmony. A service-based business is considered successful when it meets the needs of the people it serves.

An effective **dental healthcare team** can be described as a group of dental professionals, including dentists and dental auxiliaries, who work together to provide a service (Figure 1-1). This service blends technical skills with "people skills." The dental healthcare team is technically competent, compassionate, caring, fair, and well rooted in strong ethical principles. The dental healthcare team works in harmony and always places the needs of the patients first. The dental healthcare team considers patients as whole persons and attends to their needs accordingly.

YOUR ROLE AS THE ADMINISTRATIVE DENTAL ASSISTANT

Fifty years ago, the role of the dental receptionist was simplistic. The duties included greeting patients, answering the telephone, scheduling appointments, performing basic bookkeeping tasks, and occasionally filing a dental insurance claim form. As the century progressed, the receptionist's role evolved. As the duties have changed, so has the title. Today, the role of the administrative assistant is complex. The assistant may be required to manage office staff, organize a marketing campaign, be familiar with several types of healthcare delivery systems, and perform computerized tasks daily.

Because of the wide range of duties and responsibilities of the administrative assistant, dental professionals are not in agreement on the type of training that is required. Some believe that the duties of the administrative assistant are business in nature and do not require an understanding of technical dentistry. Business duties that can be expected of the administrative assistant may include:

- Knowledge of computers and several different software packages, computerized patient databases, insurance claims, word processing, accounting, electronic transfers via on-line services, Web page development, and the Internet.
- Operation of electronic business machines, such as fax machines, calculators, photocopiers, electronic credit card transmission devices, voice mail, and multiline telephones.
- Knowledge of bookkeeping practices, such as accounts receivable, accounts payable, banking, payroll, and accounting reports and records.
- Ability to communicate, both in writing and verbally, with patients, dental healthcare team members, and other dental professionals.
- Use of business management skills for staff development and supervision, marketing strategies, contract negotiations, and legal and ethical issues.

Other dental professionals believe that the duties of the administrative assistant can be carried out efficiently by a chairside dental assistant. The knowledge and skills of the chairside assistant are needed to schedule appointments efficiently, to

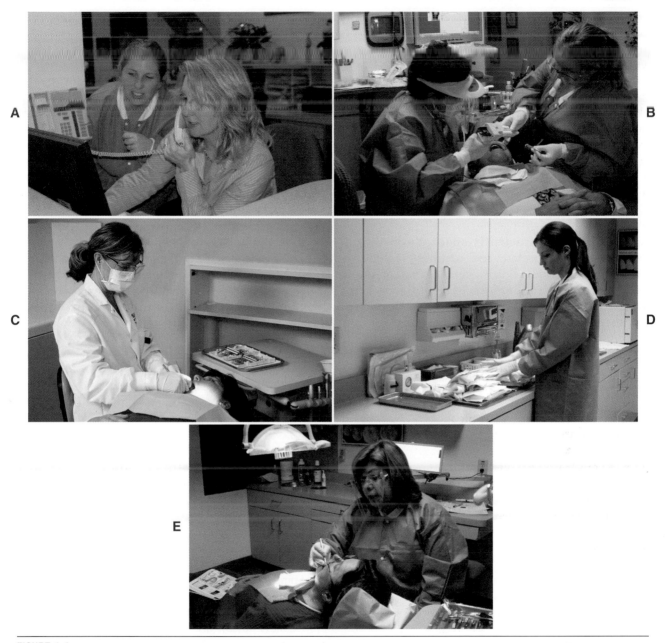

FIGURE 1-1

Dental healthcare team. **A,** The business office staff; **B,** Dentist and chairside assistants; **C,** Dental hygienist; **D,** Circulating (roving) assistant; **E,** Expanded (extended) function assistant. (**A, B, D,** and **E,** Courtesy William C. Domb, Upland, California. **C** from Bird D, Robinson D: Torres and Ehrlich Modern Dental Assisting, 8th ed, St. Louis, Saunders, 2005.)

communicate by means of dental terminology, to process dental insurance claims, to correctly code procedures for posting, to make entries in patients' clinical records, and to perform chairside assistant duties when additional help is needed in the clinical area. However, all dental professionals agree that the administrative dental assistant must be talented in patient and staff relations and must be an outstanding communicator and an active participant on the dental healthcare team.

TYPES OF ADMINISTRATIVE ASSISTANTS

The role of an **administrative dental assistant** is important, multifaceted, and complex. Depending on the size of the dental practice, the range of duties varies. In small dental practices, all of the business office duties may be assigned to one or two administrative assistants. These duties overlap and are woven into the daily activities of the business office. It is difficult sometimes to discern where one job description begins and the other leaves off. In larger dental practices, duties are divided and are given specific job titles. These titles and their corresponding duties include the following.

Office Manager

The **office manager** typically organizes and oversees the daily operations of the office staff. In a small office or a solo practice, this may be required in addition to other administrative assistant duties. In the larger, multipractitioner practice, this could be the sole responsibility of one person. The office manager's duties include:
- Formulating and carrying out office policy
- Managing business and clinical staff
- Scheduling staff
- Resolving conflicts
- Hiring and terminating business office and clinical staff
- Organizing and conducting staff development
- Being a liaison between the owner/dentist and the staff

Business Manager

In large practices, the owner of the business may be a dentist, a group of dentists, or a corporation with several locations. The business operation of the dental practice may be assigned to a **business manager.** The business manager's duties include:
- Managing the fiscal operation
- Developing marketing campaigns
- Negotiating contracts with managed care providers
- Overseeing compliance with insurance, managed care, and government programs

Receptionist

In the past, the duties of the business office were assigned to the **receptionist.** With the growth of dental practices and increased business responsibilities, the role of the receptionist has changed and is vital to the success of the dental practice.

During a patient's initial telephone call, the voice and attitude of the receptionist help determine whether the patient will have a positive or negative opinion of the dental practice. When patients arrive for their first appointment, it is the receptionist who is the first to greet them. Again, if the receptionist conveys a negative impression, in either appearance or attitude, patients may develop a negative opinion about the remainder of the staff and the quality of the dental care they are about to receive. The single most important role of the receptionist is to help the patient formulate a positive impression of the dental practice by projecting a positive and helpful attitude. Without a positive reception, patients may seek dental treatment elsewhere.

The responsibilities of the receptionist include:
- Projecting a positive attitude
- Greeting patients
- Answering the telephone
- Managing incoming and outgoing mail
- Collecting patient data
- Answering patient questions
- Being a liaison between the patient and the dentist
- Making financial arrangements

Insurance Clerk

The **insurance clerk** has one of the most important functions in the dental practice. It is the responsibility of the insurance clerk to oversee the filing of insurance claims. Before claims can be processed, the insurance clerk must gather all necessary information and documentation. In addition to filing insurance claims, the insurance clerk tracks and monitors claims to ensure that they are paid in a timely manner.

An insurance clerk's duties include:
- Collecting insurance data
- Verifying eligibility
- Determining benefits
- Communicating benefits to the patient
- Filing preauthorization forms
- Coding procedures
- Filing completed claims for payment
- Tracking the progress of insurance claims
- Collecting copayments from patients

Records Manager

The **records manager** organizes and maintains all aspects of patients' clinical charts according to preset standards. They establish and maintain an efficient filing system, ensuring that all clinical records have been placed in their correct locations.

The records manager's duties include:
- Collecting patient history
- Ensuring compliance with industry standards
- Ensuring confidentiality and accuracy
- Keeping records safe from destruction and loss

Data Processor

When a computerized system is used in a dental practice, it is necessary for the information to be keyed into the computer. The **data processor** is responsible for entering data into the computer system. This information is collected from various sources, such as patient registration forms, to create a computerized patient record.

The data processor uses various computer skills to perform different tasks, such as:
- Generating accounting reports
- Generating dental insurance claims
- Transmitting dental insurance claims electronically
- Recording chairside dental treatment
- Keeping books
- Managing patient clinical records
- Generating letters of referral to specialists
- Producing newsletters
- Maintaining a recall system
- Sending electronic mail

Bookkeeper

All bookkeeping entries must be made according to an approved method of record keeping. The purpose of bookkeeping is to track all fees, all money collected, and all money paid out. A bookkeeping system shows the amount charged for a service (fee), the amount collected for a service (income), and the amount still owed for a service (accounts receivable). It would be very difficult to understand a dental practice's financial status if it had no bookkeeping system. The Internal Revenue Service (IRS) uses bookkeeping information to calculate the amount of money owed for taxes. As is discussed in greater detail later, bookkeeping records are considered legal documents. They should never be altered or changed.

In addition to tracking the monies collected and the monies owed, the **bookkeeper** records and maintains the accounts payable. Accounts payable is a record of the money that the dental practice owes to others. These accounts include payroll, taxes, and unpaid bills. The bookkeeper maintains records of the amount of money deposited into checking and savings accounts and uses a checking system (manual check writing or electronic debt accounts) to pay vendors.

Not all dental practices hire a full-time bookkeeper. In some practices, an administrative assistant or assistants maintain the basic records and an accountant is hired to audit the records, prepare reports, and file tax returns.

The bookkeeper's duties include:
- Maintaining accounts receivable records
- Maintaining accounts payable records
- Writing checks (written or electronic transfer)
- Depositing money collected into checking and savings accounts
- Maintaining accurate and truthful records
- Paying employees
- Filing tax and payroll reports with the IRS
- Depositing tax money according to IRS and state regulations (payroll and income taxes)

Appointment Clerk

It is vital to the efficiency and success of a dental practice that appointments be scheduled so that the productivity of the dental team is maximized. Efficient scheduling minimizes the patient's stress, resulting in a positive dental experience.

The **appointment clerk's** duties include:

- Organizing and maintaining the daily patient schedule
- Assigning patients to appointment times that meet the needs of both patients and the dental practice
- Scheduling patients in a timely manner
- Maximizing the daily schedule so that personnel can work smarter, not harder
- Balancing the schedule to reduce stress among the dental healthcare team and patients
- Tracking dental treatments (determining which treatments have not been completed)
- Maintaining a recall system

PERSONAL TRAITS OF AN ADMINISTRATIVE DENTAL ASSISTANT

The administrative dental assistant's duties may be assigned to several people or to a few, depending on the size and complexity of the practice. It is clear that a successful dental practice in the 21st century will depend on careful selection of those who play key roles in the daily operation of the practice.

The personal traits of the administrative assistant are varied. The assistant should:

- Be flexible and able to do more than one job at a time
- Be multiskilled to handle both dental assisting and business needs
- Be able to work in a diverse culture and maintain patient relations
- Have a strong work ethic
- Understand and apply dental professional ethics
- Maintain good communication, both written and verbal, between patients and all members of the dental healthcare team
- Be tactful with patients, *placing patients first*
- Be productive by performing jobs quickly and efficiently
- Work effectively in a team environment
- Apply initiative
- Prioritize duties
- Make decisions and know what needs to be done without direction (but know when to ask for direction)

EDUCATION

To meet the qualifications for an administrative dental assistant in the 21st century, applicants should acquire dental assisting and business skills through a training program. Such programs enable the student to understand the complexity of a dental practice and to develop the skills necessary to become a successful member of a dental healthcare team.

No licensure is available for the duties of an administrative assistant. Those assistants who are required to take dental radiographs, perform direct patient care, or engage in infection control procedures (cleaning treatment rooms or preparing instruments for sterilization), however, must consult their state's Dental Practice Act. The **Dental Practice Act** outlines the duties that can be performed by dental auxiliaries, the type of education needed, and what licensure (if any) is required.

MEMBERS OF THE DENTAL HEALTHCARE TEAM

Dentist

General Dentistry

Heading the dental healthcare team is the dentist. He or she has completed 7 or 8 years of college, including 4 years of undergraduate studies with a strong emphasis in the biological sciences and 3 to 4 years of postgraduate studies in the field of dentistry. Those who attend an American Dental Association (ADA)-accredited dental school earn a **Doctor of Dental Surgery** (DDS) or a **Doctor of Medical Dentistry** (DMD) degree.

All dentists, regardless of training, are required to pass both a written and a practical examination, which are regulated by each state, before practicing dentistry. Dentists who receive their degree in a foreign country may require additional training before practicing in the United States. In addition to following the regulations outlined in each state's Dental Practice Act, members of organizations such as the ADA and the Academy of General Dentistry must adhere to the organizations' codes of conduct and ethical standards.

Specialization

All dentists may perform the duties described in the Dental Practice Act. When the treatment becomes too complex for the general dentist, however, he or she is required to refer the patient to a specialist. The ADA recognizes nine specialties.

Dental public health. Dentists who specialize in **dental public health** help organize and run dental programs for the general public. These programs may require knowledge of how to establish and maintain educational programs within a school system or a dental clinic in an area where people have limited access to dental care. Such a clinic can be located in an inner city, on an Indian reservation, or in a rural community.

Endodontics. **Endodontics** involves the tissues of the tooth (pulp). *Endodontists* perform root canal procedures and other surgical procedures that are needed to prevent the loss of a tooth.

Oral and maxillofacial pathology. *Oral pathologists* are specialists in **oral and maxillofacial pathology**. They diagnose and treat diseases of the mouth and oral structures.

Oral and maxillofacial radiology. *Radiologists* who specialize in **oral and maxillofacial radiology** produce and interpret images and data generated by all modalities of radiant energy (x-rays and other types of imaging) that are used for the diagnosis and management of diseases, disorders, and conditions of the oral and maxillofacial region.

Oral and maxillofacial surgery. *Oral surgeons* are specialists in **oral and maxillofacial surgery.** They perform both simple tasks, such as extractions of teeth, and complex surgical procedures, such as facial reconstruction. These specialists perform surgical procedures of the head and neck.

Orthodontics and dentofacial orthopedics. An *orthodontist* treats conditions of malocclusion (the way teeth meet) and is a member of a complex team of medical and dental doctors who have specialized in **orthodontics and dentofacial orthopedics** and who restore facial features and oral functions.

Pediatric dentistry. *Pedodontists* are specialists in **pediatric dentistry.** In all phases of dentistry, they treat patients who range in age from newborn to about 15 years. Some provide treatment in a hospital setting to patients who are under general anesthesia or who have special needs. Others provide preventive and restorative dental treatment to children.

Periodontics. *Periodontists* (specialists in **periodontics**) treat patients who have diseases of the soft tissue surrounding the teeth (periodontal disease). Periodontal disease occurs in various stages, which vary in severity. The periodontist focuses treatment on correcting and preventing progression of the disease.

Prosthodontics. *Prosthodontists* receive advanced training in **prosthodontics** and perform procedures that replace lost and damaged tooth structure. Replacement of tooth structure is accomplished by placing crowns over the remaining structures. In addition to replacement of tooth structure, prosthodontists replace teeth. Tooth replacement includes the placement of partial dentures (fixed and removable), full dentures, or crowns over implants.

An additional 2 to 4 years of education is required for a dentist to become a board certified specialist. Those who choose a specialty may do so for a variety of reasons. Some enjoy the challenge of the complexity of a given specialty, whereas others, such as those who practice pediatric dentistry, enjoy working with a select group of patients. The work of the specialist and of the general dentist in the delivery of dental healthcare must involve a team effort. The general dentist refers a patient to a specialist for complex treatment, and the specialist in turn returns the patient to the general dentist for all other phases of dentistry. Such teamwork ensures that the patient receives total quality care.

Advanced training is not limited to the nine recognized specialties; dentists can receive advanced training in all areas of dentistry. Most members of the dental healthcare team are required by the Dental Practice Act to continue their education through approved coursework.

Dental Hygienist

The **dental hygienist** provides oral hygiene instruction and oral prophylaxis to dental patients. One of the key roles of the hygienist is to instruct and motivate patients in the area of preventive dentistry. Hygienists may also perform other duties as assigned to the dental assistant by the state's

Dental Practice Act. The expanded duties of the hygienist may include:

- Administering local anesthesia
- Applying pit and fissure sealant
- Root planing, scaling, and polishing
- Processing and evaluating radiographs
- Performing all duties assigned to the dental assistant

The educational requirements for a dental hygienist vary from a 2-year to a 4-year post–high school program. Each program must be accredited by the Commission on Dental Accreditation as specified by the Council on Dental Education of the ADA. Each hygienist must pass a written and a practical examination before he or she is issued a license.

Dental Assistant

The duties of the dental assistant are essential to the efficient operation of successful dental practices. Dental assistants provide a link between the patient and the dentist. There are several types of dental assistants or **dental auxiliaries** (persons who provide a service in a dental practice other than the dentist).

Chairside Dental Assistant

The **chairside dental assistant** helps the dentist during patient treatment in such areas as maintaining a clean and clear operating field, passing instruments, and manipulating dental materials. In addition, a chairside dental assistant who is registered or certified can perform intraoral duties under the direct or indirect supervision of the dentist (according to standards outlined in the state's Dental Practice Act). In addition to direct patient care, the assistant performs many necessary adjunct duties.

Expanded (Extended) Function Assistant

The **expanded (extended) function assistant** has received additional training and education in functions that provide more independent patient care under direct or indirect supervision of the dentist. Procedures that can be performed by an expanded function assistant are outlined in the Dental Practice Act, are usually reversible, and can be redone if necessary. Some states may require an expanded function assistant to receive licensure or certification.

Circulating (Roving) Assistant

The **circulating (roving) assistant** performs a variety of duties, such as helping dentists or assistants as needed, taking dental radiographs, and maintaining responsibility for sterilization and infection control procedures.

HEALTH INSURANCE PORTABILITY AND ACCOUNTABILITY ACT OF 1996

The responsibility of enforcing the regulations and compliance issues mandated by the **Health Insurance Portability and Accountability Act of 1996** (HIPAA) in a dental office ultimately belongs to the dentist, but this is not a one-person job; each member of the dental healthcare team has a role. Most compliance issues fall under the domain of the business office; therefore, most of the responsibility falls to the administrative dental assistant. Compliance issues are numerous and include the way insurance claims are coded, how patient information is shared with others, who has access to protected health information, how records are stored, and how patients are contacted outside the dental office.

Background

In 1991, the Workgroup for Electronic Data Interchange (WEDI) was created by the US Department of Health and Human Services (HHS) to study the impact of replacing paper-generated healthcare transactions with electronically generated transactions. The purpose of the study was to find ways in which the rising costs of healthcare could be contained. The prepared report, published in 1993, stated that savings in healthcare costs would be substantial if paper-generated transactions were replaced by electronically generated transactions. This report became the foundation for the Administrative Simplification provisions incorporated into the HIPAA document that President Clinton signed in August of 1996.

As is specified in its title, the Act consists of sections on two major topics—portability and accountability. The portability section of the Act simply guarantees that a person covered by health insurance provided by an employer can obtain health insurance through a second employer should he or she change jobs. The accountability section of the Act answers the question of who and what should be accountable for specific healthcare activities. The Administrative Simplification portion of the accountability section addresses issues regarding administrative systems and the business issues of healthcare.

Administrative Simplification

Administrative simplification was designed to make the business of healthcare easier through the development of standards for transaction code sets, privacy of patient information, security of patient information, and national provider identifiers. These standard sets have been implemented over a period from October of 2002 to May of 2007. Officially, HIPAA applies to a healthcare provider who transmits any health information in electronic form in connection with a transaction identified by HIPAA. Electronic forms may include diskette, CD, and FTP (file transfer protocol). Some common transactions include electronic claims, eligibility requests, and claims status inquiries made to administrators of dental plans.

HIPAA

Four Sets of HIPAA Standards

- Electronic Transactions and Code Sets
- Privacy Rule
- Security Rule
- National Identifier Standard

Transactions and Code Sets

Almost all dental practices fall under the rules and regulations of HIPAA in one form or another. HIPAA states that any practice that electronically sends or receives certain transactions must send or receive them in a standard format. This means that all transactions and codes must be transmitted in the same format. **Transactions and code sets** are primaily a set of alpha and numeric codes used to report specific treatment, procedures, and diagnoses to insurance carriers. Before HIPAA, more than 400 different transactions and code sets could be used when medical and dental claims forms were submitted. Most insurance companies and government agencies had their own sets of codes. This high

number of code sets resulted in increased costs of medical and dental services because it was very time consuming and labor intensive to manage them. A recommendation provided by the WEDI report was that code sets should be standardized to reduce the amount of time and labor needed for processing of the claim. This change reduced not only the number of hours required to process claims on the medical and dental side, but also the workload of the insurance company or government agency that processes these claims. Today, only seven transaction code sets are used across all sectors of the healthcare industry. Another recommendation for saving costs was to make the transition from paper claims to electronic claims.

REMEMBER

HIPAA requires that all providers who do business electronically must use the same healthcare transactions, code sets, and identifiers.

Electronic Data Interchange (EDI)

The move away from paper-generated claims to electronically generated claims required the standardization of electronic data sets used to transfer and process insurance claims. Computer programs are built with these transaction data sets, which contain the information needed to code electronic transmissions. It is through these sets of codes that a computer is able to translate and process information received and transmitted. These data sets are transparent in the work that administrative dental assistants do; it is the responsibility of the computer programmer to program them into applicable systems. The final product that results from these standardized data sets is a common language that can be interpreted by all computer systems and software programs, large and small.

HIPAA also states that all codes used to report treatment must be standardized (these are the codes used by insurance clerks to identify procedures that have been completed by the dentist). The national standard for codes used to report dental treatment is the *Code on Dental Procedures and Nomenclature* **(the Code)**. The code is defined in the latest edition of *Current Dental Terminology (CDT)*, which is published by the ADA (discussed in

HIPAA

HIPAA Transactions and Code Set Standards

- Dental Codes: CDT
- Diagnosis Codes: ICD-9-CM
- Procedures Codes: CPT-4
- Physician Service Codes: CPT-4
- Inpatient Services Codes: ICD-CM
- Other Service Codes: HCPCS
- Drug Codes: NDC

HIPAA

Types of Electronic Transactions

- Submission of Dental Insurance Claims or Equivalent Encounters
- Receipt of Remittance and Payment Reports
- Query Regarding and Receipt of Claims Status From Insurance Company
- Status Reports on Enrollment and Disenrollment in a Dental Health Plan
- Query Regarding and Receipt of Patient Eligibility
- Referral Certification and Authorization
- Receipt of Coordination of Benefits Reports

detail in Chapter 11). In addition to the code for dental treatment, codes are provided for all segments of the healthcare system.

Standards for Privacy of Individually Identifiable Health Information (The Privacy Rule)

Once it was determined that the efficiency and effectiveness of healthcare could be improved through electronic transmissions, Congress expressed concern for the privacy of patient health information. The final result was that Congress incorporated into HIPAA provisions that mandated the adoption of Federal privacy protections for individually identifiable health information. After several revisions and public hearings, the HHS adopted the final Privacy Rule and ensured that it would work as intended. The intent of the rule is to protect patient health information; it applies to three types of covered entities: health plans, healthcare clearinghouses, and healthcare providers who use an electronic method of transferring information. It should be noted that the Federal Privacy Rule (compliancy date: April 13, 2003) is a minimum standard, that is, it is the least that should be done, and it does not supersede Federal, State, or other laws that grant individuals even greater privacy protections. Covered entities are free to retain or adopt more protective polices or practices.

To comply with the Privacy Rule, it will be necessary for individual dental offices (as well as other identified entities) to establish day-to-day administrative policies and procedures by which **protected health information** (PHI) can be safeguarded. PHI must be protected in all formats and in all locations; this includes the transfer of information provided in oral, written, and electronic formats and when stored (paper and electronic copies). Another component of the rule requires a written policy and procedure manual for handling PHI and the appointment of one person (**Privacy Officer**) who will be responsible to oversee the process. Some safeguards designed to control unauthorized disclosure of PHI include locking of file drawers or doors at night, assignment of computer passwords, security of passwords, and protection of patient files at all times. To keep passwords secure, a system must be established for changing passwords on a regular schedule and keeping them private. It is advised that staff members do not post or share passwords with one another. Protecting PHI in patient files may require (1) ensuring that PHI does not appear on the outside of the patient record file, (2) taking care not to leave files where they can be viewed by patients, or (3) refraining from discussion of PHI when it may be overheard by other patients.

The Privacy Rule provides patients with the following rights.

Access to Medical Records

Patients should be able to see and obtain copies of their medical records and to request corrections if they detect errors and mistakes. Providers should grant access to these patient records within 30 days of a request and may charge patients for the cost of copying and sending records.

Notice of Privacy Practices

Covered healthcare plans must provide notice to patients regarding how they may use personal medical information and their rights under the new privacy regulations. Patients also may ask covered entities to restrict the use or disclosure of their information beyond the practices included in the notice, but the covered entities would not have to agree to this request.

Limits on Use of Personal Medical Information

The Privacy Rule sets limits on how healthcare plans and covered providers may use individually identifiable health information. In addition, patients must sign a specific authorization form before a covered entity is permitted to release their medical information to a life insurer, a bank, a marketing firm, or another outside business for purposes not related to healthcare.

Prohibition on Marketing

The final Privacy Rule sets new restrictions and limits on the use of patient information for marketing purposes. Pharmacies, healthcare plans, and other covered entities must first obtain an individual's specific authorization before patient information can be disclosed for marketing purposes.

Confidential Communications

Under the Privacy Rule, patients may request that their doctors, healthcare plans, and other covered entities take reasonable steps to ensure that their communications with the patient are kept confidential.

Complaints

Consumers may file a formal complaint regarding the privacy practices of a covered healthcare plan or provider.

In addition to the privacy rules stated earlier that apply to the patient, all healthcare plans, pharmacies, doctors, and other covered entities must establish polices and procedures for protecting the confidentiality of PHI related to their patients.

Steps to Protect Patient Privacy

Written privacy procedures
- Identify staff members who have access to PHI
- Explain how PHI will be used and when it may be disclosed
- Ensure that any business associates who have access to PHI agree to the same limitations on the use and disclosure of PHI

Employee training and privacy officer
- Employees must be trained in the established privacy procedures
- Designate an individual to be responsible for ensuring that procedures are followed (Privacy Officer)
- If an employee fails to follow established procedures, he or she will be subject to appropriate disciplinary action

Public responsibilities. (Limited circumstances may require the disclosure of health information for specific public responsibilities.)
- Emergency circumstances
- Identification of the body of a deceased person, or determination of the cause of death
- Public health needs
- Research that involves limited data or that has been independently approved by an institutional review board
- Judicial and administrative proceedings
- Limited law enforcement activities
- Activities related to national defense and security

Standards for Security of Individually Identifiable Health Information (The Security Rule)

The Security Rule requires that covered providers protect the integrity, confidentiality, and availability of electronic health information. The Security Rule is divided into three standards—administrative, physical, and technical. For covered providers to meet these standards, they must perform a risk analysis and decide how to manage risks by establishing a risk management protocol, develop a sanction policy, and provide ongoing review of the established protocol to ensure compliance. The Security Rule addresses only **electronically protected health information** (EPHI) that is shared

REMEMBER

The Privacy Rule refers to what patient health information must be kept confidential. The Security Rule addresses how to keep patient health information confidential.

Confidentiality: Only authorized individuals may access electronic health information.
Integrity: The information does not change except when changed by an authorized person.
Availability: Authorized persons can always retrieve EPHI, regardless of circumstances.

electronically, in contrast to the Privacy Rule, which covers PHI provided in oral, written, and electronic forms.

National Provider Identifier Standard

The **National Provider Identifier (NPI) standard** is the final standard established under HIPAA. The NPI is given to all individual healthcare providers and provider organizations such as group practices, clinics, hospitals, and schools. The NPI, a distinctive standard identification number, is issued by the US Government and will be mandated to appear on all electronic transactions no later than May 23, 2007. The NPI will replace the Social Security Number, the Individual Tax ID, and other identifiers used with standard electronic healthcare transactions such as dental insurance claim forms.

OCCUPATIONAL SAFETY AND HEALTH ADMINISTRATION (OSHA)

The **Occupational Safety and Health Administration (OSHA)** is a government agency within the US Department of Labor that fulfills the mission of assuring the safety and health of America's workers by setting and enforcing standards. Before employees in a dental practice can perform any duty that

has been identified by OSHA to be hazardous, they must first take a safety course and pass a test administered by the employer. This information is outlined in the dental practice's Hazardous Communication Program and is available to all employees.

PROFESSIONAL ETHICS

Both laws and ethics must be observed in the daily operation of a dental practice. This responsibility is assigned to each member of the dental healthcare team. **Ethics** deals with moral judgments as determined by a professional organization. When an organization establishes a high standard of ethical and moral judgment, which is reflected in the way it treats and serves members of society, society in turn will grant the organization the opportunity to practice self-government. According to the ADA, self-government is a privilege and an obligation.

An excerpt from the preamble of the ADA's *Principles of Ethics and Code of Professional Conduct* is given on page 16, followed by the five Principles of Ethics.

LEGAL STANDARDS

In addition to the ethical standards established by a professional organization to outline the ideal standards for care, practitioners must adhere to the **legal standards** established by society to regulate all its members. Legal standards are expressed as laws and regulations. These standards are enacted by legislators and are regulated by boards and commissions. The profession of dentistry is regulated and controlled by individual state Dental Practice Acts. Each state enacts a Dental Practice Act, which outlines the duties of members of the dental profession, including dentists, dental hygienists, dental assistants, and dental laboratory technicians. Included in the Dental Practice Act are educational requirements, specific duties, and licensure requirements. Each state has its own Dental Practice Act, and all members of the dental profession who practice must uphold the state's specified standards. When a practitioner moves from one state to another, it is his or her responsibility to obtain any needed licenses and to follow the standards of the new state.

REMEMBER

When dental auxiliaries perform duties that are not assigned to them in the Dental Practice Act, they are committing a criminal act.

Licensure

Licensure is a method used to identify members of a profession who meet minimum standards and are qualified to perform the duties outlined in regulations and standards (Dental Practice Act). The **Board of Dental Examiners** is the agency that has been assigned the authority to issue state licenses. Once a license has been issued, it must be renewed at established intervals. Continued education is one requirement for license renewal. It is a condition of renewal that all requirements must have been met and documented. Renewal periods are specified in the Dental Practice Act.

Registration

Registration is a form of licensure that has been established by some states as a method of protecting the public. Requirements for registration are outlined in the Dental Practice Act. Some states mandate registration for such duties as exposing radiographs, performing intraoral tasks, and handling the expanded duties of the dental auxiliary. Registrations must be renewed periodically through additional required training.

Certification

In some states, it is a condition of licensure that the dental assistant must be a **Certified Dental Assistant**. Certification is granted by the **Dental Assisting National Board, Inc**. (DANB). To qualify for certification, the dental assistant must graduate from an **American Dental Assistants Association** (ADAA)-accredited program or must meet the work experience requirements and pass a written examination. DANB has created different "pathways" by which qualifications and requirements can be met. It offers a Certified Dental Assistant (CDA) certificate, as well as certification in various specialty areas. Administrative dental assistants receive the **Certified Dental Practice Management Assistant** (CDPMA) certificate.

PATIENT'S RIGHTS

The California Dental Association has published a Patient's Bill of Rights (*below*). It is important to know the context of this bill as it applies to the treatment of patients in the dental practice. As discussed earlier, patients want and demand to be treated in a professional manner.

Patient's Bill of Rights

You have a right to schedule an appointment with your dentist in a timely manner.

It is not acceptable for a patient to have to wait several days to a few weeks before seeing the dentist in an emergency. Scheduling is very important, and time should be allowed on a daily basis for emergency patients to be seen. Patients need to know that the dentist will see them for an emergency. The purposes of an emergency appointment are to relieve pain, eliminate the possibility of further health damage, and temporize an affected tooth structure. If further treatment is necessary, the patient will be scheduled for a later time (within a few days, not weeks) for further treatment and will receive a comprehensive dental examination. Patients who have to wait several weeks to months to be seen for routine preventive care (prophylaxis) will seek treatment elsewhere. Creative scheduling and working within the matrixed appointment book will help the administrative assistant to achieve this goal (see Chapter 9).

You have a right to see the dentist every time you receive dental treatment.

When patients are scheduled for procedures with the dental hygienist, it is necessary that the dentist also be available at that time to see the patient. If the patient is returning for scheduled treatment and has been examined by the dentist recently, it is good patient management to have the dentist step into the treatment room and ask whether the patient has any questions. Depending on the state's Dental Practice Act, the dentist may not have to be present when the patient is receiving treatment for a problem that was first diagnosed by the dentist.

Continued

Patient's Bill of Rights—cont'd

REMEMBER

Dental auxiliaries cannot diagnose and treat patients. If a patient will be seen by an auxiliary without a dentist present, the procedure must be performed according to the Dental Practice Act, and one must ask whether the patient has any questions. Depending on the state's Dental Practice Act, the dentist may not have to be present when the patient is receiving treatment for a problem that was first diagnosed by the dentist.

You have a right to know in advance the type and expected cost of treatment.

The patient must be informed of and must agree to all treatment in advance of receiving the treatment. This is accomplished when open communications exist between the dentist, the dental auxiliary, and the patient. Written treatment plans that list each procedure and its fee must be given to the patient. Consent forms outline the nature of the procedure, expectations, and possible complications.

You have a right to expect dental team members to use appropriate infection and sterilization controls.

Providing complete infection control is a duty of the entire dental healthcare team. The administrative dental assistant must ensure an adequate amount of time between patient visits to allow quality infection control procedures. The dental assistant and the dentist must follow strict infection control protocol for the protection of patients.

You have a right to ask about treatment alternatives and to be told, in language you can understand, the advantages and disadvantages of each.

Communications between the dentist, the dental auxiliary, and the patient must be spoken in a language that is understood by the patient. The dental staff must be prepared to explain all procedures with the use of common terminology.

This may be accomplished by development of scripts, use of visual aids, and provision of educational information that has been prepared for patients.

You have a right to ask your dentist to explain all treatment options, regardless of coverage or cost.

The dentist and members of the dental healthcare team must take the time to discuss and answer all questions regarding treatment.

You have a right to know the level of education and training attained by your dentist and dental team.

All dentists and dental auxiliaries should post their diplomas, certificates, and licenses in easy view of patients. Members of the dental healthcare team should be prepared to answer questions about the dentist's and the dental auxiliary's training and licensure background. A script that contains all of these details would be helpful. This information can also be transmitted to patients via newsletters, brochures, and letters of introduction about new dental healthcare team members.

You have a right to know the professional rules, laws, and ethics that apply to your dentist and the dental team.

Membership in professional organizations must be conveyed to the dental patient, along with an outline of the *Principles of Ethics and Code of Professional Conduct.* Information can be posted or placed in a portfolio. Portfolios may contain information about each member of the dental healthcare team, membership in professional organizations, and copies of ethics and professional conduct codes (unique to each professional organization). Placement of the portfolio in the reception area provides every patient the opportunity to review the information.

You have a right to choose your own dentist.

Members of the dental profession believe that every patient has the right to choose his or her own dentist. A third party should not determine the selection of a dentist.

Terms in italics are taken from the California Dental Association's Patient's Bill of Rights.
Reproduced with permission of the California Dental Association, Sacramento, California.

PROFESSIONAL ORGANIZATIONS

American Dental Assistants Association

The American Dental Assistants Association (ADAA) is a professional organization for dental assistants. It has a variety of functions, including promoting professional growth and facilitating community involvement. The ADAA provides continuing education to dental assistants through home study courses, professional journals, and local, state, and national meetings. Membership in the ADAA provides many benefits such as:

• Professional liability insurance
• Accidental death insurance
• Discounts on home study continuation courses
• Subscription to *The Dental Assistant Journal*
• Discounted membership dues for students
• Scholarship opportunities

The ADAA has adopted its own *Principles of Ethics* as a guide for its members.

American Dental Assistants Association Principles of Ethics and Professional Conduct

Each individual involved in the practice of dentistry assumes the obligation of maintaining and enriching the profession. Each member shall choose to meet this obligation according to the dictates of personal conscience. This policy is based on the premise that the profession of dentistry is committed to serving the general public.

The member shall refrain from performing any professional service that is prohibited by state law, and has the obligation to prove competence before providing services to any patient. The member shall constantly strive to upgrade and expand technical skills for the benefit of the consumer public and employer. Through active participation and personal commitment, the member should additionally seek to sustain and improve the local organization, the state association, and the American Dental Assistant Association.

Code of Professional Conduct

Members of the American Dental Assistants Association Shall:
• Abide by the Bylaws of the Association
• Maintain loyalty to the Association
• Pursue the objectives of the Association
• Hold in confidence the information entrusted by the Association
• Maintain respect for the members and employees of the Association
• Serve all members of the Association in an impartial manner
• Recognize and follow all laws and regulations relating to activities of the Association

• Exercise and insist on sound business principles in the conduct of affairs of the Association
• Use legal and ethical means to influence legislation or regulations affecting members of the Association
• Issue no false or misleading statements to fellow members or the public
• Refrain from disseminating malicious information concerning the Association or any member or employee of the Association
• Maintain high standards of personal conduct and integrity
• Do not imply Association endorsement of personal opinions or positions
• Cooperate in a reasonable and proper manner with staff and members
• Accept no personal compensation from fellow members, except as approved by the Association
• Promote and maintain the highest standards of performance in service to the Association
• Assure public confidence in the integrity and service of the Association

Statement of Ethics

The American Dental Assistants Association promotes ethical conduct throughout all aspects of oral healthcare delivery. Each individual involved in the practice of dentistry assumes the obligation of maintaining and enriching the profession to better serve the general public. The dental assistant will meet this obligation according to the dictates of personal conscience.

Reproduced with permission of the American Dental Assistants Association, Chicago, Illinois.

American Dental Association Principles of Ethics and Code of Professional Conduct, Revised January 2005

Principles of Ethics

The Association believes that dentists should possess not only knowledge, skill, and technical competence but also those traits of character that foster adherence to ethical principles. Qualities of compassion, kindness, integrity, fairness, and charity complement the ethical practice of dentistry and help to define the true professional.

Principle 1: Patient Autonomy ("self-governance"). *The dentist has a duty to respect the patient's rights to self-determination and confidentiality.*

This principle expresses the concept that professionals have a duty to treat the patient according to the patient's desires, within the bounds of accepted treatment, and to protect the patient's confidentiality. Under this principle, the dentist's primary obligations include involving patients in treatment decisions in a meaningful way, with due consideration to their needs, desires, abilities, and privacy.

Principle 2: Non-malfeasance ("do no harm"). *The dentist has a duty to refrain from harming the patient.*

This principle expresses the concept that professionals have a duty to protect the patient from harm. Under this principle, the dentist's primary obligations include keeping knowledge and skills current, knowing own limitations and when to refer a patient to a specialist or other professional, and knowing when and under what circumstances delegation of patient care to auxiliaries is appropriate.

Principle 3: Beneficence ("do good"). *The dentist has a duty to promote the patient's welfare.*

This principle expresses the concept that professionals have a duty to act for the benefit of others. Under this principle, the dentist's primary obligation is service to the patient and the public at large. The most important aspect of this obligation is the competent and timely delivery of dental care within the bounds of clinical circumstances presented by the patient, with due consideration given to the needs, desires, and values of the patient. The same ethical considerations apply whether the dentist engages in a fee-for-service, managed care, or some other practice arrangement. Dentists may choose to enter into contracts governing the provision of care to a specific group of patients; however, contract obligations do not excuse dentists from their ethical duty to put the patient's welfare first.

Principle 4: Justice ("fairness"). *The dentist has a duty to treat people fairly.*

This principle expresses the concept that professionals have a duty to be fair in their dealings with patients, colleagues, and society. Under this principle, the dentist's primary obligations include dealing with people justly and delivering dental care without prejudice. In its broadest sense, this principle expresses the concept that dental professionals should actively seek allies throughout society on specific activities that will help improve access to care for all.

Principle 5: Veracity ("truthfulness"). *The dentist has a duty to communicate truthfully.*

This principle expresses the concept that professionals have a duty to be honest and trustworthy in their dealings with people. Under this principle, the dentist's primary obligations include respecting the position of trust inherent in the dentist–patient relationship, communicating truthfully and without deception, and maintaining intellectual integrity.

Reproduced with permission of the American Dental Association, Chicago, Illinois.

HOSA (Health Occupations Students of America)

HOSA is a student organization that is sponsored by the US Department of Education and 40 other state departments of education. HOSA is a student organization whose mission is to promote career opportunities in healthcare and to enhance the delivery of quality healthcare to all people. HOSA provides a unique program of leadership development, motivation, and recognition designed exclusively for secondary, postsecondary, adult, and collegiate students enrolled in Health Science Technology programs.

Programs are started at the local school level, where members have the opportunity to participate in a wide choice of leadership and skill development activities. Most states offer local, regional, and state conferences at which members can network with healthcare professionals, participate in leadership workshops, and compete in a number of individual and team leadership and skill events. Those who rank in the top three at the state level can go on to represent their state at the National Leadership Conference (NLC). During the NLC, members represent their home state, and the top ten at each event earn national recognition. In addition to its competitive events program, HOSA annually awards more than $250,000 in scholarships to members.

KEY POINTS

- Role of an administrative dental assistant: The role of the administrative dental assistant is multifaceted and requires a broad range of skills. These assistants work in a collaborative environment with other members of the dental healthcare team. They are directly involved in patient communication and in communications with other members of the dental community. Administrative dental assistants often perform duties that are otherwise assigned to the:
  - Office Manager
  - Business Manager
  - Receptionist
  - Insurance Clerk
  - Records Manager
  - Data Processor
  - Bookkeeper
  - Appointment Clerk
- Members of the dental healthcare team: Members of the dental healthcare team work together to provide quality dental care for all patients. Members include the:
  - Dentist
  - Hygienist
  - Dental Assistant
- Subspecialties: Nine dental specialties address the various needs of patients.
- HIPAA: Each member of the dental healthcare team has a role and a responsibility to follow the rules and regulations of HIPAA. The four HIPAA standards are:
  - Transactions and Code Sets Standard
  - **Standards for Privacy of Individually Identifiable Health Information** (Privacy Rule)
  - **Standards for Security of Individually Identifiable Health Information** (Security Rule)
  - National Provider Identifier Standard
- Professional ethical and legal responsibilities: In the daily operation of the dental practice, the dental healthcare team is faced with both legal and ethical issues. Ethical issues are those that involve principles of moral judgment. Legal issues are outlined in each state's Dental Practice Act. These include:
  - ADA Principles of Ethics and Code of Professional Conduct
  - ADAA Principles of Ethics
  - Patient Bills of Rights

Web Watch

American Dental Association

http://www.ada.org

American Dental Assistants Association Home Page

http://www.dentalassistant.org

American Association of Dental Examiners State and Regional Contacts

http://www.aadexam.org

Dental Society Directory

http://www.ada.org/ADA/organizations/local.asp

Health Occupations Students of America

www.hosa.org

US Dental Organizations

http://www.dds4u.com/patiented/links.html

Principles of Ethics and Code of Professional Conduct

http://www.ada.org/prof/prac/law/code/index.asp

Journal of the American Dental Association (JADA)

http://www.ada.org/prof/resources/pubs/jada/index/asp

Job Opportunities

http://www.ada.org/prof/ed/careers/index.asp

 Log on to Evolve to access additional web links!

 CRITICAL THINKING QUESTIONS

1. How would you apply what you have learned to develop a job description for an administrative dental assistant? Use the information you have read to match the ideal traits of an administrative dental assistant with various duties. Write a brief description of each duty (receptionist, bookkeeper, insurance clerk, office manager, records manager, appointment clerk). The purpose of the description is to assist in the formulation of a brief statement for prospective employees.

2. List the various members of the dental healthcare team and briefly describe their responsibilities in the delivery of dental care.

3. What is your opinion of the Patient's Bill of Rights? Do you think it is necessary in today's society? Support your opinion.

Notes

OUTLINE

KEY TERMS AND CONCEPTS

Abutment Teeth
Amalgam
Amylase
Anatomical Chart
Anterior Teeth
Apex
Apical Foramen
Bridge
Buccal
Buccal Frena
Buccal Vestibule
Cast Crowns
Cementum
Central Incisors
Cervix
Commissures
Crown
Cusp
Dental Arch
Dental Caries
Dental Prophylaxis
Dentin
Diastema
Distal
Enamel
Endodontics
Facial
Federation Dentaire International
  Numbering System
Fluoride Treatments
Frenum
Full Dentures
Full Gold and Metal Crowns

Gag Reflex
Geometric Chart
Gingiva
Hard Palate
Incisal
Incisive Papilla
Inlay
International Standards
  Organization
Interproximal
Labial
Labial Frena
Labial Vestibule
Lateral Incisors
Lingual
Lingual Frenum
Lining Mucosa
Malocclusion
Mandibular Arch
Mandibular Left
Mandibular Right
Mastication
Masticatory Mucosa
Maxillary Arch
Maxillary Left
Maxillary Right
Mesial
Mixed Dentition
Mucous Membrane
Occlusal
Occlusion
Onlay
Oral Mucosa

Panographic X-Ray Unit
Parotid Glands
Periodontal Ligament
Permanent Dentition
Pontic
Porcelain Fused to Metal
Posterior Teeth
Primary Dentition
Proximal
Pulp Chamber
Pulpal Tissue
Quadrants
Removable Partial
Resin
Resin-Based Composite
Restorative Dentistry
Root
Root Canals
Rugae
Sealants
Sextants
Simple Extractions
Soft Palate
Sublingual Glands
Submandibular Glands
Surfaces of the Tooth
Surgical Extractions
Symbolic Numbering System
Universal Numbering System
Uvula
Veneer Crowns
Vermilion Border

2

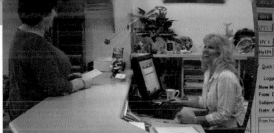

Dental Basics

LEARNING OBJECTIVES

The student will:

1. List and describe the different areas of a dental office.
2. List the basic structures of the face and oral cavity.
3. Name the basic anatomical structures and tissues of the teeth.
4. Distinguish between different tooth numbering systems.
5. Interpret dental charting symbols.
6. Categorize basic dental procedures.
7. List basic chairside dental assisting duties and identify Occupational Safety and Health Administration (OSHA) and state regulations.

INTRODUCTION

The administrative dental assistant has a unique opportunity to communicate in several "languages." You will be a translator between the dental community and the patient. As part of your job, you will represent the dentist when you communicate with other dental professionals, members of the community, and fellow team members. Patients are often unwilling or unable to ask the dentist questions directly, so they will turn to the assistants for clarification. To be an effective communicator, you must first understand the dental language.

During a typical day, you may have to explain a procedure to a patient, give postoperative instructions, review toothbrushing instructions, answer many patient questions, communicate instructions to a dental laboratory technician, speak to a pharmacist, refer a patient to a specialist, or speak to other dental professionals. In addition, you may need to clarify a treatment for a dental insurance company or other team members. Effective communication is promoted by an understanding of the language that is spoken by all diverse professionals and patients with whom you interact on a daily basis.

If you are unable to understand the dental language, it will be very difficult for you to carry out the fundamental duties of your job, such as appointment scheduling, insurance coding, clinical chart management, and billing. Therefore, it is necessary that you have a basic understanding of the dental language—the terms used to identify procedures, dental materials, and equipment. The development of a professional dental vocabulary is essential to successful communication.

REMEMBER

Tools are found in the garage.
Utensils are found in the kitchen.
Instruments are found in the dental office.

BASIC DENTAL OFFICE DESIGN

Dental offices, similar to people, come in all shapes and sizes. Although many variables may influence the architectural design of a dental office, all consist

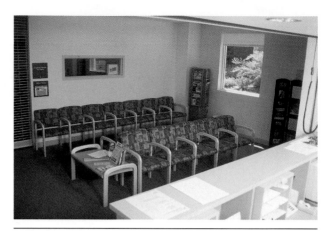

FIGURE 2-1

Typical reception area. (From Bird D, Robinson D: Torres and Ehrlich Modern Dental Assisting, 8th ed, St. Louis, Saunders, 2005, p 488.)

of the same basic work areas, which can be divided between the business of dentistry and the practice of dentistry, or the nonclinical and clinical areas.

Nonclinical Areas

Reception Area

The first area that the patient sees is the reception area (Figure 2-1). When patients enter the reception area for the first time, they begin to formulate thoughts and opinions about the dental practice. They are concerned about the cleanliness of this area because it may reflect the condition of the treatment area. Patients often perceive their dental experience in terms of the impression that they develop during the first few seconds after entering the reception area. (This is discussed further in Chapter 5.)

Business Office

The reception area usually opens into the business office (Figure 2-2). Most duties of the administrative assistant are carried out in this area. The configuration shown in Figure 2-2 is preferred by most dental practitioners, but it is not free of disadvantages. When the business area is open, all conversations can be overheard by waiting patients. For this reason, some designs include a sliding glass window in a wall between the two areas; this allows the administrative assistant to view and monitor the reception area while reducing the possibility that the patient will overhear conversations.

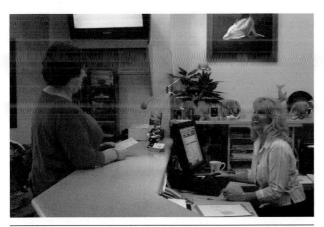

FIGURE 2-2
Administrative dental assistant performing daily tasks such as scheduling appointments, making financial arrangements, and following bookkeeping procedures. (Courtesy William C. Domb, DMD, Upland, CA.)

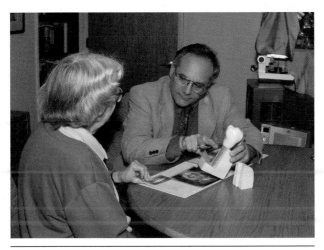

FIGURE 2-3
Dentist and patient discussing treatment options. (Courtesy William C. Domb, DMD, Upland, CA.)

Consultation Area

When privacy is needed, such as when one is interviewing patients, establishing financial agreements, or speaking with patients about private matters, an area away from other patients is recommended (Figure 2-3). Because the consultation area is used for patient contact, it should be designed with the comfort of the patient in mind. A table should be provided for the dental staff and the patient to sit down together. When all participating parties sit at a table, the environment created is nonthreatening to the patient.

This room can also double as a very comfortable work area. When equipped with a telephone, computer, and workspace, it can be used as an additional office, where phone calls and other work can be conducted without interruption.

Doctor's Private Office

A private office provides space and an area where the dentist can work quietly. This area is the private domain of the occupant, and you should not enter it unless you are specifically invited. It is advisable to ask the doctor about the status of this area and how it should be treated. Some doctors maintain an "open door" policy and welcome your entrance. Others consider this area very private and do not allow intrusion or entrance when they are not present.

Private offices may be staffed by office managers, business managers, and other specified personnel. Always respect the privacy of these areas. Papers, documents, and computer information may not be for all eyes; therefore, obtain clear direction on how these areas are to be respected.

Staff Room

The staff room is an area set aside for the exclusive use of the staff. This room can be used as a lunchroom or a meeting area. Depending on the size of the staff and the office, this room may be as simple as a very small eating area, or as large as a small apartment. Responsibility for maintaining the area is usually assigned to the dental auxiliary.

Additional Nonclinical Areas

Larger practices may provide areas for record and supply storage. These areas often include storage shelves and large file cabinets. Locker rooms provide a place for changing from street clothes into uniforms. The Occupational Safety and Health Administration (OSHA) has mandated that clothing worn during dental treatment cannot be worn outside the dental office. The dentist should provide a laundry service so that the dental assistant does not have to take contaminated uniforms home.

Clinical Areas

Dental and support activities take place in clinical areas. The dentist, dental assistant, hygienist, and laboratory technician perform their duties in these areas.

Treatment Rooms

Treatment rooms may also be referred to as "operatories." (Although the latter term is fading from use because patients associate the term with "surgical operating room," it may still be used by some dental personnel.) The treatment room is the area in which patients are treated by the dentist, dental hygienist, and dental assistant.

ANATOMY OF A TREATMENT ROOM

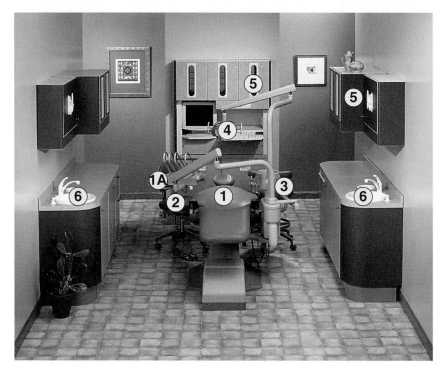

1 PATIENT CHAIR
Typically this is a lounge type chair so that the patient can be placed in a supine position. Control panels are used to place the chair in various positions. Arms are attached to the chair or to a portable unit to provide the dentist and the assistant easy access to the necessary tubing for handpieces, oral evacuation, and air-water syringe. Additional arms provide an overhead light and a tray for instrument placement.

2 OPERATOR'S STOOL
This stool is adjustable, including the backrest, and moves on rollers. It is used by the dentist, dental hygienist, or expanded function assistant while they are attending to the patient.

3 ASSISTANT'S STOOL
This stool is used by the assistant and is slightly different from the operator's stool. It typically includes a footrest because it is raised higher than the operator's stool. The abdominal arm of the stool is used for balance and to provide a rest for forearms.

4 OPERATING LIGHT
This light is either attached to the chair or suspended from the ceiling. It is high intensity and illuminates the oral cavity.

5 CABINETS
Cabinets designed for storage of equipment and supplies may be either built-in or mobile. The assistant and the dentist need areas to place the instruments they are using and to manipulate dental materials.

6 HANDWASHING SINK
A sink is placed in the room or just outside the entrance. The sink provides a place for dental personnel to properly wash and glove prior to treating the patient.

(From Bird D, Robinson D: Torres and Ehrlich Modern Dental Assisting, 8th ed, St. Louis, Saunders, 2005, p 489.)

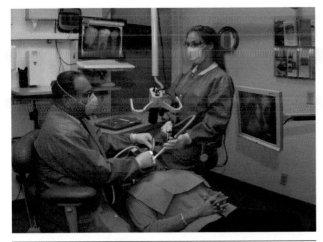

FIGURE 2-4
Treatment room featuring a video system, intraoral camera, and patient information brochures. (Courtesy William C. Domb, DMD, Upland, CA.)

Depending on the size and type of a dental practice, the basic practice will consist of two or more treatment rooms. While the dentist is attending to a patient in one room, the other room can be prepared for the next patient. In larger practices with several treatment rooms, more than one patient can be seated at the same time. Simultaneously, the hygienist may treat one patient, an expanded function assistant can finish a procedure with a second patient, and one or more dentists may be attending to their patients. Anatomy of a Treatment Room shows the basic equipment found in the treatment room. Offices may be configured slightly differently, but the goals remain the same: provide adequate equipment for use in treating the patient, allow for proper infection control, and ensure the safety of employees and patients.

In addition to basic equipment, the room may include a video system that is used to entertain and educate patients. An intraoral camera, which involves a digitized system that allows the dentist to take intraoral images (Figure 2-4), may also be present. Intraoral images are used to illustrate some problems for which dental treatment is needed that cannot be detected radiographically. These images can be stored on computers disks and are a valuable diagnostic tool.

Offices also use a variety of decorating media to enhance the beauty of the office and to create a comfortable environment for patient treatment.

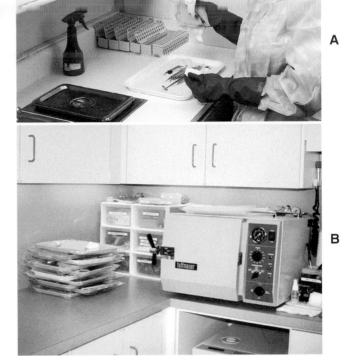

FIGURE 2-5
Sterilization area, contaminated **(A)** and clean **(B)**. (From Bird D, Robinson D: Torres and Ehrlich Modern Dental Assisting, 8th ed, St. Louis, Saunders, 2005, pp 330–331.)

Sterilization Area

In the sterilization area, contaminated instruments are cleaned, packaged, sterilized (all microorganisms completely killed), and prepared for reuse. The room is separated into two areas (Figure 2-5). The contaminated area is where cleaning, packaging, and sterilization take place. Once packages have been removed from the sterilizer, they are placed in the clean area, which is used for the assembly and storage of treatment trays. During processing and storage, sterile instruments remain packaged. To ensure sterility, they are opened only in the treatment room in the presence of the patient.

Laboratory

In the dental laboratory, the dentist and the assistant can perform duties that do not require patient contact. In small practices, this area may be used for basic laboratory functions, such as preparing

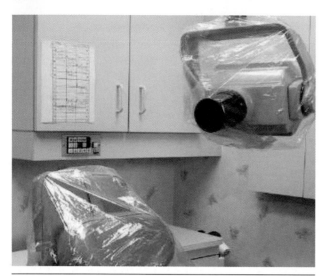

FIGURE 2-6
Radiographic area. (From Bird D, Robinson D: Torres and Ehrlich Modern Dental Assisting, 8th ed, St. Louis, Saunders, 2005, p 627.)

diagnostic casts, pouring models, and fabricating trays used for bleaching and other procedures. In larger practices that employ a dental laboratory technician, the dental laboratory would be much larger, and crowns, bridges, partials, and dentures would be made there.

Additional Clinical Areas

Radiology room. The radiology room is the place where dental x-ray films are taken. Equipment may include a standard dental x-ray machine used to take intraoral (inside the mouth) films and a **panographic x-ray unit** used to take extraoral (outside the mouth) films (Figure 2-6). Radiographic equipment may also be located in each treatment room. When digital x-ray technology is used, the room will also contain a computer system. Digital x-ray technology eliminates the need for x-ray film and the process of film development. Digital technology replaces traditional x-ray film with reusable sensors and reduces by as much as 90% the amount of radiation required.

Darkroom. Dental x-ray films are processed in the darkroom.

Patient education room. The patient education room is a separate area that is designated for use in patient education and motivation. The room includes equipment that demonstrates correct brushing and flossing techniques. A television and DVD player may also be provided in this room for use in showing videos on various aspects of dental care. Offices that are equipped with computers can provide to patients interactive educational programs via CD-ROM and various Internet sites. Brochures and pamphlets may be given to patients for home study.

BASIC DENTAL ANATOMY

Knowledge of basic dental anatomy helps the administrative dental assistant to communicate with other dental professionals, patients, and insurance companies.

Basic Structures of the Face and Oral Cavity

Skull

The skull is made up of two sections. The cranium consists of eight bones that form a protective structure for the brain, and the face consists of 14 bones (Table 2-1).

Oral Cavity

The oral cavity, or the mouth, is the anatomical area where dentistry is performed (Figure 2-7). This cavity is regarded as the beginning of the digestive system; it contains sensory receptors, is used to create speech patterns, and serves as a vehicle for human pleasure and as a weapon that can be used for defense (both verbal and physical).

Lips and Cheeks

The lips surround the opening to the oral cavity. The corners of the mouth, where the upper and lower lips meet, are the **commissures.** The **vermilion border** represents the junction of the tissue of the face with the mucous membrane of the lips (Figure 2-8). The cheeks form the side of the face. The insides of the cheeks are covered with moist **mucous membrane.** The junction of the mucous membrane of the check and the gingiva is the **buccal vestibule.** The junction of the lips and the gingiva is the **labial vestibule** (Figure 2-9).

TABLE **2-1 Bones of the Skull**

Bone	Number	Location
8 Bones of the Cranium		
Frontal	1	Forms the forehead, most of the orbital roof, and the anterior cranial floor
Parietal	2	Form most of the roof and upper sides of the cranium
Occipital	1	Forms the back and base of the cranium
Sphenoid	1	Forms part of the anterior base of the skull and part of the walls of the orbit
Ethmoid	1	Forms part of the orbit and the floor of the cranium
14 Bones of the Face		
Zygomatic	2	Form the prominence of the cheeks and part of the orbit
Maxillary	2	Form the upper jaw
Palatine	2	Form the posterior part of the hard palate and the floor of the nose
Nasal	2	Form the bridge of the nose
Lacrimal	2	Form part of the orbit at the inner angle of the eye
Vomer	1	Forms the base for the nasal septum
Inferior	2	Form part of the interior of the nose conchae
Mandible	1	Forms the lower jaw
6 Auditory Ossicles		
Malleus, incus, stapes	6	Bones of the middle ear

From Bird D, Robinson D: Torres and Ehrlich Modern Dental Assisting, 8th ed, St. Louis, Saunders, 2005, p 105.

Frenum

The **frenum** (*plural,* frena) is a strip of tissue that connects two structures. Five frena are located in the oral cavity. Two—maxillary and mandibular—are **labial frena.** These connect the tissue of the lips (labia) to the gingival tissue. Two **buccal frena** (right and left) connect the cheek to the gingiva in the area of the maxillary first molar. One **lingual frenum** connects the tongue to the floor of the

mouth (Figure 2-10). (Run your tongue around the vestibule of your mouth, and you will feel the labial and buccal frena.)

Food for Thought

> When the maxillary labial frenum is too thick or wide, it keeps the two front teeth from coming into contact. This creates a **diastema.**

Tongue

The tongue, which is covered with taste buds, is a strong muscle that aids in the digestive process and contributes to speech formation. The posterior (back) of the tongue is connected to the hyoid bone. The anterior portion is attached only to the lingual frenum.

Food for Thought

> A short lingual frenum keeps the tongue from extending as far as is needed for speech formation. This condition is referred to as "tongue tied." A simple procedure of clipping the frenum corrects the problem.

Salivary Glands

The salivary glands produce saliva, which provides moisture for the mucous membrane, lubricates food, cleans the teeth, supplies an enzyme **(amylase)** that begins the digestive process, and is the source of minerals (fluorides, calcium, and phosphate) needed for the remineralization of tooth structure. The three pairs of salivary glands are **parotid glands, submandibular glands,** and **sublingual glands** (Figure 2-11).

Hard and Soft Palates

The **hard palate,** or roof of the mouth, is covered with masticatory mucosa. Located within the hard palate are the **rugae,** or folds of tissue, behind the maxillary anterior teeth. Located straight behind (posterior) the central incisors is the **incisive papilla** (Figure 2-12). (With your tongue, press on the hard palate. Behind the anterior teeth, you should be able to feel the rugae, incisive papilla,

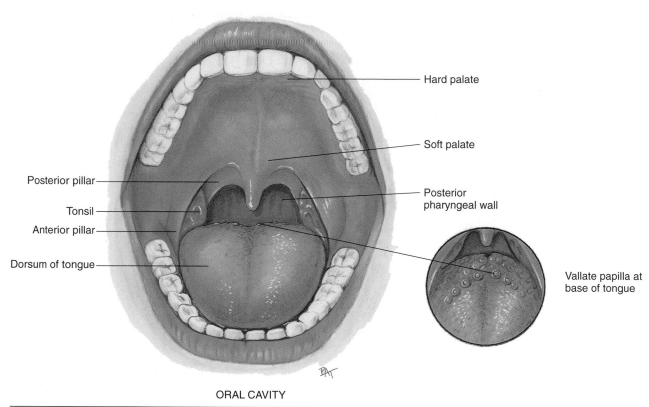

ORAL CAVITY

FIGURE 2-7

Features of the oral cavity. (From Jarvis C: Physical Examination and Health Assessment, ed 4, St. Louis, Mosby, 2003, p. 374).

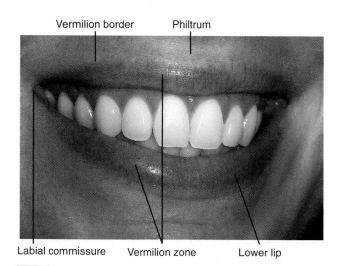

FIGURE 2-8

Landmarks of the mouth. (From Bird D, Robinson D: Torres and Ehrlich Modern Dental Assisting, 8th ed, St. Louis, Saunders, 2005, p 133.)

and the hard bony structure that forms the hard palate.)

The **soft palate** is the posterior continuation of the hard palate. The soft and flexible region located on the back (posterior) of the soft palate is the **uvula** (see Figure 2-7), which is a projection of tissue that hangs in the center of the throat. Both the soft palate and the uvula move upward during swallowing to direct food downward into the oropharynx and not upward into the nasal cavity.

During dental procedures, one must be careful not to stimulate the **gag reflex.** Tissue located in the posterior portion of the mouth, including the soft palate and the uvula, forms the gag reflex area. When this area is touched by a foreign object or is stimulated by the taste of some foods or materials, gagging can occur.

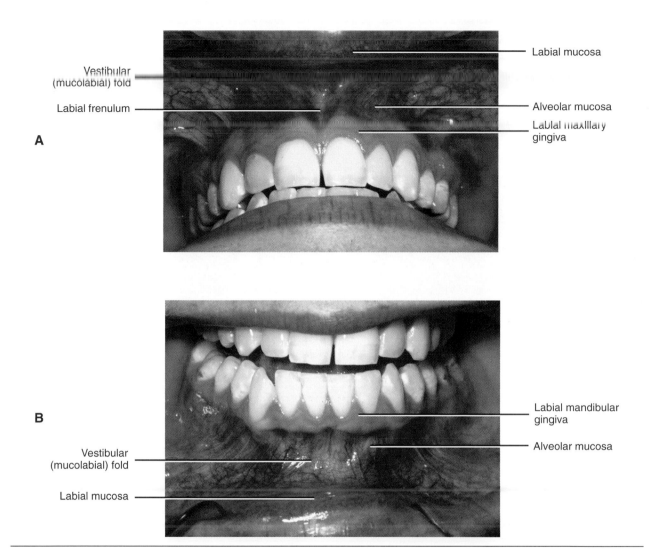

Vestibular
(mucolabial) fold

Labial frenulum

A

Labial mucosa

Alveolar mucosa

Labial maxillary
gingiva

B

Vestibular
(mucolabial) fold

Labial mucosa

Labial mandibular
gingiva

Alveolar mucosa

FIGURE 2-9
The labial vestibule and the upper and lower labial frena. **A,** Maxillary labial mucosa and attachments of the frenum. **B,** Mandibular labial mucosa and attachments of the frenum. (From Liebgott B: The Anatomical Basis of Dentistry, 2nd ed, St. Louis, Mosby, 2001, p 338.)

Oral Mucosa

The tissue that lines the oral cavity is the **oral mucosa.** Two types of oral mucosa are present. **Lining mucosa** covers the cheeks, lips, vestibule, ventral (underside) surface of the tongue, and soft palate. This tissue is very thin and can be injured easily.

Masticatory mucosa is much thicker and denser and is attached tightly to bone (with the exception of the tongue). It is designed to resist the pressure of chewing food and is not easily injured.

This tissue type forms the gingivae (gums), hard palate, and dorsum (top) of the tongue.

Gingiva

Gingiva (*plural,* gingivae) is the term that refers to the masticatory mucosa and the tissue that surrounds the teeth. Normal healthy gingival tissue is firm and is attached tightly around the teeth; in white people, it is coral or salmon pink in color. In nonwhites, the color is commonly darker.

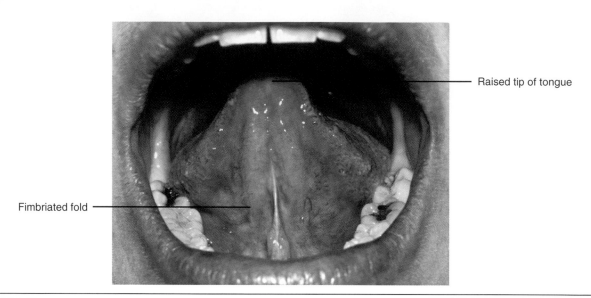

Raised tip of tongue

Fimbriated fold

FIGURE 2-10

The lingual frenum and the delicate tissues of the floor of the mouth. (From Bird D, Robinson D: Torres and Ehrlich Modern Dental Assisting, 8th ed, St. Louis, Saunders, 2005, p 138.)

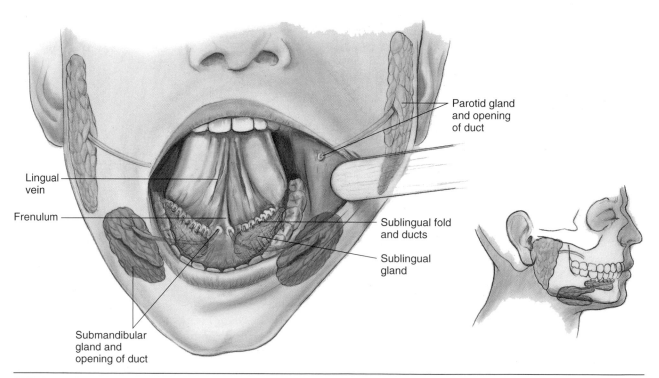

Parotid gland and opening of duct

Lingual vein

Frenulum

Sublingual fold and ducts

Sublingual gland

Submandibular gland and opening of duct

FIGURE 2-11

Salivary glands. (From Jarvis C: Physical Examination and Health Assessment, ed 4, St. Louis, Mosby, 2003, p 375.)

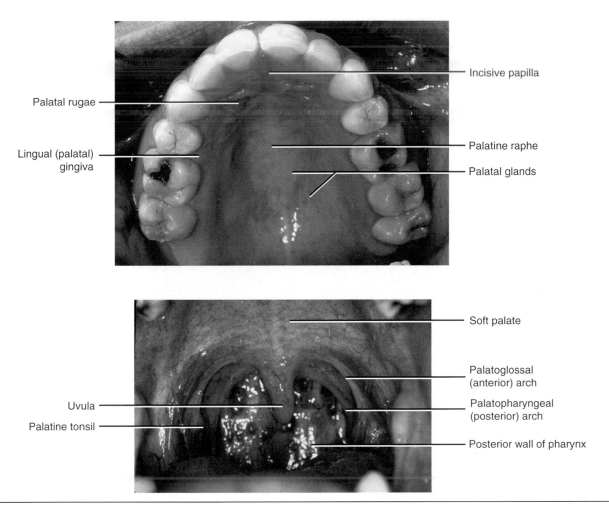

FIGURE 2-12
Tissues of the hard palate. (From Liebgott B: The Anatomical Basis of Dentistry. 2nd ed, St. Louis, Mosby, 2001, p 341.)

Food for Thought

Gingivitis is an inflammation of the gingival tissue that results in red, swollen, and bleeding gums. This condition is the result of poor brushing and flossing habits but is reversible with a regular regimen of correct brushing and flossing techniques. If gingivitis goes untreated, it will progress into periodontal disease, which is the destruction of bone and tissue. Periodontal disease, when untreated, results in tooth loss.

Basic Anatomic Structures and Tissues of the Teeth

Anatomic Structures

The shape, size, and functions of teeth vary, but teeth are made of the same component structures. In fact, each tooth consists of three anatomical structures—crown, cervix, and root (Figure 2-13). The **crown** of the tooth is covered with enamel. Crowns vary in size according to the type and function of the tooth. The **cervix,** or the neck of the tooth, is the narrow portion of the tooth at which the root and the crown meet. Each **root** is covered by a thin, hard shell called the **cementum.** Each tooth consists of one to four roots.

Tissues of a Tooth

The crown is covered with a hard, mineralized sub-stance called **enamel** (Figure 2-14). Enamel is 99% inorganic matter, and it cannot regenerate. This means that once enamel has been damaged by extensive caries or trauma, it cannot repair itself; the function of the tooth can be restored only by means of a dental restoration procedure.

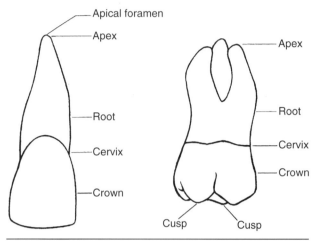

FIGURE 2-13

Anatomical structures of an incisor *(left)* and a molar *(right)*. (From Weaver TK, Apfel M: Dental Charting: Student's Manual, Austin, Texas, Center for Occupational Curriculum Development, Division of Continuing Education, The University of Texas at Austin, 1981, p 5.)

The bulk of a tooth is made of **dentin**—a living cellular substance similar in structure to bone. It is softer than the hard outer shell of the crown (enamel) and the covering of the root surface (cementum).

The **periodontal ligament** (connective fibers that help hold the tooth in the alveolar socket while providing protection and nourishment for the tooth) may attach to the tooth at the cementum—the thin, hard covering of the root surface of a tooth.

In the center of the crown is the **pulp chamber.** Within the pulp chamber is the **pulpal tissue,** which is composed of connective tissue, blood vessels, and nerves. Blood vessels and nerves enter the tooth through the **apical foramen** (a small opening) at the **apex** (tip) of the root, and they fill the **root canal** (pulp cavity).

Dental Arches

The anatomical structure of the mouth is divided into sections. The upper section is referred to as the **maxillary arch,** and the lower section is the **mandibular arch.** Each **dental arch** contains the same number of teeth.

Quadrants

The dental arches are divided into four sections, or **quadrants.** Each quadrant consists of the same number and type of teeth as the opposite quadrant.

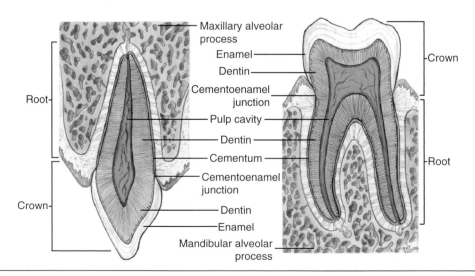

FIGURE 2-14

Longitudinal section of a tooth. (From Bird D, Robinson D: Torres and Ehrlich Modern Dental Assisting, 8th ed, St. Louis, Saunders, 2005, p 94.)

Dental Caries

Dental caries (tooth decay) is a progressive disease that demineralizes enamel, enters the dentin, and quickly reaches the pulp of the tooth. Bacteria within the mouth metabolize sugars and give off toxins (acid) that dissolve (demineralize) the calcium salts in the tooth. The process can be stopped by removing the carious lesion and replacing the lost tooth structure with a variety of dental materials (fillings). If caries are not stopped before they reach the pulp, the condition is irreversible and the tooth will die. Options available at this point include extracting (removing) the diseased tooth or performing a root canal procedure (replacing all pulpal tissue with an appropriate dental material) to save the function of the tooth.

These quadrants are **maxillary right, maxillary left, mandibular left,** and **mandibular right** (Figure 2-15, *A*).

Sextants

Dental arches are sometimes divided into **sextants** (six sections). This method of division is most commonly used in periodontal evaluations. Sextants are maxillary right posterior, maxillary anterior, maxillary left posterior, mandibular left posterior, mandibular anterior, and mandibular right posterior (Figure 2-15, *B*).

Occlusion

Occlusion is the relationship between the maxillary arch and the mandibular arch in terms of the way they meet or touch. In perfect occlusion, teeth meet at specific contact points, allowing space and room for the teeth to properly chew and grind food **(mastication).** In **malocclusion,** the teeth are out of alignment or occlusion.

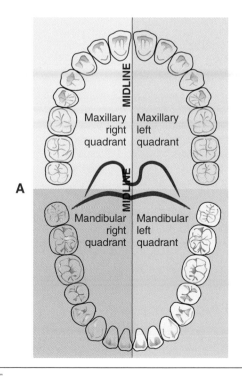

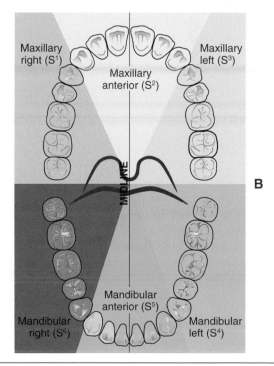

FIGURE 2-15

A, Oral cavity quadrants. **B,** Oral cavity sextants. View shown leads into the oral cavity.

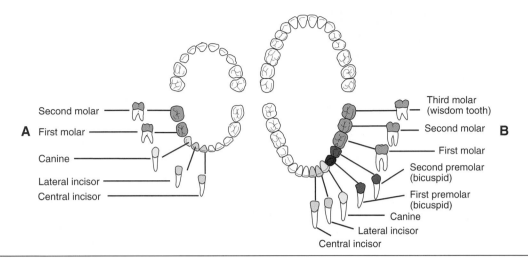

FIGURE 2-16
A, Deciduous teeth. **B,** Permanent teeth. (Modified from Applegate EG: Anatomy and Physiology Learning System: Textbook, Philadelphia, Saunders, 1995, p 331.)

Types of Teeth

Functions, sizes, and locations of the teeth are important factors in the digestive process. Each human has two sets of teeth. The first set, or **primary dentition** (Figure 2-16, *A*), consists of 20 teeth. When these teeth are lost or shed, they are replaced with **permanent dentition,** which consists of 32 teeth (Figure 2-16, *B*). Not all of the primary teeth are lost and replaced at the same time. The presence of both primary and permanent dentition is referred to as **mixed dentition** (Table 2-2).

Anterior Teeth

The size and function of teeth vary according to where they are located in the dental arch (see Figure 2-16). **Anterior teeth** (toward the front) consist of **central incisors, lateral incisors,** and cuspids (canines). Incisors are characterized by thin, sharp, incisal edges that aid in food cutting. Cuspids, which are very strong and have a sharp point **(cusp),** are designed for grasping and tearing food.

Posterior Teeth

Posterior teeth (toward the back) consist of first premolar, second premolar (bicuspid), first molar, second molar, and third molar (wisdom tooth). These teeth have flat surfaces with rounded projections and are used for grinding and crushing.

TABLE 2-2 Ages at Which Teeth Erupt and Are Shed

Tooth Type	Age at Eruption	Age at Shedding
Deciduous Teeth		
Central incisors	6-8 months	5-7 years
Lateral incisors	8-10 months	6-8 years
First molars	12-16 months	9-11 years
Canines	16-20 months	8-11 years
Second molars	20-30 months	9-11 years
Permanent Teeth		
First molars	6-7 years	
Central incisors	6-8 years	
Lateral incisors	7-9 years	
Canines	9-10 years	
First premolars	9-11 years	
Second premolars	10-12 years	
Second molars	11-13 years	
Third molars	15-25 years	

Surfaces of the Teeth

Each tooth is divided into sections, which are referred to as the **surfaces of the tooth** (Figure 2-17). Each surface has a name that is used by the dental professional to describe the exact location of tooth decay, restorations, and other conditions:

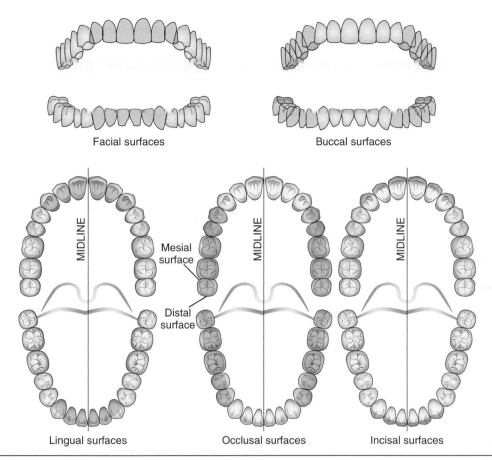

Facial surfaces   Buccal surfaces

MIDLINE

Mesial surface

Distal surface

MIDLINE

MIDLINE

Lingual surfaces   Occlusal surfaces   Incisal surfaces

FIGURE 2-17
Surfaces of the teeth. *Top,* Facial and buccal surfaces. *Bottom,* Lingual, occlusal, mesial, distal, and incisal surfaces.

- **Proximal** refers to the surfaces (distal and mesial) that are adjacent or next to another surface of a tooth.
- **Interproximal** is the space created by two proximal surfaces.
- **Mesial** refers to the proximal surface (of a tooth) that is facing toward the midline (vertical line that divides the face into two sections, running between the eyes, down the center of the nose, and between the right and left centrals).
- **Distal** refers to the proximal surface that faces away from the midline.
- **Buccal** refers to the surfaces of posterior teeth that face or touch the cheeks.
- **Lingual** refers to the surfaces of teeth that face the tongue, or the inside of the mouth.
- **Occlusal** refers to the broad, flat chewing surface of posterior teeth (premolars and molars).

- **Incisal** refers to the sharp cutting edges of the anterior teeth (incisors and cuspids).
- **Labial** refers to the surfaces of anterior teeth that face or touch the lips.
- **Facial** is an interchangeable term used to describe the buccal and labial surfaces.

Without knowledge of these surfaces, the dental assistant is unable to interpret directives given by the dentist during clinical examinations and dental procedures. It is the responsibility of the administrative dental assistant to transfer information about these conditions from the clinical record to other forms and to correctly bill the patient and the insurance carrier.

In addition to singular surfaces, names for combinations of surfaces further identify and locate dental conditions and restorations. When two surface names are combined, the *-al* of the first

TABLE **2-3** **Tooth Surface Abbreviations**

B	Buccal
D	Distal
F	Facial
I	Incisal
L	Lingual
M	Mesial
O	Occlusal
BO	Bucco-occlusal
DI	Distoincisal
DL	Distolingual
DO	Disto-occlusal
LO	Linguo-occlusal
MI	Mesioincisal
MO	Mesio-occlusal
MOD	Mesio-occlusodistal
MODBL	Mesio-occlusodistobuccolingual

surface name is replaced with an -*o*-, which is followed by the second surface name in full (e.g., distolingual). When more than two surface names are combined, the -*al* is replaced with -*o*- for all names, except the last (e.g., mesio-occlusodistal). Note that when the surface name *occlusal* follows another -*o*-, a hyphen must be inserted between the two *o*'s. Table 2-3 provides a complete list of surface name combinations and their corresponding abbreviations.

NUMBERING SYSTEMS

Universal Numbering System

The **Universal Numbering System** was developed in the United States to ensure consistency in identification of individual teeth (Figure 2-18). Instead of calling out the name of a tooth, such as maxillary right second molar or mandibular right second premolar, the dentist can simply call out tooth numbers 2 and 29. This system begins with the maxillary right third molar and assigns number 1 to this tooth and continues across the maxillary arch, ending with tooth number 16 (maxillary left third molar). Numbering of the mandibular arch is continued by assignment of number 17 to the mandibular left third molar tooth and of number 32 to the mandibular right third molar.

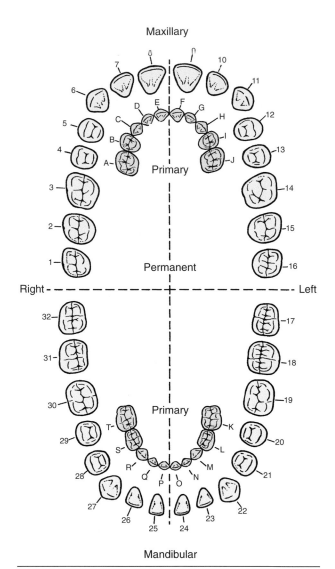

FIGURE 2-18

Universal Tooth Numbering System. (From Weaver TK, Apfel M: Dental Charting: Student's Manual, Austin, Texas, Center for Occupational Curriculum Development, Division of Continuing Education, The University of Texas at Austin, 1981, p 11.)

International Standards Organization Designation System

The **International Standards Organization** (ISO) numbering system is also called the **Federation Dentaire International (FDI) Numbering System** (Figure 2-19). This system is widely used in countries other than the United States. In this system, the quadrants and sextants are assigned

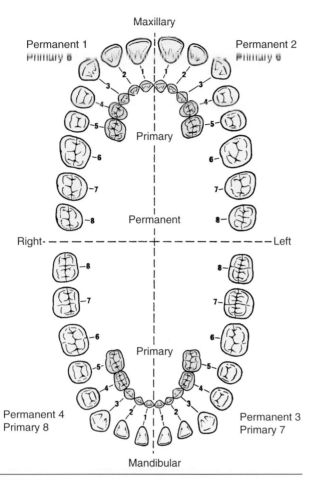

FIGURE 2-19
International Tooth Numbering System. (Modified from Weaver TK, Apfel M: Dental Charting: Student's Manual, Austin, Texas, Center for Occupational Curriculum Development, Division of Continuing Education, The University of Texas at Austin, 1981, p 10.)

numbers. Each configuration is a two-digit number that consists of a 0 and the numbers 1 through 8. Instead of calling out the name of the quadrant or sextant, the dentist refers to the numbers (as shown in Table 2-4). Each number is pronounced individually, for example, 10 is pronounced "one zero," and so forth.

In addition their use in identifying quadrants and sextants, numbers are used to identify individual teeth. Numbering is the same for each quadrant; therefore, identical teeth have the same name and the same number. For example, central incisors are assigned number 1, laterals number 2, and so forth; third molars are assigned number 8. The com-

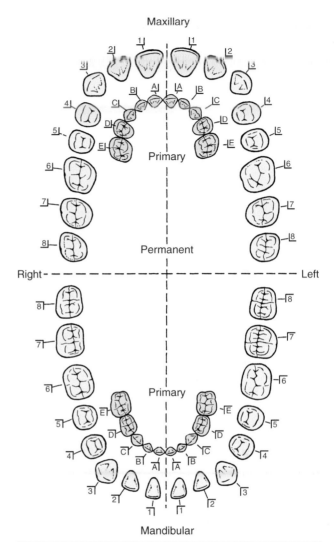

FIGURE 2-20
Symbolic (Palmer) Tooth Numbering System. (Modified from Weaver TK, Apfel M: Dental Charting: Student's Manual, Austin, Texas, Center for Occupational Curriculum Development, Division of Continuing Education, The University of Texas at Austin, 1981, p 12.)

bination of the quadrant number and the tooth number gives each tooth an individual number configuration.

Symbolic Numbering System (Palmer System)

In the **Symbolic Numbering System,** each tooth in a quadrant is assigned a number, and quadrants are differentiated by a symbol (Figure 2-20). The

TABLE **2-4 International Standards Organization Designation System**

00	Oral cavity
01	Maxillary arch
02	Mandibular arch
10	Maxillary right quadrant
20	Maxillary left quadrant
30	Mandibular left quadrant
40	Mandibular right quadrant
03	Maxillary right posterior sextant
04	Maxillary anterior sextant
05	Maxillary left posterior sextant
06	Mandibular left posterior sextant
07	Mandibular anterior sextant
08	Mandibular right posterior sextant

numbering system begins with the central incisor as number 1 and ends with the third molar as number 8 (permanent dentition). Each quadrant is represented with a symbol, and the number or letter is placed within the bracket:

Maxillary right	**Maxillary left**
8 7 6 5 4 3 2 1	1 2 3 4 5 6 7 8
8 7 6 5 4 3 2 1	1 2 3 4 5 6 7 8
Mandibular right	**Mandibular left**

Primary teeth are assigned letters, beginning with the central incisor as A and ending with the second primary molar as E.

Maxillary right	**Maxillary left**
E D C B A	A B C D E
E D C B A	A B C D E
Mandibular right	**Mandibular left**

This symbolic system is used primarily in orthodontic and pediatric dentistry.

CHARTING METHODS

The primary objective of charting is to express, through symbolism, various conditions that involve individual teeth, or groups of teeth, in their respective arches. Such symbolic writing is referred to as dental shorthand. The charting process allows existing restorative conditions to be easily recognized; work that needs to be completed is easily identified as well. Charting involves several components, such as color coding, symbolization, and type of chart used to record the information.

Color Coding

Red indicates dental conditions that require treatment:
- Dental caries
- Extractions, tooth impactions
- Existing restorations that must be replaced
- Periodontal abscesses
- Fractures
- Endodontic treatment (uncompleted)

Blue indicates existing dental restorations or conditions that do not require treatment at this time:
- Amalgam and composite restorations
- Crowns and bridges
- Completed endodontic treatment
- Impacted teeth
- Extracted teeth

Charting Symbols

Information is recorded on a dental chart with a combination of symbols and color. Unlike the numbering systems, which have been standardized, charting conventions still vary widely among practices. It is necessary for all members of the dental healthcare team to follow a standardized method of charting within their own practice to ensure consistency. An example of common charting illustrations is provided.

Types of Dental Charts

Two different types of dental charts are used to record dental conditions. One is the **anatomical chart,** which uses an anatomical representation of the teeth within the dental arches. The other type is the **geometric chart,** on which circles are used to represent teeth and are divided into sections that represent the surfaces of the teeth.

In each of the charting methods, the teeth are arranged in the same configuration as they are in the mouth. In most systems, when you look at the chart, it is as though you are looking at the patient. The patient's right is located on your left, and the patient's left is located on your right. Occasionally, doctors choose to reverse the chart, in which case,

Common Charting Symbols

The following matrix and the three different chart examples (anatomical, geometric, and computer generated [see charts on pp. 41–42]) of the same patient's clinical chart symbolize dental procedures and conditions.

The matrix is divided into five columns. The first column categorizes **Dental Procedures** according to the categories listed in the CDT. (See Chapter 11 for detailed information on the CDT.) The second column, **Description,** represents the subcategories of the CDT. The third column, **Charting Instructions,** explains how to illustrate the identified dental procedure or condition on the patient's clinical chart. With proper illustration of procedures and conditions and use of correct color coding and symbolization, the dental healthcare team will be able to correctly interpret the patient's clinical chart. The fourth column, **Charting Example,** identifies the tooth number on the charting examples (anatomical, geometric, and computer generated). All charts, although they differ in design, present the same information. The fifth column, **Black's Classification,** identifies the corresponding classification and tooth surface.

Dental Procedures and Condition	Description	Charting Instructions	Charting Example	Black's Classification
Restorative Procedures	Amalgam	Dental caries are outlined and filled in with red. Completed amalgam restorations are colored solid blue or black.	Tooth #2 Tooth #18	Class II MO Class I O
	Resin-Based Composite	Dental caries are outlined in red. Completed restorations are filled with blue or black dots.	Tooth #7 Tooth #29 Tooth #4	Class III M Class II MOD Class V B
	Inlay/Onlays Cast metal	Work to be completed is outlined in red and diagonal lines are drawn. Completed restorations are drawn over in blue or black.	Tooth #31	MOD Inlay
	Inlay/Onlay Resin-Based	Work to be completed is outlined in red. Completed restoration is filled in with blue or black dots.	Tooth #14	DOL Onlay
	Crown Cast metal	Work to be completed is outlined in red and diagonal lines are drawn. Completed crown is drawn over with blue or black.	Tooth #30	
	Crown Porcelain fused to gold	Work to be completed is outlined in red on the buccal surface or facial surface, and diagonal lines are drawn on the occlusal and lingual surface (posterior teeth) and the lingual surface (anterior teeth). Computer-generated chart draws diagonal lines on all surfaces. Completed crown is drawn over in blue or black.	Tooth #19 Tooth #21 Tooth #15	
	Crown Porcelain or Resin-Based	Work to be completed is outlined in red. Completed crown is filled with blue or black dots (computer-generated chart outlined in blue).	Tooth #13	
	Stainless Steel Crown	Work to be completed is identified by writing **SS** in red on the crown of the tooth (computer-generated chart outlined in red). Completed crown is identified by writing over the SS in blue or black (computer-generated chart outlined in blue).	Tooth #3	
	Veneer bonding	Work to be completed is outlined in red on the facial surface only (computer-generated chart filled facial surface in red). Completed veneer is filled in with blue or black dots (computer-generated chart filled facial surface in blue).	Tooth #8 Tooth #9	

Continued

Common Charting Symbols—cont'd

Dental Procedures and Condition	Description	Charting Instructions	Charting Example	Black's Classification
Restorative Procedures (cont'd)	Post and Core Build-up	A red vertical line is drawn through the root (approximating the root canal) and a small inverted triangle is drawn in the gingival third of the crown (approximating the pulp chamber of the tooth). Completed post and core is filled in with blue or black.	Tooth #30	
Endodontic Procedures	Endodontic Therapy (root canal)	When therapy is indicated, a red vertical line is drawn through each root (approximating the root canal). Completed treatment is drawn over in blue or black.	Tooth #28	
	Periapical Abscess	A small red circle is drawn at the apex of the root of the infected tooth.	Tooth #27	
Implant Services	Implant	When an implant is indicated, horizontal red lines are drawn across the root of the replaced tooth. When an implant is present, blue or black lines are drawn (computer-generated chart outlined root).	Tooth #13	
Prosthodontics Fixed	Fixed Bridge	Follow the charting instructions for the type of crown to be used in the construction of the bridge. In addition, connect the teeth involved with two horizontal lines, and draw an **X** through the roots of the missing teeth. When the bridge has been inserted, color over in blue or black.	Tooth #19 Tooth #20 Tooth #21	(Retainer) (Pontic) (Retainer)
Oral Surgery	Extraction	A single angled red line is drawn through the tooth (/) (computer-generated chart drew two lines II).	Tooth #1 Tooth #32	
	Extracted or missing tooth	A blue or black **X** is drawn through the tooth.	Tooth #16	
	Impacted or unerupted tooth	A red circle is drawn around the tooth (crown and root).	Tooth #17	
Other Conditions	Rotated tooth	Place a red semicircular line at the root of the tooth with an arrow pointing in the direction of the rotation.	Tooth #17	
	Drifting tooth	Place a red line above the crown of the tooth with an arrow indicating the direction of the drift.	Tooth #31	
	Fractured tooth	Place a red zigzag on the tooth surface where the fracture occurred. If the root is fractured, place the zigzag on the root.	Tooth #24	Class IV
	Diastema	When there is more space than normal between two teeth, place two vertical red lines between the teeth.	Teeth #8, 9	

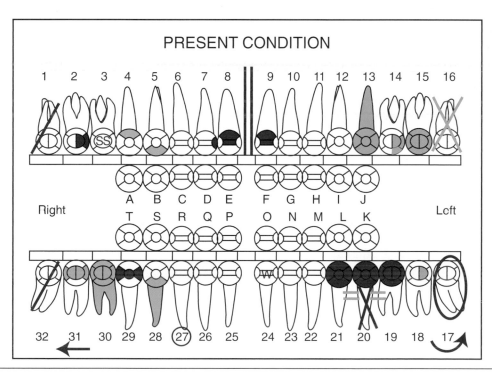

Anatomical chart.

PRESENT CONDITION

Geometric chart.

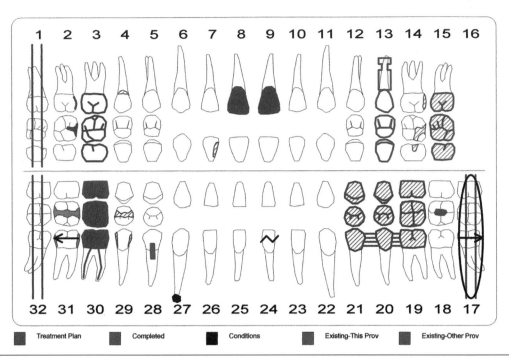

| Treatment Plan | Completed | Conditions | Existing-This Prov | Existing-Other Prov |

Computer-rendered chart.

the patient's right is located on your right and the patient's left is on your left (the numbering system *will not change;* the maxillary right third molar will always be tooth #1 [Universal Numbering System]).

DENTAL PROCEDURES

It is necessary for the administrative dental assistant to have an understanding of dental procedures if he or she is to be an effective and efficient member of the dental healthcare team. Administrative dental assistants perform several tasks daily that require the identification and understanding of dental procedures. These tasks include:

- Scheduling appointments
- Billing insurance companies and patients
- Corresponding with dental specialists
- Communicating with patients and other dental healthcare team members
- Planning treatments

Basic and Preventive Dental Procedures

The following procedures are just a few of the many that may be performed in a dental practice.

Initial Examination

Initial oral examination is performed during the patient's first visit to the dental practice. Diagnostic aids are used during the examination to help the dentist identify existing conditions and restorations, as well as the dental needs of the patient. These aids may consist of radiographs—both intraoral and extraoral—diagnostic models, and an intraoral camera to digitally document conditions within the oral cavity. In addition to performing the oral examination, the dentist evaluates other tissues and structures of the head and neck to help determine whether any other medical conditions may exist. Included in this procedure is the recording of vital signs, as well as occasionally, the drawing of blood for use in laboratory testing.

Prophylaxis

During **dental prophylaxis,** the dentist or dental hygienist removes stains and deposits and polishes teeth. In addition to this cleaning, the patient may receive brushing and flossing instructions, nutritional counseling, and home care instruction. **Fluoride treatments** (to strengthen enamel and protect teeth from developing carious lesions) are normally performed after children's teeth are cleaned.

Restorative Procedures

Restorative Dentistry

During **restorative dentistry,** the dentist removes caries from the tooth. After the caries have been removed, the tooth is prepared to receive a material that will replace the lost tooth structure. The type of restorative material used depends on the location and the size of the restoration.

Amalgam Restorations

Restorative materials fall into two basic categories—amalgam and resin-based composite. **Amalgam** is an alloy of different metals that is silver in color and is used to restore the function of posterior teeth. Because of the color of the restoration, amalgam is used only in posterior teeth or on the lingual surfaces of some anterior teeth. This metal is strong and lasts for 5 to 20 years. Amalgam is inexpensive and its use is covered by most insurance companies.

Resin-Based Composite Restorations

Resin-based composite restorations are tooth colored and are used primarily on anterior teeth. New hybrid resin–based composites that are now becoming popular are much stronger than the original composites and are being used in posterior teeth as well.

Cast Crown Restorations

Cast crowns are needed when a large amount of tooth structure is removed. Because the design and functions of teeth may vary, if a large amount of tooth structure is removed, amalgam or resin-based composite may not be strong enough to restore the tooth to full function. In these cases, it is necessary to use

material that can withstand the stress and force of normal tooth function. Gold is the closest replacement for tooth enamel. Because of the color of gold, it is used only on posterior teeth, especially in the maxillary arch, which is not normally visible. (In some cultures, visible gold teeth are a status symbol.)

A cast restoration is a two-step procedure. On the first visit, the tooth is prepared for the crown, impressions are taken, and a temporary crown is fabricated. Impressions are sent to the dental laboratory, where a technician prepares the casting according to the directions of the dentist (instructions are given on a prescription called a lab slip). There are different types of cast restorations:

Full gold and metal crowns are cast from gold alloy and other metals and are categorized according to the amount of gold used: high noble, noble, low noble, and nongold (similar to the karat system for gold jewelry: 18k, 14k, and 10k).

- **Porcelain fused to metal** or gold is a cast crown with a porcelain cover (tooth colored).
- **Veneer crowns** offer thin coverage on the facial surface with only a cast composite or resin material.
- An **inlay** offers partial coverage of a tooth, usually on the same surfaces as amalgam restorations. It is cast from gold or composite materials.
- An **onlay** offers partial coverage of a tooth, similar to the inlay, except that an onlay includes more tooth structure, and a cusp is replaced. An onlay is cast from gold or composite.

Prosthetic Procedures

Prosthetic procedures include replacing missing teeth with an artificial tooth or teeth. When a tooth is missing, it can be replaced with a removable or fixed prosthetic appliance. The construction of crowns, bridges, partials, and dentures requires more than one appointment and must be coordinated with the dental laboratory.

Fixed Prosthetics

A fixed prosthetic, or fixed partial denture, is commonly referred to as a **bridge.** A bridge requires that teeth on either side of the missing tooth must be crowned. These teeth are called **abutment teeth.** Abutment teeth form the anchor for the **pontic,** which is the artificial replacement for the missing tooth or teeth. The pontic is soldered to the abutment teeth. When abutments are permanently cemented, the new bridge is strong and is permanently in place.

Removable Prosthetics

The opposite of a permanent bridge is a removable partial. The **removable partial** replaces missing teeth, but, unlike the bridge, it can be removed and is held in place by a metal framework of acrylic and clasps that wrap around abutment teeth. A partial is used when several teeth are missing. The number of teeth to be replaced, the health of surrounding gingival tissue, and the cost are factors to be considered in the decision of whether a partial should be used instead of a bridge.

Full Dentures

Full dentures replace all of the teeth in an arch. They are constructed of acrylic and are custom-fitted for each patient. Care should be taken to match the size, shape, and shade of replacement teeth as closely as possible to those of the natural teeth. It is possible to retain some or all of the natural teeth in one arch while all of the natural teeth in the opposite arch are replaced.

Surgical Procedures

Simple Extractions

Simple extractions involve the removal of one or more teeth without the need to remove bone or cut tissue.

Surgical Extractions

Surgical extractions are more involved and involve the cutting of tissue and the possible removal of bone to facilitate the removal of a tooth. Besides extractions, several other types of dental surgery may be provided. Routine extractions and surgical procedures can be performed by a general dentist. Extensive procedures that necessitate the use of general anesthesia may be referred to an oral maxillofacial surgeon.

Endodontic Procedures

Endodontic, or **root canal,** procedures are performed to replace the pulp. When pulp becomes diseased, it must be removed. Once pulp tissue has been removed, the tooth is no longer vital (alive), but it can remain in the dental arch and can be functional. (The only other option is extraction.) The process includes removing the diseased tissue, cleaning the pulp chamber and root canal, and sealing it with a replacement material. Once a root canal procedure has been performed, the tooth becomes brittle and will weaken over time. It may become necessary to reinforce the tooth with a post or build-up and place a crown to protect the tooth from the possibility of fracture.

When endodontic treatment is billed, the number of canals that have been treated determines the fee for the service. Molars have three to four canals, premolars and anterior teeth have one canal, and maxillary first premolars have two canals.

Other Common Procedures

Sealant application is a procedure that is done to cover the chewing surface of a tooth with a thin coating of resin. The purpose of this treatment is to seal and protect the tooth from the effects of acid attacks, which cause demineralization of enamel and lead to carious lesions. This procedure is performed on newly erupted permanent teeth, and the effects will last until a child reaches the late teens or early adulthood. Sealants, regular dental check-ups, and the use of fluorides reduce the number of cavities.

As an administrative dental assistant, you must know about the different types of dental procedures, and you must be able to determine the amounts of time they will take and the number of appointments that will be needed for their completion. This information is essential for effective scheduling and for correct coding of insurance claims forms to optimize the benefits of patients' insurance coverage. Each procedure has a specific code and fee that is based on the number of surfaces involved and the material used. It is the responsibility of the administrative dental assistant to ensure that the correct procedures have been billed to the patient and the insurance company. It is easy to forget or to overlook procedures, especially if you do not understand the language that is used in patients' charts. It is up to you to learn the dental language. Never be afraid to ask questions when it is not clear which procedures have been completed.

1. Check the room to see that it has been properly cleaned (cleaning the room requires knowledge of infection control).
2. Prepare the dental chair for the patient.
   Cover the chair with a protective barrier.
   Position the back of the chair in an upright position.
   Lift the armrest on the side of the chair on which the patient will be entering.
   Move the tray table, light, and other equipment away from the chair (to provide easy entry for the patient).
3. Check the pathway from the door to the chair and make sure that all hoses and equipment have been moved (to ensure patient safety).
4. Place the patient's chart on the counter, open the chart to the treatment page, and place any radiographs on the view box.
5. Place a patient napkin and napkin chain on the counter for draping the patient.
6. Go to the reception area and greet the patient. Ask the patient to follow you to the treatment area. A special area should be provided for the patient to hang a coat or place other items.
7. Instruct the patient to be seated. (Make sure that the patient is seated all the way back in the chair.)
8. Place the napkin on the patient. (During some procedures, long plastic drapes may also be used to protect the patient's clothing.)
9. Ask the patient to remove any lipstick (provide a tissue) and any jewelry that may interfere with the treatment. (A small container can be used to store jewelry safely.) Remind the patient to ask for the jewelry before leaving the office.
10. After the patient has been seated, advise the patient when the dentist will be entering the room, ask if there are any questions, and provide a magazine or turn on the television. (It is at this point that the patient can view educational videos.)
11. Notify the dental assistant or the dentist that the patient has been seated.

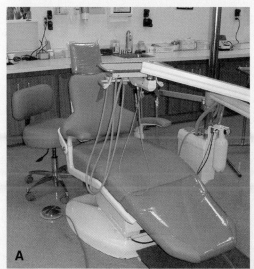

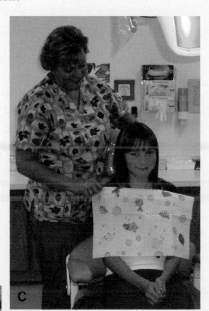

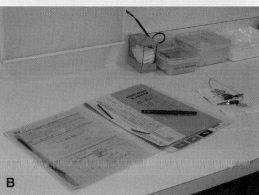

FIGURE 2-21

Seating a patient. **A,** Check the room to see whether it has been properly cleaned and set up for the next patient. **B,** Place the patient chart on the counter along with the patient napkin. **C,** Seat the patient.

BASIC CHAIRSIDE DENTAL ASSISTING DUTIES

In the everyday operation of a dental practice, it may be an assigned or an occasional duty of the administrative dental assistant to help fellow team members in performing the functions of the back office. Current trends in dentistry and in other businesses require that employees must be able to perform multiple tasks. In the dental profession, this means that dental auxiliaries must be trained in more than one aspect of assisting. With cross-training, the administrative dental assistant can, when needed, perform basic chairside duties, and the chairside assistant can perform common functions in the front office. Multitasking also helps to increase career opportunities.

Seating and Dismissing a Patient

A basic procedure that may be asked of the administrative assistant is to seat or dismiss a dental patient. It is not necessary for the assistant to put on gloves before performing this task.

If the dentist requires the administrative dental assistant to perform functions of the chairside assistant, the assistant must be properly trained and must have been given the option of obtaining the hepatitis B vaccination series. The value of administrative dental assistants to the dentist increases if they are able to perform other duties, but they must fulfill all of the same licensure and training requirements of the chairside assistant, even if they perform the task only occasionally.

REMEMBER

This procedure does not include setting the room up for the treatment. This is the job of the dental assistant, and unless you are trained in chairside assisting and have received OSHA training in the safe handling of equipment and instruments, you should not proceed beyond simply seating the patient.

Radiographs

Most states regulate the taking of dental radiographs by requiring a certificate, license, or passage of an examination. No national license is available; therefore, it is necessary for interested individuals to check their state's Dental Practice Act to find out the requirements that must be met in the state in which they work.

Occupational Safety and Health Administration (OSHA)

OSHA is a national government agency that was created to protect workers from workplace injury. OSHA regulates all areas of employment. Most states also have their own version of OSHA, which in some cases is stricter than the federal agency. It is the function of OSHA to develop specific guidelines for specific occupations. Dentistry has very specific regulations concerning the safety of dental employees.

It is the legal responsibility of the dentist to inform each and every employee of all safety hazards. New employees must receive training within 10 days of hire. All employees must receive training and testing yearly.

OSHA has established categories that outline an employee's potential for exposure to toxic or hazardous materials or blood-borne pathogens. Dental office employees may be classified as Category I or Category II according to their job description. An administrative dental assistant who *will never* be assigned to work in the clinical area may fall into Category III.

Most of the tasks performed by a dentist, dental assistant, hygienist, and laboratory technician fall into Category I. Administrative dental assistants who may assist in the clinical area by cleaning treatment rooms, handling contaminated instruments, and preparing laboratory cases are assigned to Category II. Both Category I and Category II classifications require that the employer must provide proper training, protection, and immunization (against hepatitis B) to employees who fall into these categories.

Infection Control

Infection control measures are taken to protect patients from contracting an infectious disease in the dental office. It is the duty and obligation of the dental healthcare team to protect patients at all times.

Protection from disease is ensured with proper cleaning and sterilization of instruments and equipment. It is essential that the patient be protected from cross-contamination by other patients or by members of the dental healthcare team. Proper infection control protocol must be followed at all times. If administrative dental assistants accept the responsibility of helping dental assistants in the clinical area, they must take it upon themselves to be fully trained in the proper infection control protocol. It is not a valid excuse to be negligent in this area just because someone told you to do a job that you have not been trained to perform. Each and every member of the dental healthcare team has the moral, legal, and ethical responsibility to be fully trained before performing assigned duties.

KEY POINTS

- Basic dental office design divides the dental office into two main areas. Nonclinical areas are where most of the duties assigned to the administrative dental assistant take place:
  - Reception area
  - Business office
  - Consultation area
  - Private offices
  - Staff room
- Clinical areas are used by the dentist, dental assistant, and hygienist for tasks related to patient treatment:
  - Treatment rooms
  - Sterilization area
  - Laboratory
  - Radiology room
  - Darkroom
- Administrative dental assistants must know basic dental anatomy and terms so they can effectively communicate with patients and dental professionals about aspects of dental treatment.
- By interpreting dental charts and charting symbols, the administrative dental assistant translates information from the clinical chart for use in daily tasks.

- All assistants who wish to be cross-trained in other aspects of dental assisting require additional knowledge and must be trained in OSHA standards and infection control protocol. Other duties that may be asked of an administrative assistant include:
  - Seating and dismissing a patient
  - Processing radiographs
  - Setting up and cleaning treatment rooms

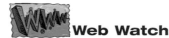 **Web Watch**

Human Anatomy Online

http://www.innerbody.com/htm/body.html

OSHA (Occupational Safety and Health Administration)

http://www.osha.gov

Recommended Infection Control Practices for Dentistry

http://www.hivdent.org/dtc/dtc.htm

    Log on to Evolve to access additional web links!

 Critical Thinking Questions

1. Summarize the various areas within the dental office and outline which activities occur in each area.
2. Draw and label the following structures and tissues of a tooth:
   - alveolar process
   - apical foramen
   - cementum
   - cervix
   - crown
   - dentin
   - enamel
   - gingivae
   - periodontal ligament (membrane)
   - pulp and pulp cavity
   - root
   - root canal

3. Develop a comparison chart of the different numbering systems: Universal Numbering System, International Standards Organization Designation System, and Symbolic Numbering System. Identify the name of the tooth, the quadrant where it is located, and the corresponding number that should be assigned.

4. Translate the following abbreviations:
   - B
   - BO
   - D
   - DO
   - F
   - I
   - L
   - M
   - MI
   - MO
   - MOD
   - MODBL

Notes

_____
_____
_____
_____
_____
_____
_____
_____
_____
_____
_____
_____
_____
_____
_____
_____
_____
_____
_____
_____
_____

OUTLINE

KEY TERMS AND CONCEPTS

Channel
Conference Calls
Credibility
Emotions
Feedback
Interpersonal Communication
Jargon
Loudness

Medium
Message
Noise
Nonverbal Messages
Pitch
Receiver
Semantics
Sender

Sincerity
Smiles
Speed
Stereotyping
Tone
Touch
Verbal Messages
Voice Mail

3

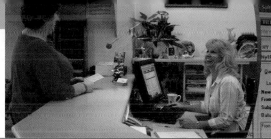
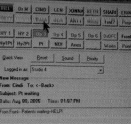

Communication Skills and Telephone Techniques

LEARNING OBJECTIVES

The student will:

1. Identify the five elements of the communications process.
2. Differentiate between verbal and nonverbal messages and describe how the two are used to send and receive messages.
3. Demonstrate how the dental healthcare team sends nonverbal cues.
4. Categorize the different types of interpersonal communication and describe how they are used in the dental profession.

5. Discuss the barriers to effective communication and express how members of the dental healthcare team can remove these barriers.
6. List the responsibilities of the sender that contribute to effective communication and list the responsibilities of the receiver in effective communication.
7. Identify and describe professional telephone manners.

INTRODUCTION

Communication is a two-way process in which information is transferred and shared between a sender and a receiver. Communication can occur between individuals or groups. During the communication process, information is transferred from one person or group to another through a system of symbols (written and spoken language), behaviors (tone of voice), and actions (nonverbal gestures). Transfer is effective only when information is shared and understood. Communication may seem like a very natural and simple task, but during transfer of information, several barriers can interfere with it. It is important for the dental healthcare team to understand and practice effective communication skills.

ELEMENTS OF THE COMMUNICATION PROCESS

The process of communication includes reading, writing, speaking, and listening. During the process, five elements link together to complete the exchange of information between the sender and the receiver:

- The **sender** has an idea that must be shared with another person or group.
- The idea is translated into a **message.**
- The message is placed on a **medium** or **channel.**
- The medium is sent by various channels and is received by the **receiver.**
- The receiver reacts to the message and provides **feedback.**

Transfer of information begins with the sender. The sender has an idea that must be sent and shared. The sender formulates the idea in the form of a message. The message may consist of information, directions, questions, or statements. The message must be placed on a medium and transferred to the receiver. The medium can be verbal (oral or written words) or nonverbal (symbols, gestures, facial expressions, body language, and proximity). The receiver reacts to the message by following instructions, answering questions, or asking questions. This reaction, called feedback, is the method used by the sender to determine whether the message the sender sent was received and understood by the receiver. When the receiver reacts to the message, he or she becomes the sender,

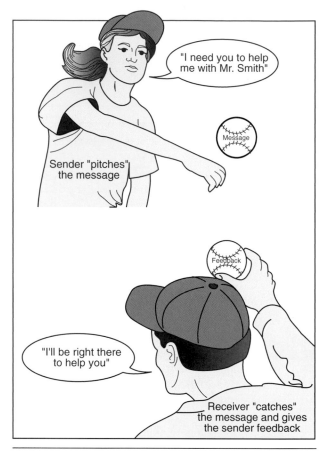

FIGURE 3-1

The communication process. When the sender "pitches the ball," the message is sent. When the receiver "catches the ball," the message is received. Feedback occurs when the receiver throws the ball back.

sending verbal or nonverbal cues; thus, the process goes back and forth until the message or series of messages is sent and received and understanding is established and agreed upon (Figure 3-1).

MEDIUMS OF COMMUNICATION

When the message is sent, it must be placed on or in a format that can be understood by the receiver. The medium can be verbal, nonverbal, or a combination of the two.

Verbal Communication

Verbal messages (messages using words) can be divided into two categories: spoken and written.

Spoken verbal messages may be delivered face to face or transferred electronically (by telephone, voice mail, or video conferencing). Written communication includes letters, memos, faxes, e-mails, newsletters, and several other forms of printed information.

The need for feedback determines the type of medium that will be used to send a message. When the sender needs immediate feedback, the message will be sent via a spoken medium. The spoken medium allows for real-time feedback and the exchange of ideas. When the message includes information and directions (postoperative instructions, treatment plans, financial plans), written communication can be used.

Nonverbal Communication

Nonverbal messages (body language) communicate many things without the use of words. Facial expressions can express different emotions (happiness, sadness, puzzlement, pain). Body gestures (pointing, hand signals) can indicate direction. Tone of voice can give added meaning to a message (anger, joy, importance). Proximity to the receiver and eye contact also add meaning to a message.

Imagine a patient who has left work, spent 20 minutes in heavy traffic, and rushed for a dental appointment, only to find that the dentist is running about 30 minutes behind schedule. The patient's tone of voice, along with crossed arms and frown, indicates irritation when he responds, "I understand." He has just told you he understands verbally, but you know by his nonverbal message that he is very irritated.

Learning to read a **nonverbal communication** aids in interpreting messages. During a visit to the dentist's office, patients often communicate several different nonverbal messages: tenseness, embarrassment, anger, and fearfulness.

Tenseness

Tenseness can be expressed nonverbally in the way a patient sits. Tenseness can be seen in the reception area, where patients anxiously wait to be called. They may sit with their legs tightly crossed and ankles wrapped. Their hands may tightly clutch the arms of the chair. As a member of the dental healthcare team, you should try to relax the patient when you see this message. This effort may be as simple

as saying a few kind words of understanding. You can also ask patients how their vacation was, offer them refreshment while they wait, or share a new magazine to provide subtle diversion.

Embarrassment

Embarrassment can cause patients to cover their mouths. This may be because they have anterior teeth that are less than perfect (caries, missing teeth, malocclusion, or poorly constructed dentures). Patients may try to conceal an imperfection by tightly closing their lips or by placing a hand or tissue over their mouths.

Anger

Anger, disapproval, and defensiveness can be deduced when patients cross their arms, clench their fists, and sit in a very tight manner (legs tightly crossed, arms crossed). This may happen when patients feel they are not being taken care of properly, or if they have to wait for the dentist, are being ignored by members of the dental healthcare team, or are unhappy with the treatment they have just received. It is the responsibility of team members when they receive these nonverbal cues to identify the problem and correct it as quickly as possible.

Patients may feel ignored when they are not recognized as they enter the office, when conversations are taking place between team members while they wait, and when team members are talking on the telephone (even when it is with another patient). Care should be taken to address problems quickly and to identify areas that need attention. A simple smile as a patient enters the reception area acknowledges that the patient has been recognized. When talking on the phone, you should complete the call as soon as possible.

Nonverbal Cues From the Dental Healthcare Team

Members of the dental healthcare team also send nonverbal messages. Caution should be taken to send only positive cues.

Smiles

Smiles always communicate a positive thought. They can be used to ease a patient's apprehension, send a warm greeting to a child, or acknowledge the arrival of a patient. Smiles can even be "seen" over the telephone because they change the tone of your voice. When you are busy on the telephone or are involved in a professional conversation with another team member, a quick wave or smile acknowledges that you will be with the patient as soon as possible.

Touch

Touch can convey a message of warmth, reassurance, understanding, and caring. Patients will recognize the message when they are lightly touched or patted on the shoulder, back of the hand, or arm. Although some patients will welcome the gesture, others will not. Use this method cautiously.

Sincerity

Patients can recognize **sincerity** when members of the dental healthcare team remove barriers. Barriers can take the form of desks and other objects that come between the team member and the patient. For example, during a consultation, when the dentist sits behind a desk, he or she is unable to convey openness. If the desk is removed, patients may feel as though they are on the same level as the dentist and that one is not superior to the other. This allows patients to participate in the conversation on an equal status with the dentist.

INTERPERSONAL COMMUNICATION

Interpersonal communication takes place when the sender and the receiver exchange information in real time. This includes face-to-face, telephone, and video conferencing conversations. Interpersonal communication is the method most often used to communicate in the dental office. The telephone is used by patients and assistants. Face-to-face conversations take place in the dental office during scheduling procedures, treatment planning, and setting up financial arrangements. During interpersonal communication, the flow of information is transferred from one person to another.

The direction of communication varies depending on the type of transfer and the intended receiver. In the dental office, this process can be divided into four broad categories.

The first type of communication transfer occurs when a patient transfers (sends) information to a member of the dental healthcare team. Typically, this is a request for information about the dental practice, fees, the type of treatment offered by the dental practice, availability of appointments, and the type of dental insurance accepted. The patient will ask the team member questions and will expect answers in return (discussed further in Chapter 5).

Patient to Dental Healthcare Team

- Information seeking
- Questions
- Directions
- Telephone conversations
- Appointment scheduling

The second type of communication transfer is passed from the dental healthcare team (sender) to the patient (receiver). This information commonly takes the form of spoken directions and written communications. The information transferred may relate to treatment planning, financial arrangements, appointment scheduling, postoperative care, motivation, and education. When important information is shared with a patient, the dental healthcare team will follow the spoken word with the written word. The medium changes to help facilitate the message. Patients who have just undergone extensive dental treatment may not remember or think to ask questions about the postoperative instructions they have just received. The dental assistant will follow the oral instructions with written instructions, thereby increasing the chance that the patient will remember and follow postoperative instructions [make a note in patient's clinical chart].

Dental Healthcare Team to Patient

- Planning treatment
- Making financial arrangements
- Scheduling appointments
- Giving oral instructions
- Answering questions
- Sharing information
- Motivating
- Informing

The third type of communication transfer takes place between members of the dental healthcare team. This communication is necessary in the everyday operation of the dental practice and is discussed further in Chapter 6.

Team Member to Team Member

- Directional
- Organizational
- Informational
- Professional
- Personal

The fourth type of communication transfer takes place between professional members of the healthcare system, dental specialists, medical doctors, laboratory technicians, and pharmacists. Members of the dental healthcare team transfer information via interpersonal communications and written communications (discussed in Chapter 4).

Professional to Professional

- Referral
- Inquiry
- Consultation
- Direction

BARRIERS TO EFFECTIVE COMMUNICATION

We cannot communicate effectively if the receiver is not receiving the message that is sent. It is like speaking two different languages; we may be saying what we want to say, but the receiver is not hearing and understanding the message as it is intended. It is necessary that the sender and receiver both speak the same language. This includes not only the same vernacular but also the same terminology, lingo, and dialect.

Semantics

Semantics is a change in the meaning of a word. For example, a word used in the context of dentistry may not have the same meaning when it is used outside of the dental field (see Positive Dental Terms on page 59). For example, when dental personnel use the word *drill,* they mean a very small instrument used to remove teeth or shape tooth structure. A drill is a very important instrument in the everyday operation of dentistry. When patients hear the word *drill,* the first thing they picture is the drill that is used in construction work. This drill is large; its use in the mouth is an unpleasant thought. By exchanging the word *handpiece* for *drill,* dental personnel do not trigger the preconceived mental picture of a large drill because the word is less threatening. Therefore, it is important for the dental professional to select words carefully when communicating with patients. When semantics enters into the communication process, the meaning according to the sender may not be the same as that interpreted by the receiver.

Jargon

Each profession and specialty group has its own jargon. **Jargon** refers to specialized words, acronyms (groups of initials), and other sayings that are unique to the profession. The meaning of the message is lost when the sender uses jargon that is unfamiliar to the receiver.

Credibility

Credibility is the weight that is put on a message according to the status, or qualifications, of the person who is sending the message. For example, the dentist who tells a patient what type of treatment is planned has greater credibility than a dental assistant who conveys the same information. Barriers to the message can be created when the receiver believes that the sender does not have the credibility needed to send the message. Levels of credibility also can change the meaning of the message. For example, a patient with periodontal disease is told by his wife that if he does not floss and brush his teeth, he will lose them. Although the message is understood, the receiver doubts the severity of the problem. When the dental assistant sends the same message, it is received and carries greater impact, but still not enough for the patient to make changes. When the dentist sends the same message, the patient believes the message because the dentist has sufficient credibility. The patient receives the message in the context in which it was intended.

Preconceived Ideas

A major barrier to communication arises when **preconceived ideas** change or block the way a message is received. Information that has already been received and is considered true can block a message. For example, the patient with periodontal disease has come to believe that all adults will lose teeth and will have to wear dentures. This assumption is based on past experiences and information. When he is told about the need for brushing and flossing, he doubts the credibility of the message. Once the message has been established as truthful, the patient's idea is changed, and the new information is considered factual.

Nonverbal information may lead to preconceived ideas about people. Consider, for example, the patient who is presented a treatment plan that is costly. When presenting the information, the dentist notices that the patient is wearing inexpensive, outdated clothes. He hesitates to mention the ideal treatment because he is not sure that the patient will be able to afford the fee or will want the treatment. However, because the dentist believes that all treatment options should be presented without regard to the ability to pay, he presents all of them. As it happens, the patient is not only willing to have the work done but also wants to pay cash in advance to take advantage of the pretreatment discount given by the dentist. Because the patient wears outdated, inexpensive clothing, it was presumed that he did not have money. The fact was that he was very wealthy and just was not concerned about his outward appearance.

Other Barriers

Emotions

Emotions play an important role as barriers to communication. When people are upset, angry, or even happy, they sometimes do not hear the message. The ability to interpret nonverbal cues will help dental healthcare team members to adjust the message according to the needs of the patient, thereby avoiding negative response.

Stereotyping

Stereotyping blocks effective communication because assumptions are made on the basis of non-factual information or preconceived ideas about a person, idea, or procedure.

Noise

Noise may alter the message if the sender and the receiver cannot hear the message. When conversations take place around machinery or large, noisy groups of people, the message that is being sent may not be completely received. When the receiver reacts to the message, the sender may not hear the feedback.

REMEMBER

Dental offices have areas that are very noisy, such as treatment rooms, the area near the laboratory, and the business office area, where several activities could be occurring at once.

Conflicting Interpretation

Conflicting interpretations of nonverbal communications can alter or change the meaning of a message. People from different cultures and backgrounds will interpret nonverbal signals in different ways. Care should be taken to avoid these types of signals in the dental office.

How meaning is communicated is an important cornerstone of effective communication. We can choose the message carefully, but the true meaning may be lost in the tone of voice we use or in other nonverbal cues. Tone of voice accounts for 38% of the interpretation of a message and body language or nonverbal communication, 55%.

Barriers to Communication

- Semantics
- Jargon
- Credibility
- Preconceived ideas
- Emotions
- Stereotyping
- Noise
- Conflicting nonverbal communication

IMPROVING COMMUNICATION

Communication can be improved when the sender and the receiver follow a few basic rules of communications.

Responsibilities of the Sender

The sender has the responsibility to ensure that the proper message is sent and that the receiver understands the content of the message. This can be accomplished when the sender formulates the message in such a way that the true meaning or intent is not lost in the translation. This is a simple task when all barriers have been removed. Unfortunately, the sender may not be aware of all the various barriers that can prevent the receiver from understanding the message. However, we can be prepared to listen to the responses of the receiver and to interpret the feedback (verbal and nonverbal).

Selecting the Medium

Selecting the proper medium for the message is the responsibility of the sender. Predetermine the type of message to be sent and the type of medium that will help to minimize misunderstanding. For example, patients who have just spent 3 hours in the dental chair undergoing extensive dental treatment are not likely to remember everything they are told. Following spoken instructions with written instructions provides confirmation for the patient.

REMEMBER

To document transfer of information to the patient, give the patient a copy of the instructions, and make an entry in the patient's clinical chart.

Timing

Timing the transfer of information, which is the responsibility of the sender, is a key component of effective communication. Not all messages are received and understood when the receiver is angry, busy, tired, preoccupied with others, or in pain. This does not mean that the sender does not send the message unless the conditions are just right; what it does mean is that it is important for the sender to understand the receiver and to know how the receiver reacts under less than ideal conditions. When conditions are such that the receiver will not respond to the message, the sender may consider waiting, rephrasing the message, or selecting a different medium.

Checking for Understanding

Check for understanding by listening to the questions and responses of patients and interpreting nonverbal cues. If the meaning of the message is not understood in the context in which it was sent, it is the responsibility of the sender to rephrase or change the message and to work with the receiver until the message is understood. Most often, during poor communication, this step is not followed. Sometimes, the sender believes that the message is so simple that it has to be easily understood and does not check for understanding. For example, when patients are given instructions on how to brush their teeth, it is often forgotten that they may have been doing the process incorrectly. They in turn realize that they should know how to brush their teeth and are too embarrassed to ask for clearer instructions. It is the responsibility of the sender to check for understanding and to work with the receiver until the message is understood in the context that the sender has in mind.

Responsibilities of the Sender

- Formulate a message (clear, concise, complete).
- Select the proper type of medium (verbal, nonverbal).
- Use an appropriate transfer method (interpersonal, written).
- Understand the receiver (interpret possible barriers).
- Listen to feedback to ensure that the message was received and understood.

Responsibilities of the Receiver

Responsibility is shared by the sender and the receiver. The receiver has the responsibility to be attentive during the transfer of information. The receiver should block outside and internal distractions.

Listen to the Complete Message

One of the greatest barriers to effective communication occurs when the receiver evaluates the message before it is completed. When the receiver hears only a portion of the message and then begins to formulate a response or make a judgment, the remainder of the message is not heard. In addition, the receiver will sometimes try to guess what the remainder of the message is before the entire message is delivered. When the receiver does not listen attentively to the complete message, a portion or all of the message will not be heard or understood.

Characteristics of a poor listener

- Interrupts the sender
- Comes to a conclusion before the complete message is sent
- Finishes sentences for the speaker
- Maintains poor posture
- Changes to a different subject
- Shows negative nonverbal signals (eyes wander, arms are crossed)
- Gives poor feedback (uh huh, ok, mmm)
- Tells the sender to "get on with it" (verbal and nonverbal messages)
- Loses emotional control
- Shows distraction physically (taps fingers or feet, paces)

Qualities of a good listener

- Maintains good posture; stands or sits upright
- Maintains eye contact with the sender
- Listens to the complete message (without external or internal distractions)
- Provides feedback (asks complete questions, summarizes the message, follows directions)
- Completes a message transfer before changing the subject (message sent, received, and understood)

Be sensitive to the sender. Place value and importance on the message. Help make the message clear if the sender is having difficulty understanding it. Indicate an appropriate medium, and state preferences for how to receive messages.

Initiate feedback. It is the responsibility of the receiver to initiate feedback. Feedback can be provided through verbal and nonverbal cues. Ask questions if the message is not clear, state your interpretation of the message, or summarize.

Responsibilities of the Receiver

- Be a good listener.
- Be sensitive to the sender.
- Indicate an appropriate medium.
- Initiate feedback.

In later chapters, communication skills are applied to written communications, patient relations, and dental healthcare team communications.

TELEPHONE TECHNIQUES

Communication over the telephone requires a different technique and strategy than those used in face-to-face communications. The ability to read nonverbal cues visually is replaced with listening for nonverbal cues. Developing a pleasing telephone voice is necessary if the correct message is to be conveyed.

People cannot see the person with whom they are speaking on the telephone. Therefore, they formulate impressions that are based on the tone of voice and the mannerisms of the person on the other end

 HIPAA

Privacy Rule

- Take appropriate and reasonable steps to keep a patient's personal health information (PHI) private.
  - Do not discuss PHI with anyone other than the patient [unless authorization has been given by the patient and is on file in the patient record].
  - Share PHI only with authorized healthcare providers.
  - Has the patient authorized the sharing of PHI with persons other than healthcare providers?
- Follow the patient's request for notification.
  - Does the patient wish to be called somewhere other than at home?
  - Has the patient requested that information be sent in an envelope and not on a postcard?

Positive Versus Negative Dental Terms

Positive	Negative	Positive	Negative
Dentures	False teeth	Injection	Shot
Reception area	Waiting room	Empty your mouth	Spit
Remove	Pull	Prepare your tooth	Drill your tooth
Treatment area	Operatory	Examination	Check-up
Instrument	Tool	Consultation	Case presentation
Dentistry	Work	Continued education	Convention
Discomfort	Pain	Change in schedule	Cancellation
Statement	Bill	Investment	Cost
Confirm	Remind	Condition	Acid etch
Fee	Price		

What patients may visualize with negative terms

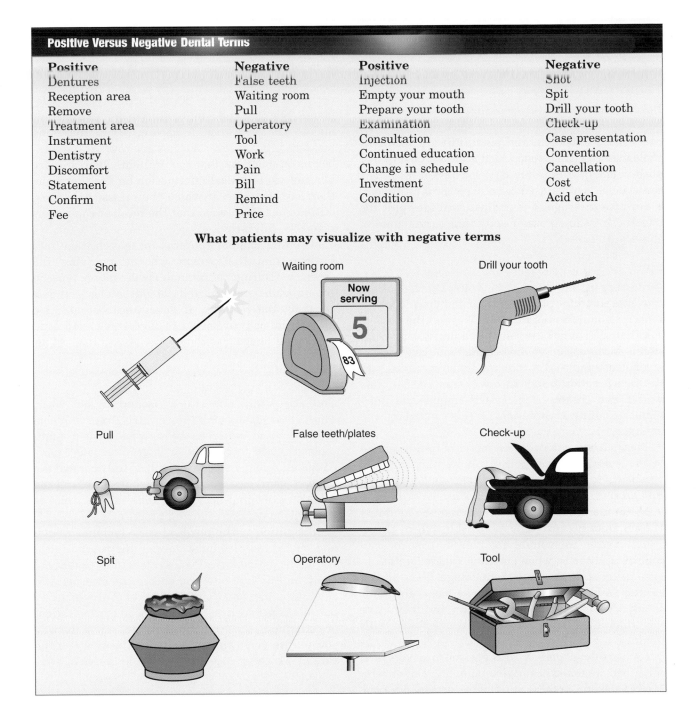

Shot

Waiting room

Drill your tooth

Pull

False teeth/plates

Check-up

Spit

Operatory

Tool

of the line. This image is a combination of several cues that are projected during the conversation.

Developing a Positive Telephone Image

Developing a positive speaking image requires a pleasing tone of voice. Physical voice includes loudness, speed of speech, and pitch. Physical and psychological conditions combined create a negative or positive image that is based on the tone of voice. The same words can be used to send either a positive or a negative message. The receiver will interpret the meaning of the message according to the tone of voice.

Loudness

Loudness is the volume of the voice. During normal conversation, the volume goes up and down slightly, reflecting on different words. It is when the volume is either too loud or too soft that a negative impression is formed. The volume of the voice can become so uncomfortably loud that the listener has to hold the receiver of the telephone away from the ear. This distraction creates a negative image and may result in misinterpretation of the context of the message.

Many things can cause an increase in the volume of the voice. Physically, the volume may increase because of a hearing problem. When senders have a cold or permanent hearing loss or are working in a noisy environment, they may increase the loudness of their voice because they are unable to hear themselves clearly. The volume can also increase for psychological reasons, when emotions (anger, agitation, and excitement) play into the message. Some people assume (falsely) that a person who has a disability or poor speech pattern cannot hear, and they raise the volume of their voice when speaking with them.

Conversely, a person who speaks in a very low voice also creates a negative image. The person who is often asked to repeat statements or who does not receive the correct responses from patients should consider whether the listener is hearing the full message. One reason why people speak in a low voice is lack of self-confidence. If this is a problem, people need to work on improving their self-image; in turn, their telephone image will improve.

Speed

The **speed,** or rate, of speech refers to the quickness with which a message is spoken. When the speaker speaks fast, the receiver may not understand a portion of the message. Several of the types of telephone calls that the administrative dental assistant makes are repetitive in nature. When the same message is given several times in a row, the message begins to sound mechanical. Patients, however, are hearing the technical information for the first time; therefore, the rate at which the message is transmitted must be slow, so that the receiver can understand the full message.

When developing your rate of speech, take into consideration the person who is receiving the message. During a normal conversation, speech should sound natural and should be easily understood by the receiver. If your voice becomes too mechanical or your speech is too fast, you will send a negative image.

Pitch

Tone, or **pitch,** refers to the sound of your voice. Those who speak in a low pitch have a deep, gravelly voice, whereas those who have a high-pitched voice speak in a high, squeaky tone. Although it may be very difficult to fully change the pitch of your voice, you should be able to control the sound. Developing a pleasing tone in your voice is key. This may take time and practice.

In addition to the physical voice (volume, speed, and pitch), you also must develop the psychological voice. The psychological voice refers to the quality of what you say and how you choose the message you send. Although you do not intend to convey nonverbal messages such as depression, anger, agitation, or excitement, these emotions can be seen in the way you phrase your words, the tone of your voice, the rate at which you speak, and the loudness of your voice.

Vocabulary

Proper word usage adds to the quality of a message. Often, patients develop a mental picture on the basis of the words we use. These words or phrases may be very common to the dental profession but may represent something different to the patient.

Developing an Active Script

Instead of saying	Practice saying . . .
Are you a new patient?	When was your last visit to our office?
I don't know the answer; I am just the receptionist.	Sharon is our insurance clerk, and she will be able to answer that question for you. Would you like to hold while I transfer your call?
We don't do that in this office.	In this office, we see patients for general dentistry. Would you like the telephone number of the dental society that has a list of dentists in the area who perform that procedure?
I don't know where he is.	He is unavailable at this time.
It's crazy here today.	It seems several of our patients need us today.
I can't.	I won't be able to because _____.
You're wrong.	Let me see if I can clarify this situation.
I have to check on that.	I will be happy to check on that.
What is this in regard to?	Is there any information that would be helpful for Dr. Edwards to have before she returns your call?
I don't know.	May I check on that for you and call you back?
We can see you today, but you will have to be here by 3:30.	Yes, we can see you today. Can you be here by 3:30?
No, we cannot see you at 5:30.	Mr. Smith, I wish we could see you at 5:30, but our time to see emergency patients today is at 3:30. If you like, we could see you tomorrow at 10:00 AM or 4:00 PM. Which day and time is convenient for you? [Paraphrase. Tell what you can do and why.]
There is no way. We cannot do that for you.	I'm sorry, but we are unable to _____. [If conceivable, give more than one option. This returns control back to the patient. If you are unable to offer solutions, ask the patient if you can call back later. Research the problem, develop a plan, and return the call as soon as possible.]

Active Scripts

It is necessary for dental personnel to develop an active script that creates a positive image and avoids misunderstandings. Practice some of the following phrases and develop them into normal conversations that take place in the dental office. Practice is the only way that correct phraseology can be incorporated on a daily basis. When developing a professional voice, you will need to learn new phrases, words, and ways in which to communicate. As you grow in your profession, you will develop your own voice and apply it to the workplace. At first, some of the terms and phrases will seem unnatural, but as you practice them, they will begin to sound natural and you will become an effective communicator.

In addition to the telephone script, several dental practice management consultants suggest that

scripts should be used in different areas of the dental practice. They should be used with new patients to ensure that all necessary information is collected. Scripting helps the dental healthcare team to ask questions that will elicit the answers they are looking for. As discussed in Chapter 5, each patient is different and has different thoughts and opinions about dentistry. Scripting helps staff to obtain answers to many questions by asking them in a logical, concise, and well-organized sequence.

Before a script is used, whether for telephone conversations, appointment scheduling, financial arrangements, or case presentation, it is necessary that it be practiced until it becomes a natural and normal procedure. To help facilitate the outcome, practice sessions are scheduled. In these sessions, a variety of techniques are used, including role playing and audio and video recording. These techniques are numerous, and all sessions should be perceived as learning experiences. Even assistants and dentists with several successful years of experience are finding the use of scripts helpful and rewarding. Once scripts are developed for an office, they should be monitored for effectiveness and adjusted when needed.

Answering the Telephone

When the telephone rings, we have no idea who is on the other end of the line. It could be a prospective patient looking for information, a personal friend of the dentist, another dental professional, an angry patient, an emergency caller, and so forth. Each call must be answered in the same professional manner. A few simple rules should be followed for all telephone calls. Once the caller has been identified, proper responses can be provided.

Professional Telephone Manners

- Answer the telephone within three rings.
- Identify the dental practice by name.
- Identify yourself by name.
- Speak in a clear, distinct voice that conveys a smile.
- Use appropriate terminology [no slang].
- Give your full attention to the caller.
- Use good listening skills.
- Do not place the caller on hold [if necessary to do so, thank the caller].
- Speak directly into the telephone receiver.
- Thank the caller.
- Hang up after the caller does.

It is necessary from time to time for you to take a message for the dentist or for another team member. Be prepared to take a message by having a message pad and pencil next to all telephones used for incoming calls. Message pads come in a variety of sizes and formats. Each has space in which the same basic information can be inserted: the name of the caller, who the message is for, the telephone number to call, the time and date of the message, and a space for notes. Message pads that make a duplicate copy are preferred because a record of the original message is kept (which can save time used to look for lost messages).

When you take a message, make sure that all information is recorded, the names are spelled correctly, and the return telephone number is correct.

Record any additional information if necessary, and note the type of response that is requested (return the call, wait for a call back, none because the purpose was only to convey information). Once the message has been taken, the next step is to deliver the message to the correct person. This can be accomplished in several ways; a preset protocol must be established and followed. (Is there a central location for all messages? Are they delivered personally to the individual? Are they placed on the dentist's desk? Are they left with the receptionist and picked up later?)

Placing Outgoing Telephone Calls

During the course of a business day, the telephone is used to receive and place calls. Outgoing telephone calls may involve confirming scheduled dental appointments, scheduling recall appointments, speaking with insurance companies and other dental professionals, or ordering supplies. Several steps should be followed when a telephone call is placed:

HIPAA

Privacy Rule

- Place calls in a private area if the call contains the private health information (PHI) of the patient.
- Do not leave PHI in a voice message.
- You can leave a message as long as it does not contain PHI.

---

1. Gather all necessary documents (patient chart, recall list, referral forms, order forms) that you will need to refer to.
2. Plan the call so that you will not be interrupted. Provide privacy if the call will require discussion of confidential information.
3. When using a multiline telephone system, select an open line before you pick up the receiver.
4. Before dialing, check for a dial tone.
5. Take care to dial the telephone number correctly.
6. Know the extension number of the person you are calling.
7. When the phone is answered, identify yourself and the dental office: "Hello, this is Diane from Canyon View Dental." Briefly state the reason

you are calling: "I am calling regarding a mutual patient, Rose Budd." Stop at this point, and wait for the response of the answering party; he or she may transfer you to a different department.

8. At the end of the conversation, summarize the outcome of the call: "I will send you a release of information form, and you will then send Dr. Edwards a report. We can expect the report to be in our office next Friday, is that correct?" If the answer is yes, say, "Thank you. Goodbye."

9. Make sure that the conversation has ended before you hang up. This is usually signaled with a simple "goodbye."

10. If you call the wrong number, apologize for the error and verify the number. Never ask receiving parties their telephone numbers; instead, you should repeat the number you called.

Conference Calls

Occasionally, it may be necessary for the dentist to receive or place a conference call. **Conference calls** allow several people to be present on the telephone line at one time. The purpose of a conference call is to hold a meeting without having everyone in the same location. Conference calls are planned in advance to be held at a predetermined date and time. Anyone who is expecting a conference call should notify the administrative dental assistant as soon as possible. Once the date and time have been set, the appointment schedule needs to be adjusted to ensure that scheduled parties will be available.

A third party conference call is initiated and managed by a service other than the dental office. The call is arranged with the service, contact information is given for each party joining in on the call, and at the time of the prearranged conference, the call is placed by the service. When all parties have been contacted, they are connected to a single line and can begin their conference. If a party is not available at the time the operator calls, the operator will leave a telephone number and a conference number to be used when the party does call in, at which time the party will be connected to the conference call.

Another type of third party conference call gives each conference attendee a telephone number and access code. When it is time for the conference to begin, each attendee personally initiates the call. This type of call is usually less expensive and can be accessed by the attendee from any telephone (elimi-

nating the need for the attendee to be at a given number at the arranged time). Some telephone equipment also allows for conference calling that can be initiated without the assistance of a third party.

HIPAA

Privacy Rule

Take appropriate and reasonable steps to keep a patient's protected health information (PHI) private.

Voice Mail

When you place calls to patients and others, it may be necessary to leave a message in their **voice mailbox.** The person called can access the mailbox at a later time and retrieve the message. When you leave a message, be sure to identify yourself and the dental office, speak slowly, keep the message brief, leave a return number (given in a slow, distinct, clear voice), and specify the type of response you want:

Hello. This is Diane from Canyon View Dental. I would like to place an order for dental supplies. Please return my call before 5:30 today. The office number is 909-555-2345. [Give the number slowly so that the receiver can write it down as you speak.] Talk to you later, thanks.

Personal Calls

Personal calls are never appropriate during working hours. From time to time, it may be necessary to place a personal call during working hours. When this happens, make the call during your break or lunch time. Always follow the protocol of the office. If absolutely no personal phone calls are allowed, abide by the rule. If an emergency arises and you have to place a call, notify the dentist or the office manager first and ask permission. Receiving personal calls during the day is also not acceptable. If an emergency arises, callers should identify themselves and state that it is an emergency call.

KEY POINTS

• Communication is a two-way process in which information is transferred between a sender and a receiver. The five elements of the communication process are:

- Sender
- Message
- Medium or channel
- Receiver
- Feedback
- Verbal communication occurs through words, spoken and written. Nonverbal communications do not use words. Messages are sent through facial expressions and body gestures. The administrative dental assistant uses verbal and nonverbal communication on a daily basis to communicate with patients, dental team members, and other professionals.
- Telephone communication requires a set of skills needed to convey a positive image. These skills include:
  - Developing a pleasing tone of voice
  - Using positive dental terms
  - Referring to an active script
  - Speaking with professional telephone manners
  - Taking appropriate and reasonable steps to keep a patient's protected health information (PHI) private

Web Watch

Improving Verbal Skills

http://www.itstime.com/aug97.htm

Let Them Hear You Smile: Telephone Techniques

http://www.onlinewbc.gov/docs/market/mk_appear_
phone.html

Your Communication Style Preference

http://www.onlinewbc.gov/docs/market/style_pref.html

Nonverbal Communication

http://www.onlinewbc.gov/docs/market/mk_appear_
nonverbal.html

Telephoning Skills

http://ec.hku.hk/epc/telephoning

Virtual Presentation Assistance

http://www.ku.edu/cwis/units/coms2/vpa/vpa.htm

 Log on to Evolve to access additional
web links!

 Critical Thinking Questions

1. How would you apply what you learned about the communication process to ensure that the message that you send is received and understood by the receiver? Identify the process and give an example.
2. Make a distinction between patients who are tense, angry, or embarrassed by describing the way they are sitting in the reception area while waiting to be seen. Explain the nonverbal cues that you recognize for each condition.
3. Evaluate your telephone voice:
   How would you change or improve the way you currently speak on the telephone?
   What would you do to ensure that you are projecting a positive telephone image?

Notes

OUTLINE

KEY TERMS AND CONCEPTS

Administrative Management
  Society
Attention Lines
Blocked
Body of Letter
Closing
Company Signature
Completeness
Complimentary Closing
Computerized Letter Template
Concise
Date Line
Dual Addressing
Enclosure Reminder
Express Mail
First-Class Mail
Full-Blocked
Incoming Mail

Inside Address
Introduction
Letterheads
Line Spacing
Logical
Main Body
Modified Blocked
Notation Line
Office Letter Portfolio
Open Punctuation
Organization
Outgoing Mail
Outlook
Paragraphing
Postage
Postal Cards
Priority Mail
Reference Initials

Reference Line
Referral Letter
Return Address
Salutation
Semi-blocked
Signature Identification
Simplified
Square-blocked
Standard Mail (A)
Standard Mail (B)
Standard Punctuation
Stationery
Subject Line
Tone
Type
White Space

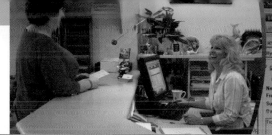

CHAPTER

4

Written Correspondence

LEARNING OBJECTIVES

The student will:

1. Discuss the four elements of letter writing style and compose a letter.
2. Describe letter style appearance as it applies to a finished business letter.
3. Recognize the different parts of a business letter.
4. Evaluate a completed business letter by identifying letter style format, judging letter style appearance, and assessing letter writing style.
5. Identify when HIPAA Privacy and Security Rules apply to written communications.

67

INTRODUCTION

Written correspondence is no longer limited to the letters sent to patients and other professionals. Today, the progressive dental practice uses written communication to perform a wide variety of tasks. Computers are useful in a dental practice. They can be used to develop patient brochures and monthly newsletters, create office manuals for employees, store databases and sample letters, and perform merge techniques to mass mail an assortment of letters and notices. Even with all the available resources for producing communications, you must still understand the basic letter styles that are used in the business world. This chapter reviews the basic letter writing skills necessary to create a well-organized, appealing, and effective business letter.

Types of Written Correspondence

- Letters
- Insurance company correspondence
- Laboratory instructions
- Prescription orders
- Newsletters
- New patient information letters
- Recall notices
- Collections letters
- Thank you letters
- Birthday cards
- Special recognitions
- Employee manuals
- Office policy
- Office philosophy

LETTER WRITING STYLE

Writing style is a combination of elements that, when arranged properly, help to communicate a message. The style selected to communicate the message varies according to the type of message and the receiver.

Tone

Tone is very similar to "tone of voice" in spoken communication. It is intended to clarify meaning. When people speak, they change the tone of the message by adjusting their voice. In written communications, the tone can be changed through the selection of words and phrases. Tone should set the mood of the letter and should sound natural.

As per your request, please find enclosed herewith the radiographs of Traci Collins.

Unnecessary phrases such as *as per* and *herewith* do not add to the message. The writer sounds forced and unnatural. Include words that are natural and that fit the intended tone of the letter (formal or informal).

As you requested, I am enclosing the radiographs for Traci Collins.

The above statement sounds natural and is easy to read.

Phrases to Avoid in Letter Writing

- According to our records
- Acknowledge receipt of
- As to, with reference to, with regard to, with respect to
- At hand, on hand
- Attached please find, attached hereto, enclosed herewith, enclosed please find
- Beg to inform, beg to tell
- Duly
- For your information
- Hereby, heretofore, herewith
- I have your letter
- I wish to thank, may I ask
- In due time, in due course of time
- In receipt of
- In the near future
- In view of
- Our Girls
- Permit me to say
- Thank you again
- Thank you in advance
- Thereon

Outlook

Another important element in business communication is outlook. **Outlook** refers to presentation of information in a positive form, even when the letter contains unpleasant subject material. Because

Phrases to Use in Letter Writing	
Instead of	Use
Advise, inform	Say, tell, let us know
Along these lines, on the order of	Like, similar to
As per	As, according to
At an early date, at your earliest convenience	Soon, today, next week
At this writing	A specific date
Check to cover	Check for
Deem	Believe, consider
Due to the fact that, because of the fact that	Because
Favor, communication	Letter, memo
For the purpose of	For
Forward	Send
Free of charge	Free
In accordance with	According to
In advance of, prior to	Before
In compliance with	As you requested
In re, re	Regarding, concerning
In the amount of	For
In the event that	If, in case
Kindly	Please
Of recent date	Recent
Party	Person (a specific name)
Said	Not to be used as an adjective
Same	Not to be used as a noun
Subsequent to	After, since
The writer, the undersigned	I, me
Up to this writing	Until now

(Modified from Geffner A: Business Letters, The Easy Way. 3rd edition. New York, Barron's Educational Series, Inc., 1998, pp 1, 2.)

patients are customers and we should strive for customer satisfaction, it is important to remain diplomatic and considerate. The objective is to convey to readers that they are your first priority. Simple terms like *please* and *thank you* help project a positive image.

Instead of:

We have received your payment of $100.00.

Try:

Thank you for your payment of $100.00. (positive)

Instead of:

We have not received your payment of $100.00.

Try:

Please send your payment of $100.00.

Avoid being impersonal:

A check of our records confirms that an error was made on your March statement.

Add a positive personal statement, which will help smooth any negative feelings the patient may have developed because of an error in the March billing:

We hope that you have not been seriously inconvenienced by the error in your March statement.

Letters that deal with unpleasant subject matter should be checked carefully to ensure that the correct message is being sent. We may want to say *pay now,* but we will not get results if we sound as if we are attacking an individual. For example, avoid:

Because you have been delinquent in paying your account, it is necessary to report your delinquency to a credit reporting agency.

Try a more positive approach:

Because the balance on your account is now over 90 days past due, your credit rating may be at risk.

Because the second statement is not a personal attack on the reader, it will probably be read and accepted as information.

Personalizing Letters

It is important to use the "you" technique. This technique, which personalizes the letter for the reader by using the word *you,* conveys courtesy and concern for patients and gains their attention. Care should be taken not to overuse the reader's name in the body of the letter; this tactic, when overdone, may make the message sound condescending.

Instead of:

Please accept our apologies for the error on your March statement.

Try:

We hope that you have not been seriously inconvenienced by the error on your March statement.

This statement lets the patient know that you care.

The "you" technique does not eliminate the need to use *I* and *we* in letters. When you use these pronouns, remember some key points in their proper use:

- *I* refers to the person who is signing the letter.
- *We* refers to the company (dental practice) that is sending the letter.

REMEMBER

Do not use the company name or the doctor's name in the body of a letter signed by the company or the doctor. This is the same as using your name instead of *I* or *me* in a letter you sign. You can refer to the doctor by name in a letter that you sign (because the doctor is not sending it).

Organization

The final element in letter writing style is organization. **Organization** is a process through which you identify what you want to say and the results you hope to attain. The end product must be logical (make sense), complete (state everything you want to say), and concise (not say too much).

Logical

Before you write the letter, make a list of the information you wish to convey to the reader. Start with the reason, list the facts, and give any explanations that may be needed. Next, arrange the list in a **logical** order. This will help the reader understand the message you are sending.

Complete

Always check for **completeness.** This step is completed in the organizational stage. When checking, make sure that you have included all of the information, facts, and explanations that the reader needs. You will want to say everything you can to obtain the desired response from the reader. It is not uncommon to include a phrase that appeals to the reader's emotions or understanding.

Concise

The final consideration in organization is being **concise.** You want to say just the right amount without overusing words and phrases. Developing this skill takes practice. We often think that we need to say more than is necessary to convey the idea to the reader. One way that letters are overwritten is the reiteration of points. One example is ending a letter with:

Thank you once again.

If you have thanked the reader once, it is not necessary to thank him or her again. This type of statement breaks the logical flow of the letter and distracts the reader.

Adding information at the close of a letter that is not related to the main point of the letter lessens the desired effect. Consider how you would feel if you received a collection letter from a dental office that concludes:

Just a friendly reminder that you are due for your 6-month recall appointment. Please call our office today to schedule your appointment.

Do not give readers more information than they need. Unnecessary information only confuses readers and dilutes the desired effect.

Redundancy is another block to effective letter writing. Redundant words and phrases distract from the correspondence:

Dr. Jones and Dr. Smith will cooperate together in the treatment of their mutual patient, Patty Payne.

Cooperate means *working together;* drop *together.* Because we know that they are working together, drop the phrase *of their mutual patient:*

Drs. Jones and Smith will cooperate in the treatment of Patty Payne.

Developing Letter Writing Style

- Tone . . . Select pleasant, natural-sounding words and phrases.
- Outlook . . . Be courteous and polite (use *please* and *thank you*).
- Positive approach . . . Use words that emphasize good points instead of bad.
- "You technique" . . . Use the word *you,* and direct information to the reader personally.
- Organization . . . Be logical, complete, and concise.
- Plan . . . plan . . . plan. . . .

LETTER STYLE (APPEARANCE)

The appearance of correspondence is as important as the writing style. It is necessary to gain the attention of the reader before the letter is read. If the letter is neat, well formatted, and written on appealing stationery, it has a better chance of being read.

Appearance

The first impression of your correspondence will be formulated by its physical appearance. Factors that contribute to the first impression are type of paper, color, font (print style), placement of type, and use of a logo.

Stationery

Stationery is a collection of similar-looking paper products that are used in a variety of correspondence. Effective professional communication is a combination of selected stationery and the message. Stationery comes in a variety of sizes and styles (Figure 4-1). **Letterheads** are placed at the top of the paper and include the name of the dentist or dental practice and the address. Additional information may include the telephone number, fax number, and e-mail address.

Although the letterhead is typically centered at the top of the paper, it can be attractively placed in other locations at the top. In addition to names and addresses, it may include a logo. Occasionally, the information is divided between the top and the bottom of the page, with the logo and the practice name at the top and the address and telephone number at the bottom. Once the dentist has selected a style and a logo, these will be used on all corresponding stationery. The key to the placement of information included in the letterhead is appearance. The letterhead should be attractive and balanced on the page.

Types of Stationery

- Standard-sized paper ($8^1/_2 \times 11$ inches)
- Note-sized paper ($6^1/_4 \times 9^1/_4$ inches)
- Appointment cards
- Standard #10 envelopes (standard paper)
- Note envelopes (note-sized paper)

Stationery is made in papers of different weights (thickness), color, and style. Professional stationery is made from a combination of different natural products, such as cotton, linen, and flax. Each material or combination of material adds to the appearance of the paper. The paper may be lightly textured and may contain a watermark (light mark on the paper that identifies the type or manufacturer of the paper)

Stationery is available in a variety of colors. The color selected should project a professional image. Common colors available for stationery are beige, ivory, white, blue, and other subtle tones. The style and color of the print should harmonize with the overall desired appearance of the letterhead. Type used in the letterhead will be of one or two colors and can be raised or flat.

REMEMBER

The finished product will be used for communicating with patients and professionals.

Type

The **type** is single spaced in the body of the letter, with double spacing between paragraphs. Type is black (dark) and neat. When a typewriter is used, errors can usually be erased with tape. It is not good style to erase or use correction fluid. When a computer is used, the document must be carefully checked for mistakes before it is printed. If an error is discovered after the letter has been printed, return to the original document, make the correction, and reprint the letter.

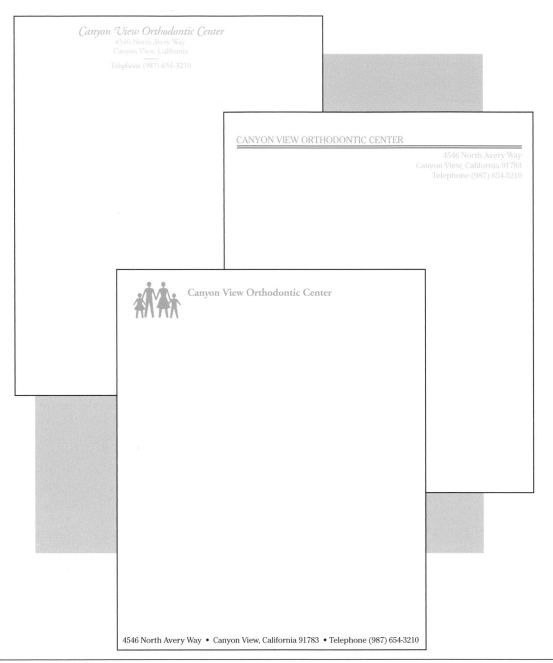

FIGURE 4-1
Assortment of stationery and letterhead formats.

Paragraphing

Paragraphing is the method used to insert natural breaks in the flow of information. Care should be taken to create paragraphs of equal lengths. When a short paragraph is followed by a very long paragraph, the document appears to be unbalanced, and this distracts from the appearance of the letter.

White Space

White space is the empty areas surrounding the text of the letter. This surrounding space should be

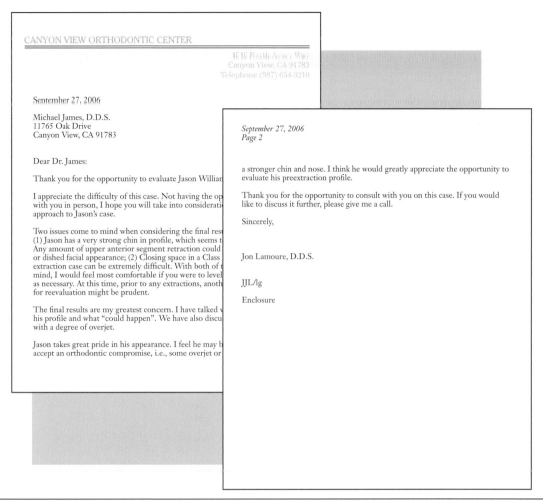

FIGURE 4-2

The second page starts at the top of a blank page and is not centered down on the page. (Modified from SmartPractice: The Complete Dental Letter Handbook: Your Fingertip Resource for Practice Communication, Phoenix, Semantodontics, 1989.)

uniform and balanced. A short letter should be started farther down on the paper than usual so that there is approximately the same amount of white space above and below the text. Longer letters may require the addition of a second page. When a second page is started, it is always started at the top of a blank page (no letterhead) and is not centered down on the page (Figure 4-2). When a second page is used, care should be taken to include one full paragraph or several lines. It is poor style to end a letter on a second page with just one line.

Line Spacing

Line spacing is the number of empty lines between the different elements of a letter. Typically, a line,

or space, is created when the return key is struck. For example, if you wanted to create a double space, you would strike the return key twice; for a single space, you would strike it once.

LETTER STYLE (FORMAT)

Five basic letter styles are used in business correspondence:
1. Full-blocked
2. Blocked
3. Semi-blocked, or modified blocked
4. Square-blocked
5. Simplified or AMS (Administrative Management Society)

Style is selected according to the type of letter and the preference of the dentist. (The two types of punctuation that can be used, open and standard, are explained later.) Within each style, spacing and margins can be adjusted to allow for flexibility in producing a visually appealing letter.

In the **full-blocked** format, all letter sections begin at the left margin. The spacing outlined earlier is applied between sections (Figure 4-3).

Line Spacing	
Date line	2 to 6 inches below the letterhead (adjust for the length of the letter)
Inside address	3 lines below the date line
Attention line	2 lines below the inside address (optional)
Salutation line	2 lines below the inside address (or attention line when used)
Reference line	2 lines below the salutation line (optional)
Body of the letter	2 lines below the salutation line or reference line (when used). Text is single spaced; a double space is used between paragraphs
Complimentary	2 lines below the last line of text closing
Company signature	2 lines below the complimentary closing (optional)
Signature	4 lines below the complimentary closing or company signature (allows space identification for signature)
Reference initials	2 lines below the signature identification
Enclosure reminder	1 line below the signature identification
Notation line	1 line below the enclosure reminder

In the **blocked** format, all sections begin at the left margin, except the line, complimentary closing, company signature, and writer's identification, which all begin at the horizontal center of the page (Figure 4-4, *Bottom*). Variations can be used. The date line can be justified right (end at the right margin), and the attention and subject lines can be centered or indented five or ten spaces.

The **semi-blocked,** or **modified blocked,** format is the same as the blocked format with one change. Paragraph beginnings are indented five spaces (see Figure 4-4, *Top*).

The **square-blocked** format is very similar to the full-blocked format. The date line is on the same line as the first line of the inside address and is justified right. Reference initials and enclosure reminder are typed on the same line as the signature and signer's identification and are justified right. This style allows for squaring of the letter and is used when space is needed (Figure 4-5, *Bottom*).

The **simplified,** or **Administrative Management Society** (AMS), style is fast and efficient. The style is the same as full-blocked, with the following changes:
- Open punctuation is used.
- No salutation or complimentary closing is included.
- A subject line must be used, in all capital letters, with the word *subject* omitted.
- The signer's identification is provided in all capital letters.
- Lists are indented five spaces. If a numbered list is used, the period is omitted and the list is not indented.

The simplified, or AMS, style does not include personal identification of the reader. It is therefore recommended that the reader's name be mentioned at least one time in the body of the letter (see Figure 4-5, *Top*).

PUNCTUATION STYLES

Punctuation marks within the body of the letter are used according to the same rules in any formal document. The punctuation style used in the salutation and complimentary closing can be either open or standard. In **open punctuation,** no punctuation is used in the salutation and complimentary closing (punctuation *is* used in the body of the letter) (see Figure 4-5, *Top*). In **standard punctuation,** the salutation is followed by a colon (:), and the complimentary closing is followed by a comma (,) (see Figures 4-2, 4-3, and 4-4).

Text continued on p. 79

Canyon View Orthodontic Center

April 28, 2006

Jo Ann Grant
27 South 3rd Street
Canyon View, CA 91783

Dear Ms. Grant:

We look forward to seeing you again on May 21st at 10:30 a.m.

Enclosed is the information you requested on orthodontic treatment. If you have any additional questions, I will be happy to answer them before we begin orthodontic treatment.

At this appointment, we will review your treatment plan. You should expect to spend at least 30 minutes with us.

We will then set up other convenient times for you to complete banding. This process will take one or two additional appointments.

Sincerely yours,
Canyon View Orthodontic Center

Martha James
Treatment Coordinator

MJ
Enclosure
CC: Mary A Edwards, D.D.S.

TYPE:	Full blocked
PURPOSE:	Pretreatment
PUNCTUATION:	Standard

Canyon View Dental Associates

June 8, 2006

Gary Thompson, D.D.S.
2134 South Marshall Canyon
Canyon View, CA 91783

Dear Dr. Thompson:

On May 24 I completed an oral-dental examination without radiographs on Marcie Lynn. Radiographs taken within the past year are being forwarded to our office from her previous general dentist.

Marcie's dental status was within normal limits, except for her primary orthodontic condition. Specifically, she has a severe Class II skeletal malocclusion and anterior open bite, resulting from an underdeveloped mandible, exacerbated by a nocturnal finger-sucking habit. At her young age, this malocclusion could very likely inhibit her speech pattern development.

I have recommended to her parents that they consult with you for further orthodontic advice, as well as a speech pathologist.

It is always a pleasure to consult with you.

Yours truly,

Mary A. Edwards, D.D.S.
MAE/lg

TYPE:	Full blocked
PURPOSE:	Referral
PUNCTUATION:	Standard

FIGURE 4-3

Full blocked style. **A,** Pretreatment letter/diagram. Referral letter. (Modified from Limoli Portion! The Complete Dental Letter Handbook: Your Fingertip Resource for Practice Communication, Phoenix, Semantodontics, 1989.)

Canyon View Dental Associates

April 28, 2006

Mr. and Mrs. Fred Collins
35901 E. 10th Street
Flora, CA 91782

Dear New Neighbors:

WELCOME GIFT

We have a gift for each member of your family. We would be delighted to
have you stop by our office between 9:00 a.m. and 5:00 p.m., Monday
through Thursday to pick up your complimentary dental kits.

All of us at Canyon View Dental Associates really take pride in our
friendly, gentle atmosphere. We listen and are sensitive to your dental
needs. If you have any dental need or emergency, we'll be available to
help.

Welcome to the community! It will be great to meet you and your family.

Sincerely yours,
Canyon View Dental Associates

Mary A Edwards, D.D.S.

MAE/lg
Enclosure

TYPE:	Semi-blocked/Modified block
PURPOSE:	Welcome to the Community (Direct Mail)
PUNCTUATION:	Standard

Canyon View Dental Associates

September 7, 2006

Blue Cross of California
P.O. Box 3254
Flora, CA 91783

To Whom It May Concern:

Re: Rose Budd, Group 8476, ID# 123-45-6789

Ms. Rose Budd's tooth #3 was extracted on 7-23-98 because of prior
unsuccessful endodontic treatment, which caused chronic periapical and
intraradicular infection. The endodontic procedure was not done in my
office and I have no prior radiograph of the tooth.

To prevent mesial drift and occlusal trauma, I am recommending a
permanent three-unit porcelain bridge from tooth #2 to #4 for Ms. Budd. I
am enclosing a preextraction periapical radiograph and a post-extraction
panograph for your review.

Thank you.

Sincerely yours,
Canyon View Dental Associates

Mary A. Edwards, DDS

MAE/lg
Enc. 2

TYPE:	Blocked (dateline and attention line options)
PURPOSE:	Insurance correspondence
PUNCTUATION:	Standard

FIGURE 4-4

Top, Semi-blocked/modified block, "welcome to the community" letter (direct mail); *Bottom,* Blocked, insurance correspondence. (Modified from SmartPractice: The Complete Dental Letter Handbook: Your Fingertip Resource for Practice Communication, Phoenix, Semantodontics, 1989.)

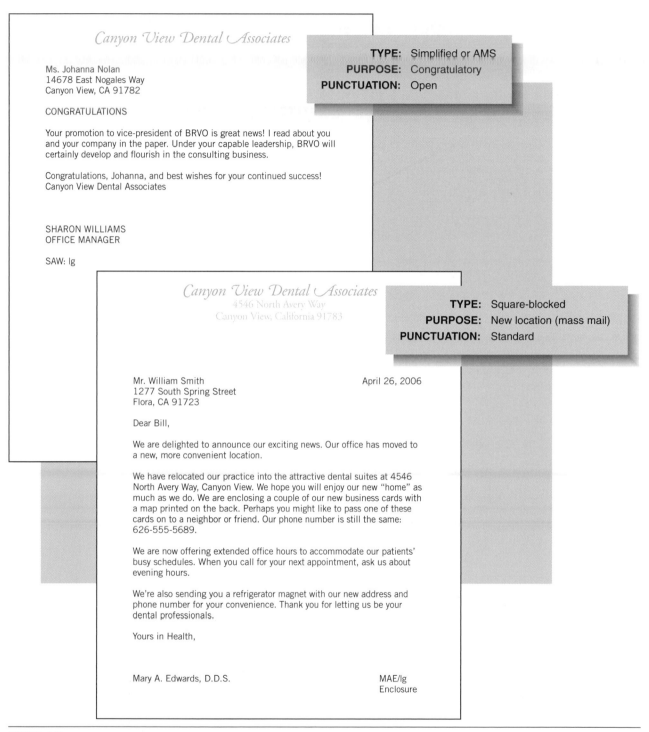

Canyon View Dental Associates

Ms. Johanna Nolan
14678 East Nogales Way
Canyon View, CA 91782

CONGRATULATIONS

Your promotion to vice-president of BRVO is great news! I read about you
and your company in the paper. Under your capable leadership, BRVO will
certainly develop and flourish in the consulting business.

Congratulations, Johanna, and best wishes for your continued success!
Canyon View Dental Associates

SHARON WILLIAMS
OFFICE MANAGER

SAW: lg

TYPE:	Simplified or AMS
PURPOSE:	Congratulatory
PUNCTUATION:	Open

Canyon View Dental Associates
4546 North Avery Way
Canyon View, California 91783

TYPE:	Square-blocked
PURPOSE:	New location (mass mail)
PUNCTUATION:	Standard

Mr. William Smith   April 26, 2006
1277 South Spring Street
Flora, CA 91723

Dear Bill,

We are delighted to announce our exciting news. Our office has moved to
a new, more convenient location.

We have relocated our practice into the attractive dental suites at 4546
North Avery Way, Canyon View. We hope you will enjoy our new "home" as
much as we do. We are enclosing a couple of our new business cards with
a map printed on the back. Perhaps you might like to pass one of these
cards on to a neighbor or friend. Our phone number is still the same:
626-555-5689.

We are now offering extended office hours to accommodate our patients'
busy schedules. When you call for your next appointment, ask us about
evening hours.

We're also sending you a refrigerator magnet with our new address and
phone number for your convenience. Thank you for letting us be your
dental professionals.

Yours in Health,

Mary A. Edwards, D.D.S.   MAE/lg
                                                     Enclosure

FIGURE 4-5

Top, Simplified or Administrative Management Society (AMS) style, congratulatory letter. *Bottom,* Square-blocked style, "new
location" letter (mass mail). (Modified from SmartPractice: The Complete Dental Letter Handbook: Your Fingertip Resource for Practice
Communication, Phoenix, Semantodontics, 1989.)

ANATOMY OF A BUSINESS LETTER

(1) **CANYON VIEW**
DENTAL ASSOCIATES   *4546 North Avery Way*
Canyon View, CA 91783

(2) April 28, 2006

(3) Canyon View Medical Group
2908 Circle Drive
Canyon View, CA 91783
(4) Lynn Saunders, M.D.
Director of Pediatric Medicine

(5) Dear Dr. Saunders:

(6) Subject: NURSING BOTTLE SYNDROME

(7a) Keeping smiles is our business and recently we have treated several young children with rampant decay. We are treating cavities caused by nursing bottle syndrome.

(7b) As you know, this is caused by giving a baby a bottle with milk, formula, or juice at bedtime. The sugars in these liquids feed the mouth bacteria-producing acids that dissolve tooth enamel in a relatively short period of time.

Babies and young children should be given only water at bedtime or before a nap. If a child falls asleep with a bottle containing anything else, the potential for nursing bottle syndrome increases.

(7c) Thanks for passing this information to the parents of your young patients. If you need more information or pamphlets, please call us at 626-555-5689. (7)

BODY OF THE LETTER

(8) Sincerely,

(9) Canyon View Dental Associates

(10) Mary A. Edwards, D.D.S.

(11) MAE/lg
Enclosure (12)

(13) cc:

(1) **LETTERHEAD**
Identifies the company or dental practice sending the letter. The letterhead style will vary in color, font style, and size. The name and address of the dental practice (company) are included, but telephone number, fax number, e-mail address, web address, or company logo are optional. Traditionally the letterhead is placed at the top of the paper, but this may vary. Letterheads are used only on the first page.

(2) **DATELINE**
The date the letter was written is placed a few lines below the letterhead (if the letterhead is at the top of the page). Rules for spacing the dateline are flexible, to allow for a well-balanced, appealing letter.

(3) **INSIDE ADDRESS**
The same as the address on the outside of the envelope. When addressing the letter to an individual, several different methods can be used:

1) The name of the intended reader is listed, followed by the company name and address.
2) The company name and address is listed, followed by an attention line to identify the intended reader.

These styles vary and may be determined by the type of computer software being used. Most software packages can print envelopes with information from the inside address.

(Modified from SmartPractice: The Complete Dental Letter Handbook: Your Fingertip Resource for Practice Communication, Phoenix, Sexmantodontics, 1989.)

(4) ATTENTION LINES

Used to draw attention to the person you wish to read the letter. The full name should be typed and underlined, or typed in all capital letters. Do not include redundant titles such as Dr. Mary A. Edwards, DDS. A person's company title can be placed on a second line, for example:

Lynn Saunders, M.D.
Director of Pediatric Medicine
2908 Circle Drive
Canyon View, CA 91783

(5) SALUTATION

Greets the reader. When the reader's name is known, it is best to use the name: Dear Ms. Jones, Dear Tom Smith. If the reader is familiar with you and this is a less formal letter, Dear Tom is appropriate. If the reader is unknown, general titles may be used: Dear Sir, Dear Madam, Dear Sir or Madam, Dear Ladies and Gentlemen, Gentleman, To Whom It May Concern.

(6) SUBJECT LINE

Draws attention to the subject of the letter. Its use is optional. It can be underlined or typed in all capital letters.

(7) BODY OF THE LETTER

Within the body of the letter there are three sections, the introduction, the main body, and the closing.

(7a) The **introduction** is the first paragraph and states the reason you are writing. This section is one paragraph long and should contain a brief list of the important points you will cover in the main body of the letter.

(7b) The **main body** gives details of the points that you stated in the introduction. This section is one or two paragraphs long, depending on the number of points that you cover. This section should be concise and to the point.

(7c) The **closing** paragraph describes the next step or expected outcome. Clearly state what action will be taken. For example, if you are sending a letter of referral to a specialist introducing a patient, inform the dentist what the patient will do next (call for an appointment, wait for the dental office to call and set up an appointment, or explore options and then decide what to do). The closing paragraph should enable the reader to determine what to do next.

(8) COMPLIMENTARY CLOSING

Closes the letter courteously. Typical complimentary closings are Yours truly, Truly yours, Sincerely yours, and so on. The type of complimentary closing should follow the overall intent of the correspondence. For example, you would not close a collection letter with Best wishes.

(9) COMPANY SIGNATURE

Identifies the company of the person who is sending the letter and is optional. It is used when the sender of the letter represents the company.

(10) SIGNER'S IDENTIFICATION

Occurs four lines below the previous item (complimentary close or company signature) to allow room for a signature. Type the signer's name and appropriate title (if needed).

(11) REFERENCE INITIALS

Identify the sender and the typist of the letter. Type the sender's initials in capital letters, followed by a slash (/) or a colon (:) and the typist's initials in lower case. The purpose is to identify the preparer.

(12) ENCLOSURE REMINDER

Alerts the reader that there is more to the letter. Use a reminder line when attachments or enclosures are included with the letter.

(13) COPY NOTATION

Notifies the reader that a copy of the document is being forwarded to another party. CC is the notation used. It stands for "carbon copy" or "computer copy" and states that a copy of the letter has been forwarded to the recipient whose name follows the CC notation.

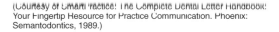

(Courtesy of Smart Practice! The Complete Dental Letter Handbook: Your Fingertip Resource for Practice Communication. Phoenix: Semantodontics, 1989.)

REMEMBER

Be consistent in the use of open and standard punctuation. If the salutation is punctuated with a colon, the complimentary closing must be followed by a comma. The salutation is never followed by a comma in business letter writing; this is used only in personal correspondence.

Punctuation and Grammar Basics

- Start every sentence with a capital letter.
- Make sure every sentence has a subject and a verb.
- Use commas to separate three or more words or phrases in a series.
- Use commas to separate two or more adjectives in a description.
- Use a comma between city and state names.
- Do not use contractions (for example, don't) in formal business writing.
- Put commas and periods within quotation marks at the end of a quotation.
- Do not put colons or semicolons within quotation marks at the end of a quotation.
- Use quotation marks to set off exact quotations from other sources. Do not use quotation marks when you paraphrase.
- Spell out numbers from one to nine, and use numerals for numbers 10 and above.

TYPES OF CORRESPONDENCE USED IN DENTISTRY

Dental professionals use a number of different types of letters in their correspondence with patients and other professionals. Letters are used for marketing and public relations, patient recall, professional correspondence (referring patients to specialists), and prescriptions for laboratory work. Often these types of communications will contain protected health information (PHI) that must be kept confidential. A key to following HIPAA (Health Insurance Portability and Accountability Act) Privacy and Security

Rules is to ask the following questions when processing written communications:

- Does the communication contain PHI?
- What is the office policy for handling PHI?
- Which office personnel have been identified in the office policy as "needs to know"?
- How do you alert the addressee that the communication contains PHI?
- Has the patient requested that PHI not be shared with others?

Letters to Patients

Welcome to Our Practice

Welcome letters are used effectively to communicate a variety of items to new patients. The practice philosophy is stated, office hours are listed, and what to expect at the first visit to the dental practice is described briefly. A simpler form of the welcome letter simply thanks the patient for making the appointment, restates the day and time of the appointment, and briefly states the office philosophy. This letter can be adjusted for adults and children. Follow-up letters can be sent after the first visit to thank the patient.

Thank You

Thank you letters are used to thank patients for referring new patients, family, and friends. A thank you card shows appreciation.

REMEMBER

Most patients choose a new dentist on the basis of word of mouth information (talking with other patients). A card or letter of thanks encourages patients to continue referring others.

Direct Mail Promotion

Direct mail promotions are sometimes used to introduce a dental practice to a large number of potential patients. A letter of introduction sent along with a practice brochure or newsletter is an excellent way to build a practice. This method is used in rapidly growing communities and by the new dentist who is just starting a practice (see Figure 4-4, *Top*). Before you send out direct mail, it is advised that you check with the state dental board and the American Dental Association to make sure that your letter and brochure coincide with all legal and ethical regulations.

Introduction of a New Associate or Other Team Member

A letter can be sent to all patients to introduce a new dentist, associate, or other team member. This letter is intended to give background information about the new member and serves as a formal introduction.

Birthday and Holiday Greetings

Letters and cards can be sent to patients to acknowledge birthdays and to send holiday greetings. Holiday greeting cards must be appropriate to the holiday that the patient celebrates (for example, Easter or Passover, Christmas or Hanukkah). It is easy to generate mailing labels, lists of birthdays, and even personalized cards with computers and databases.

Congratulatory Occasions

Congratulatory letters are a wonderful way to acknowledge the accomplishments of patients, young and old (see Figure 4-5, *Top*). The newspaper serves as a resource tool. Articles about patients can be clipped from the paper and enclosed with a brief message.

Other Types of Letters to Patients

- Abandonment of patient
- Advertisements
- Bills and collection
- Consent
- Expanded hours
- Financial arrangement letter
- Financial policy
- Newsletters
- Postexamination information
- Posttreatment information
- Recall

Letters Between Professionals

Referral letters are used to send information about patients to other professionals (see **Figure 4-3**, *Bottom*). The purposes of the **referral letter** are to introduce the patient and to state the purpose of the referral. When the dental practice refers patients on a regular basis, a template can be designed that will facilitate the writing of referral letters.

HIPAA Privacy Rule: Protected patient health information is anything that ties a patient's name or social security number to that person's health, healthcare, or payment for healthcare, such as x-rays, charts, laboratory reports, or invoices.

Several different types of letters may result from one referral letter. These include letters to specialists to refer a patient and letters to patients to confirm referrals. In addition, the specialist may write to acknowledge the referral or to present clinical information. As you can see, there are several different types of correspondence just between a dentist, specialist, and patient.

REMEMBER

The dentist and the dental specialist work together as a team when they have mutual patients. This is accomplished by following ethical and professional standards. Written correspondence plays a key role in communication between the general dentist and the dental specialist.

Other areas of the dental practice also require written correspondence. These areas are discussed in greater detail throughout this book.

Other Types of Letters to Dental Professionals

- Consent forms to obtain records
- Insurance correspondence
- Specialist referrals
- Thank you to a specialist
- Personal, professional, dental society, and other professional organization correspondence

Correspondence Between Staff Members

Different types and formats of written correspondence are used between dental healthcare team members (see Chapter 6).

Correspondence Between Staff Members

- Interoffice memo
- Office policy and procedures
- Performance reviews
- Professional goals

WRITING RESOURCES

Today, it is possible for you to access a multitude of resources to help you perfect your letter writing skills. Those who may lack the skills or knowledge to write a flawless letter can consult specific resources that may help. The first step is to identify what type of letter will be generated and then check for appropriate resources. Several publications furnish different form letters that can be copied and customized. In this case, you simply retype the letter on the dentist's letterhead, change the name and the date (given in the example), and customize the letter for your needs. If you use a word processing software package, you can save the letter in a file and reuse the letter as often as is needed (making changes if needed). This is what is known as a **computerized letter template.**

An **office letter portfolio** organizes samples of letters that can be used for different occasions. The portfolio is similar to the computerized templates except that the letters are saved on hard copies and are placed in a notebook. When a letter is needed, the administrative assistant refers to the portfolio, selects the type and style of the letter, and retypes.

Newsletters can be produced with the help of public relations firms and other publishers. Information supplied to the publisher is formatted and printed as a newsletter. With the help of desktop publishing software, some offices publish their own newsletters. These newsletters are sent to patients and other members of the community.

Resources for Letter Writing

- Publications of sample letters
- Computerized templates (from software packages)
- Public relations firms
- Online resources

MAIL

Mail is classified into several categories, each requiring a special handling process. Mail to a dental office is delivered by a postal worker and is placed in a mailbox, or is picked up at the post office by the dentist or the dentist's employee. Once the mail has been received, it is sorted according to the correct protocol and is distributed to appropriate persons for further processing.

HIPAA

Privacy Rule: Confidential Communications

- If a letter arrives and is marked *confidential* do not open and deliver the sealed envelope to the addressee.
- All mail should be quickly removed from sight of patients or unauthorized personnel to protect patient confidentiality.
- Open mail may need to be placed in a file folder to protect confidential information in lab reports or other correspondence

Incoming Mail

Incoming mail must be sorted. It is separated according to category and is routed to the correct person or department. Mail can be separated into the following categories:
- Payments (insurance and patient)
- Requests for information, insurance company correspondence, transfer of records, referrals
- Professional journals (for example, *Journal of the American Dental Association*), new product information, articles, state and local dental society publications

- Personal mail, investment reports, accounting information, professional correspondence
- Laboratory cases
- Requests for payment, invoices, billing statements
- Magazines, newsletters, and publications for the reception room
- Catalogs, ordering information, advertisements (dental)
- Junk mail

Each of these categories requires special handling to ensure that the correct party receives the correct mail. Not all mail should be opened before it is delivered. It may be the protocol to stamp the mail with the date it was received and then route it unopened to the correct person. If the mail is to be opened before it is stamped, carefully open the letter with a letter opener (an instrument used to cut an envelope by placing the blade under the flap of the envelope and slicing) and deliver it without taking the letter out of the envelope.

REMEMBER

Procedures for handling incoming mail vary from office to office. Care should be taken to respect the privacy of all mail to ensure that the HIPAA (Health Insurance Portability and Accountability Act) Privacy Rule is applied; any information seen should be held in strictest confidence.

When mail that contains payments is handled, care should be taken to route the mail to the correct party as quickly as possible; checks should never be left lying on a countertop or on a desk. When you separate the check from the envelope, make sure that all documentation is removed, including the top portion of a statement that contains accounting information about the patient or the Explanation of Benefits (EOB) from insurance companies. This saves time when payments are made and ensures that payments will be credited to the correct account.

Quick and efficient handling of the mail helps eliminate the possibility that mail will be lost or misplaced. Efficiency will be measured in how quickly and accurately the mail is routed, how efficiently payments are processed, and how soon mail is answered.

Outgoing Mail

A variety of items will require the administrative dental assistant to send **outgoing mail.** Types of outgoing mail include the following:

- Insurance claims
- Patient statements (bills)
- Professional correspondence, referral letters, transfer of records, professional letters, letters to patients, promotional letters
- Recall notices
- Mass mailings of newsletters and promotional items
- Laboratory cases
- Sharps containers

The type of mail determines the method needed to deliver the mail in the fastest, most economical way. General categories of delivery are overnight delivery, priority mail, and bulk mailing. Each service is designed for different special handling requirements. A number of private companies provide mailing services. For bulk mailings and special handling needs, obtain specific instructions from the company that you will be using.

The US Postal Service also offers a wide variety of services, including some that generate documentation that a letter or package was sent and received:

- **Express Mail** is the fastest service offered by the US Postal Service. Express mail is guaranteed overnight delivery, 365 days a year.
- **Priority Mail** offers faster delivery time than First Class at a reasonable rate. A Priority Mail letter or package must be clearly marked and must weigh under 70 pounds. The postal service will provide Priority Mail stickers, labels, envelopes, and boxes. A 2-pound flat rate envelope can be used by the dental office when batches of insurance forms are mailed.
- **First-Class Mail** is used for sending letters, postcards, and greeting cards that weigh less than 11 ounces. First-Class Mail is usually delivered overnight to local areas, in 2 days to locally designated states, and in 3 days to all other areas. Additional services such as certified and registered mail can be added to First-Class Mail at an additional charge. When a letter weighs more than 11 ounces, it should be mailed Priority Mail.
- **Standard Mail (A)** is used by retailers, cataloguers, and other advertisers to send out mass mailings. Churches and other charitable organizations may take advantage of the nonprofit rates. Standard Mail (A) and Nonprofit Standard Mail are designed for large-volume mailing (200 pieces or 50 pounds). When you use this service, be sure to follow the guidelines of the postal service, which will inform you about how to separate and bundle the mailing.
- **Standard Mail (B)** is used for sending parcels that weigh less than 70 pounds. Parcels are usually delivered in 2 to 9 days. If a faster service is needed, use First-Class, Priority, or Express Mail.

Postage

Postage is the amount of money that is required to mail an item. Postage can be purchased in several different ways. One way is to buy postage stamps. Stamps can be purchased from the post office through different methods. Stamps can be ordered by mail, over the phone with a credit card, from the post office directly, or via private services (which may charge a service fee in addition to the postage fee). Postage meters are another form of purchasing postage. Postage is purchased at the post office, and the amount purchased is recorded in the meter. The meter weighs the item and prints the correct amount of postage on a label or directly onto an envelope. When the prepaid postage is gone, additional postage can be purchased and recorded in the meter. The use of a postage meter expedites the stamping process and eliminates the need to weigh each item manually and affix a postage stamp.

The size and weight of the item being mailed determine the postage. First-Class postage is used for standard envelopes and business envelopes that do not weigh more than 1 ounce. Additional postage is required when items do not meet standard size and weight. For Minimum Size Standards, pieces of mail will be returned if they do not meet the following requirements:

- Pieces must be less than $1/4$ of an inch thick when they are rectangular.
- They must be at least $3\frac{1}{2}$ inches high but not more than $6\frac{1}{8}$ inches high.

- They must be at least 5 inches long but not more than $11^{1}/_{2}$ inches long.
- They must be at least 0.007 inch thick (about the thickness of a postcard) but not more than $^{1}/_{4}$ inch thick.

Mail that does not fall within the standards stated above will be assessed a surcharge for special handling because it cannot be read electronically. The purposes of the surcharge are to cover the added expense of hand processing the item and to encourage the use of standard or business-sized envelopes.

Preparing an Envelope for Mailing

Special instructions are available for addressing an envelope. The use of abbreviations is emphasized in the US Postal Service Guidelines (Table 4-1). Mail is processed at large processing centers by electronic readers that have a difficult time reading script. The use of bar codes and zip codes expedites processing. When mail has to be read by a person, the processing time is longer.

Use the following formatting guidelines:
- Capitalize all letters. Use plain block (UPPER CASE) letters and place the address information in a block format (Figure 4-6).
- Do not use punctuation (except for the hyphen in the ZIP+4 code).
- Use the abbreviations listed in Table 4-1.
- Use correct ZIP codes.
- Place special delivery information, such as ATTENTION or CONFIDENTIAL, below the return address or above the delivery address only (see Figure 4-6).

The delivery address is formatted as follows:
- Line 1: Recipient's name
- Line 2: Name of company, if applicable
- Line 3: Street address, post office box, rural route number and box number, or highway contract route number and box number
- Line 4: City, state (see Table 4-1), ZIP code

Dual addressing is use of a post office box and a street address in the same destination address. The address listed directly above the city, state, and ZIP code line is where the mail will be delivered.

The **return address** is placed in the upper left-hand corner of the envelope. The same type of information is included as in the destination address. The return address can be preprinted, printed on a label, or placed with a stamp.

REMEMBER

The ZIP code of the street address may be different from the ZIP code of the post office box.

Folding the Letter

A correctly folded letter adds professionalism. A standard business letter ($8^{1}/_{2} \times 11$ inches) is folded in thirds. The bottom of the paper is brought up one third (minus $^{1}/_{4}$ of an inch) of the way and creased. The middle and bottom thirds are then folded up over the top one third of the letter, leaving a $^{1}/_{4}$-inch tab. When a letter is correctly folded, the letterhead and inside address are on that third of the page that the reader lifts and looks at first. The letter is inserted into the envelope in such a way that when it is removed by pulling on the $^{1}/_{4}$-inch tab, it will unfold and be ready to read (Figure 4-7). The same method can be used with a smaller envelope and paper. It is never good business practice to place a full-sized sheet of paper into a small envelope. If this must be done, the letter is folded in half, from top to bottom, and then folded into thirds, side to side, and placed in the small envelope.

Postal Cards (Postcards)

Postal cards (postcards) are used to send short messages. Recall cards and appointment reminders are commonly used in the dental profession. When correspondences, such as birthday greetings, thank you notes, and congratulatory, welcome, and get well messages, are sent to patients, preprinted postal cards can be used instead of letters. Simply order several cards of each type. Cards can be customized to fit the needs and style of the dental practice. Keep a supply on hand ready to use when the need arises.

A postcard comes in two different formats. The first is a colorful card with a picture on one side and the address and message on the other side. This type of card is used effectively to remind patients that it is time to return to the dental practice for an examination and cleaning (prophylaxis). The message and address side of the card is divided vertically. The right side of the card is used for the address, and the left-hand side of the card is used for the message.

TABLE **4-1** **Official Postal Service Abbreviations**

AL	Alabama	VT	Vermont
AK	Alaska	VA	Virginia
AS	American Samoa	VI	Virgin Islands, U.S.
AZ	Arizona	WA	Washington
CA	California	WV	West Virginia
CO	Colorado	WI	Wisconsin
CT	Connecticut	WY	Wyoming
DE	Delaware		
DC	District of Columbia	AA	Armed Forces the Americas
FM	Federated States of Micronesia	AE	Armed Forces Europe
FL	Florida	AP	Armed Forces Pacific
GA	Georgia	Ave	Avenue
GU	Guam	Blvd	Boulevard
HI	Hawaii	Ctr	Center
ID	Idaho	Cir	Circle
IL	Illinois	Ct	Court
IN	Indiana	Dr	Drive
IA	Iowa	Expy	Expressway
KS	Kansas	Hts	Heights
KY	Kentucky	Hwy	Highway
LA	Louisiana	Is	Island
ME	Maine	Jct	Junction
MH	Marshall Islands	Lk	Lake
MD	Maryland	Ln	Lane
MA	Massachusetts	Mtn	Mountain
MI	Michigan	Pky	Parkway
MN	Minnesota	Pl	Place
MS	Mississippi	Plz	Plaza
MO	Missouri	Rdg	Ridge
MT	Montana	Rd	Road
NE	Nebraska	Sq	Square
NV	Nevada	Sta	Station
NH	New Hampshire	St	Street
NJ	New Jersey	Ter	Terrace
NM	New Mexico	Trl	Trail
NY	New York	Tpke	Turnpike
NC	North Carolina	Vly	Valley
ND	North Dakota	Way	Way
MP	Northern Mariana Islands		
OH	Ohio	Apt	Apartment
OK	Oklahoma	Rm	Room
OR	Oregon	Ste	Suite
PW	Palau		
PA	Pennsylvania	N	North
PR	Puerto Rico	E	East
RI	Rhode Island	S	South
SC	South Carolina	W	West
SD	South Dakota	NE	Northeast
TN	Tennessee	NW	Northwest
TX	Texas	SE	Southeast
UT	Utah	SW	Southwest

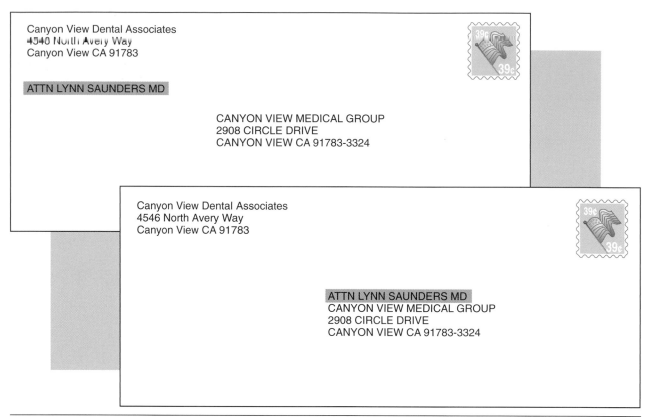

FIGURE 4-6

Envelope addressing styles. *Top,* Envelope with confidential line below the return address. *Bottom,* Envelope with attention line above the delivery address.

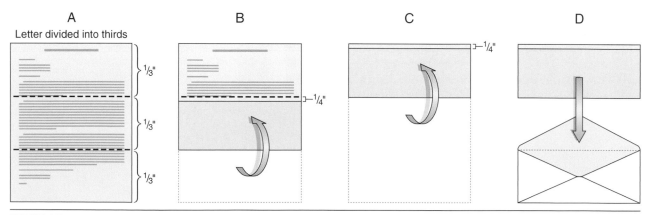

FIGURE 4-7

Folding a business letter. **A,** Divide the letter visually into thirds. **B,** Fold the bottom third up over the middle third (minus $^1/_4$ inch). **C,** Fold the middle and bottom thirds up over the top third of the letter, leaving a $^1/_4$-inch tab. **D,** Insert the letter into the envelope so that it can be removed by pulling the $^1/_4$-inch tab at the top of the letter.

The size of the card is $3\frac{1}{2} \times 5$ inches. Another style of postcard has the address on one side and the message on the other. Advantages of using postcards instead of letters include their size, the cost of postage, and the colorful graphics, which attract the attention of the person receiving the card.

Electronic Mail (E-Mail)

Correspondence can now be sent electronically from one computer to another. This method is referred to as e-mail and requires a slightly different format in the production of the letter. E-mail is intended for use in sending brief messages quickly. E-mail can be used to communicate within an organization, or it can be used to communicate with others who have computers. A few things need to be remembered when e-mail is used. First, e-mail is not a secured method of transferring information; therefore, any document that needs to be kept confidential should not be sent via e-mail. Second, if you send a personal message, make sure that it does not contain information that would embarrass you if someone else reads it.

Guidelines for Sending E-Mail

- Use business letter format.
- Keep the length of the letter to one page (screen).
- Use professional or trade jargon.
- Use abbreviations.
- Keep sentences short.
- Include only questions that can be answered in one or two words.
- Let your reader know from the beginning the subject of the message and what you want done.

DICTATION

Some reports and correspondence may require the use of dictation machines. These machines are recorders into which the originator of the message dictates (speaks). The machine may be physically present or can be accessed by telephone. The recording is then given to a transcriber, who translates the spoken message into a report or letter. This method is used for lengthy medical and dental reports. Typically, the transcription is done by an outside service, and the transcriber works in another office or at home. Once the message has been transcribed, the finished report is sent to the doctor to be proofread and signed.

KEY POINTS

- Written forms of communication are used for a variety of tasks in the dental office. The creation of business letters requires basic letter writing skills to create a well-organized, appealing, and effective letter.
- **Letter writing style** includes the following elements:
  - **Tone:** The way words and phrases are used to convey a message
  - **Outlook:** Presentation of information in a positive form
  - **Personalizing letters:** A means of gaining the reader's attention by conveying courtesy and concern (e.g., use of the pronoun *you*)
  - **Organization:** A process used to identify what you want to say and the results you hope to achieve in a logical, complete, and concise manner
- **Letter writing, appearance:** To make a positive impression on the reader, the letter must be neat, well formatted, and written on appealing stationery
- **Letter style, format:** Following a specific format helps make the letter look neat:
  - Full-blocked
  - Blocked
  - Semi-blocked or modified blocked
  - Square-blocked
  - Simplified or AMS
- Processing of mail consists of receiving and sending mail. Mail received at the office needs to be classified and delivered to the correct department or person in accordance with the office protocol for protection of PHI. Considerations for outgoing mail are delivery time and which company to use (US Postal Service, FedEx, UPS, and so forth). Correct postage is also important for expediting delivery.

Web Watch

Business Letter Writing

http://www.business-letter-writing.com/index.html

Business Writer's Free Library

http://www.mapnp.org/library/commskls/cmmwrit.htm

Common Errors in English

http://www.wsu.edu/brians/errors/

Effective Written Communications

http://www.itstime.com/nov2000.htm

Elements of Style (by William Strunk, Jr.)

http://www.bartleby.com/141/

Guide to Grammar and Writing

http://grammar.ccc.comment.edu/grammar

Professional Writing Handouts and Resources

http://owl.english.purdue.edu/handouts/pw/

 Log on to Evolve to access additional
http://evolve.elsevier.com   web links!

 Critical Thinking Questions

1. On the letter on p. 89, label the different elements.
2. Retype the letter on p. 89 in a different format. Identify the style you chose. Identify the punctuation style you used.
3. In the letter on p. 89, highlight and label passages that are examples of:
   • Tone
   • Outlook
   • Personalized statement
4. How would you compare the points stated in the chapter on organization of a letter with the letter on p. 89? Select passages or sections of the letter to support your opinion.

Canyon View Dental Associates
4546 North Avery Way
Canyon View, California 91793

Mr. William Smith   April 26, 2006
1277 South Spring Street
Flora, CA 91723

Dear Bill:

We are delighted to announce our exciting news. Our office has moved to a new, more convenient location.

We have relocated our practice into the attractive dental suites at 4546 North Avery Way, Canyon View. We hope you will enjoy our new "home" as much as we do. We are enclosing a couple of our new business cards with a map printed on the back. Perhaps you might like to pass one of these cards on to a neighbor or friend. Our phone number is still the same: 626-555-5689.

We are now offering extended office hours to accommodate our patients' busy schedules. When you call for your next appointment, ask us about evening hours.

We're also sending you a refrigerator magnet with our new address and our phone number for your convenience. Thank you for letting us be your dental professionals.

Yours in Health,

Mary A. Edwards, D.D.S.   MAE/lg
                                                        Enclosure

(Modified from SmartPractice: The Complete Dental Letter Handbook: Your Fingertip Resource for Practice Communication, Phoenix, Semantodontics, 1989.)

OUTLINE

KEY TERMS AND CONCEPTS

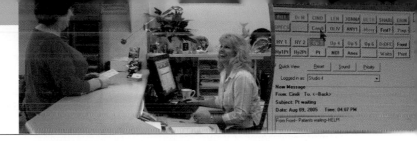

5

Patient Relations

LEARNING OBJECTIVES

The student will:

1. Compare and contrast the humanistic theory according to Maslow and Rogers. Relate the theory to patient relations.
2. List the different stages that present a positive image for the dental practice.
3. Describe the elements of a positive image and give examples.
4. Demonstrate different problem-solving techniques.
5. Examine different methods of providing outstanding customer service.
6. Discuss team strategies and personal strategies for providing exceptional patient care.

INTRODUCTION

Patient relations involve empathy, understanding, concern, and warmth for each patient. These emotions can be demonstrated in the way we communicate with patients, in the type of service we provide, in how members of the dental healthcare team relate to each other, and in how problems are solved. Every aspect of the dental practice should be conducted with the understanding that the patient is "number one."

REMEMBER

Most patients have a choice of when and where they will seek dental treatment.

Dentistry is considered a service-based business (a business that provides a service to customers). All service-based businesses have the same common element: they provide a direct service to customers (patients). Customers, in turn, can usually choose the providers of these services. Customers, when given a choice, will select a business that meets their personal needs. Conditions that contribute to a positive image include the attitude of team members, professionalism, friendliness, and so forth.

PSYCHOLOGY: HUMANISTIC THEORY

Numerous articles and books have been written about and research conducted to study the psychology of human beings—what they want, why they react, what makes them happy, and how they relate to others. Theories are interpretations and observations that provide a framework of general principles. The works of Abraham Maslow (1908–1970) and Carl Rogers (1902–1987) have contributed to the humanistic theory.

Maslow: Hierarchy of Needs

Maslow believed that each individual has to reach a level of physiologic need before he or she is motivated to seek the next level. These levels range from the basic needs of life (food, shelter, safety) to the higher needs of love, belonging, and self-esteem to the highest, self-actualization. For example, homeless people living on the street have to struggle to meet their daily needs of food and shelter. It takes all of their energy to fulfill those needs. Homeless people are not motivated to seek safety, love, or self-esteem until they are assured that their basic needs have been met (Figure 5-1).

According to Maslow, people who have grown up well fed, loved, and respected are more likely than those who have not done so to reach the self-actualization or self-fulfilled stage. This stage is normally achieved in later life and can be seen in those persons who devote time and energy to discovering the meaning of life and to understanding their unique purpose.

Rogers: Fully Functioning Human Beings

Rogers concurred with Maslow that all healthy people are constantly trying to obtain their potential. Rogers termed the concept *"fully functioning human beings"* (Rogers: On Becoming a Person: A Therapist's View of Psychotherapy. Boston, Houghton-Mifflin, 1961). Rogers theorized that each healthy individual believes in an ideal self and that he or she is constantly trying to achieve the ideal self as much as possible. Working toward the ideal self is a two-step process. The first step is to improve the real self, and the second step is to modify the concept of the ideal self to be realistic. By adjusting the concept of the ideal self, a person can assume a wider variety of emotions and behaviors that fit into real life.

People need the help of those around them to become fully functional human beings. These people around them are considered "significant others"—parents, marital partners, and close friends. They offer **unconditional positive regard,** which is perceived to be total love and respect, no matter what the problem. For example, consider the child who complains that he or she did poorly on a test. Parents express unconditional positive regard when, instead of becoming angry and criticizing, they help the child to understand why he or she did poorly and then help to correct the problem. Rogers states that unconditional positive regard is simplified by a **phenomenological** approach to others, which is the ability to view a situation from the other person's point of view. Rogers' humanistic approach of

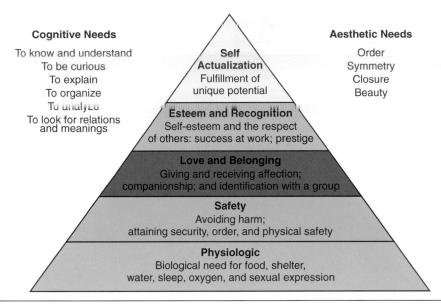

Cognitive Needs
To know and understand
To be curious
To explain
To organize
To analyze
To look for relations
and meanings

Aesthetic Needs
Order
Symmetry
Closure
Beauty

Self Actualization
Fulfillment of
unique potential

Esteem and Recognition
Self-esteem and the respect
of others: success at work; prestige

Love and Belonging
Giving and receiving affection;
companionship; and identification with a group

Safety
Avoiding harm;
attaining security, order, and physical safety

Physiologic
Biological need for food, shelter,
water, sleep, oxygen, and sexual expression

FIGURE 5-1
Maslow's hierarchy of needs.

unconditional positive regard is founded on the theory that we must respect each person's human worth and dignity.

Humanistic Theory in the Dental Office

In the dental office, we can use **humanistic theories** to help us understand the needs of our patients and team members. Young parents who are struggling to provide food and shelter for their children may not see the need for extensive orthodontic care. Their motivation may change once they have provided for the basic needs of their family. Instead of becoming angry and disapproving of patients' decisions regarding healthcare, the dental healthcare team should provide unconditional positive regard, with respect for their decisions and dignity.

Meeting the needs of patients and understanding their motivation are not always easy. It is difficult to understand the motivation of a patient who has money, status in the community, and knowledge of good oral health but refuses treatment. Once the dental healthcare team has informed the patient of a dental need, answered all questions, and educated the patient, it becomes the choice of the patient to continue treatment; this decision must be respected, even when we do not agree.

POSITIVE IMAGE

Have you ever wondered how a person selects a dentist, manicurist, or hairdresser, or a particular store in which to shop? What images can be projected that will present a positive image? These questions have long been the basis for countless seminars and workshops. A basic understanding of the needs of people tells us that all people want to feel safe and to feel that they are important. We are all individuals and will make selections according to our own needs, goals, and objectives. Individuals pass through several stages when they are formulating an impression of a dental practice.

Investigation Stage

Name of the Dental Practice

What is in a name? If the dental practice is a group, the selection of the name can be very important. Things to consider in the selection of the name are the message it conveys, where it will be located in the telephone book (alphabetically), and whether the name has been used before. Names that may have a negative connotation should not be used. For example, two brothers with the last name of Payne

---

Elements That Contribute to a Prospective Patient's Impression

Investigation Stage

- Is the name of the dental practice pleasing and memorable?
- What insurance plans are accepted?
- Are the advertisements (telephone directory, mailings, signage) appealing?
- What do others say about the dental practice?

Initial Contact Stage

- How is the telephone answered?
- How are questions answered?
- Is a sufficient amount of information given?
- Do the answers to questions match the individual's needs?

Confirmation of Initial Impression Stage

- Is the office easy to find?
- How does the outside of the office appear?
- Is there a sign on the door?
- How does the reception area appear?
- What is the greeting by the administrative dental assistant like?
- How much time is spent waiting?

Final Decision Stage

- How did the first appointment go?
- Did the financial arrangements meet the patient's needs?
- Was the patient's insurance plan accepted?
- What types of communication skills do the staff and dentist have?
- Did the dental team's attitudes and professionalism meet the patient's expectations?

---

who want to open a dental practice should not name it "Payne Dentistry." They may be proud of their accomplishments and name, but the name also suggests an unpleasant association.

Generic names should also be avoided. "Family Dentistry," "Gentle Dental Care," and so forth can easily be confused with other practices.

Insurance Plans

Patients may base their decision to visit a new dentist on the type of dental insurance the practice accepts. A list of plans with specific information should be kept near the telephone to help the assistant answer questions about insurance policies.

Advertisements

Some dental practices want to let others know about their practice. Advertisements can take the form of yellow page ads, mass mailings, a sign on a building, or graphics on an office window. According to the American Dental Association (ADA) Code of Ethics, advertisements must present realistic statements and slogans. Care should be taken to check state Dental Practice Acts and the ADA for specific guidelines.

Asking Others About the Dental Practice

How do other patients describe their experience with your dental practice? If you want your patients to refer others and to speak highly of you, then it is necessary to develop and maintain the image you wish to convey, not just during the first visit but during all visits. The patient has to feel that he or she is "number one." Patients want schedules to be kept and staff to be friendly, and they want to feel that the staff is working together for the benefit of patients (not themselves).

Initial Contact Stage

Once prospective patients decide whom they are going to call, the next step is to place the call and ask questions. If successful communications have taken place, the patient will decide to make an appointment.

The first few seconds that prospective patients are in contact with the dental practice can determine whether they will make an appointment. Patients have several different concerns, from infection control to the types of insurance plans accepted. Assistants who answer the telephone must be skilled in communication. They must be ready to answer questions and to tell why their dental practice is unique.

Whether the conversation will continue is based in part on the tone of voice and the greeting used when the telephone is answered. The tone of voice should be friendly and light.

The greeting should contain a welcome, identify the dental practice, and identify the person answering the telephone: "Thank you for calling Canyon

View Dental. This is Diane. How may I help you?" The script selected can vary, but the three main ingredients—welcome, practice identification, and assistant identification—remain the same. Some practices prefer that assistants identify themselves with their full name, whereas others are comfortable with just the first name. If two assistants or staff members have the same first name, then it is advisable to use the first and last name. Practice the script until you are comfortable with it. It may take some adjustment to fit your tone and presentation. Each person who answers the telephone should use the same or a similar script.

A script can also be developed to maintain constancy in dealing with several different situations. The use of telephone information forms (see p. 140) helps to maintain consistency in answering questions and obtaining necessary information.

Factors That Influence a Patient's Impression

- Was the telephone answered quickly (within three rings)?
- Did the patient receive the full attention of the assistant during the conversation?
- Was the voice of the person answering the phone pleasant?
- Were questions answered with ease?
- Was the patient's name used correctly during the conversation?
- Were the patient's needs identified and met?

How Long It Takes to Answer the Phone

Telephones must be answered within three rings. If the assistant is on the telephone and receives a second call, it may be necessary to place the first caller on hold. When this happens, follow the correct protocol; ask permission, and thank the patient. When answering the second call, open with the correct script and obtain the following information: name of the person calling, the reason for the call, and whether you can put the caller on hold. You may

find at this time that the patient simply wants to know if his or her appointment was at 10:00 or 10:30. It will take only a few seconds to answer the question and return to your first call. When you have to place patients on hold for more than 1 minute, ask if they would prefer if you returned the call as soon as possible.

Attention to the Patient During the Conversation

Patients and others will not feel that they are receiving the attention they deserve if they are not given full attention during a conversation. Patients on the telephone should not be placed on hold unless it is absolutely necessary. Some telephone systems will tell callers that the party they wish to speak with is unavailable to answer the telephone and will give instructions to leave a voice mail message. This works well for the party who is on the telephone, but it is poor practice. Patients who are not able to speak with an assistant and have to call back or leave a message may feel that they have not been given full attention.

Telephone Voice

Smile and never seem rushed. Patients like to have your full attention when they are calling. If they feel rushed, they may perceive that their dentistry will be handled in the same manner. Conversely, do not take more time than necessary. Be efficient.

Questions Answered With Ease

Be prepared to answer common questions such as the hours that the dentist sees patients, directions to the office, types of insurance plans accepted by the dentist, different types of payment plans available, and infection control protocol followed. When you are not familiar with a question, tell callers that you will find out the answer and get back to them, or that you will have another team member who can answer the question take the call. Rehearsing scripts will help you to answer questions with speed and ease.

It is a good idea to write scripts for commonly asked questions and place them in a notebook near the telephone. When a patient calls and asks questions, the assistant can refer to the answers in the script book to ensure speed and ease in answering the question. (Caution: Do not sound like you are reading from a book.) This works well for training a new assistant or using temporary help, or when an assistant who normally does not answer the phone is helping in the business office. Patients may never suspect that the assistant they are speaking with is not the assistant who usually answers the phone.

Patient's Name Used Correctly During the Conversation

When you address patients, it is vital that you give them the courtesy of addressing them properly. Unless otherwise instructed, address all adults using the correct form: Mr., Mrs., Ms., or Miss. For example, a new patient calls and tells you her name is Rose Budd. When ending the call, thank Ms. Budd for calling (you have not been instructed to refer to her by her first name). Once a patient relationship has been established, the patient may request that you use his or her first name.

REMEMBER

Members of different cultures and generations have very strict rules on how they are addressed. Using the incorrect name may be interpreted as disrespect for the patient. When dealing with a culturally diverse patient population, it may be wise to seek the assistance of an expert in cultural relations before you establish office protocol.

Patient's Needs Identified and Met

How will you know when patients have identified their needs and you have answered their questions? Communication is key, and you have to be a good listener. Research has shown that you cannot be an effective communicator if you do not listen. When you listen, you must give full attention to the speaker. Look at the person (when on the telephone, do not work on other tasks) and concentrate on what is being said. Do not start to formulate an opinion or try to answer the question while someone is still speaking. As soon as you start to think about an answer, you will not hear the remainder of the conversation. Patients expect to know what fee is going to be charged, if they will be required to pay at the time of service, what treatment will be performed, and approximately how long they will be in the office.

Patients will make an appointment only if they believe that their needs will be met.

Confirmation of Initial Impression Stage

After patients arrive for their appointment, they continue to take into account several factors that will confirm or change their first impression.

Office Location

Patients do not want to drive around for a long time trying to find the dental office. If the office is difficult to find, give clear directions and describe the area. For example, if the office is located behind a fast food restaurant or another identifiable landmark, let the patient know this.

Outside Appearance

The appearance of the dental practice is very important. Think about going to a restaurant for the first time. Your friends tell you about a wonderful new restaurant where the food is good and the service is outstanding. You decide that you want to try the new restaurant and ask your friend for directions. On your way to the restaurant, you have a difficult time finding the correct building (it is behind another and is not seen easily from the street). Once you locate the building, you notice that it is not maintained well. As you walk up to the door, you look inside and see only one other couple seated for dinner. At this time, you are going to make a choice about whether to enter or find another restaurant where you would feel more comfortable. Most people at this point will make a decision to find another restaurant based only on the fact that they do not feel comfortable. The situation is the same for dental offices. If the office is difficult to locate and does not send out a warm welcome, patients may choose to seek care elsewhere.

Sign on the Door

It confuses patients when they arrive for an appointment and the dentist they have an appointment with is not listed on the front door. When only the name of the dental practice is listed, for example, Canyon View Dental Associates, then the names of individual dentists should be attractively posted in the reception area.

Appearance of the Reception Area

After the patient enters the office for the first time, the condition of the reception area is the next most influential factor. A positive image will be formulated when the reception area is clean and organized and provides current reading material (Figure 5-2). Once a negative factor is discovered, such as a stain on the carpet, patients will look for other negatives.

Greeting

The administrative dental assistant should identify patients as soon as they enter the reception area. Plan on spending the first 60 seconds giving a new patient your undivided attention. Reconfirm the reason for the visit (emergency, examination, consultation). Explain what the patient can expect: "Mrs. Potter, this is your first visit to our office. I have forms for you to complete. Dr. Edwards will examine the area where you are having discomfort. Once a diagnosis is made, she will discuss treatment options. Our goal today is to relieve your discomfort."

Time Spent Waiting

Many dental practices are judged by the amounts of time patients spend waiting. New patients should not have to wait for longer than a few minutes. There are always ways to fill time before a patient sees the dentist for the first time. Forms can be reviewed, or a tour of the office can be conducted. Patients who must wait longer than 10 minutes during a subsequent visit should be given options: "Mrs. Potter, Dr. Edwards will be ready for you in about 20 minutes. If you would like, there is a coffee house around the corner where you could wait, or you are more than welcome to stay here. We have water or coffee available for you." When you give patients options, they accept the wait more easily. You have made it clear that their time is valuable.

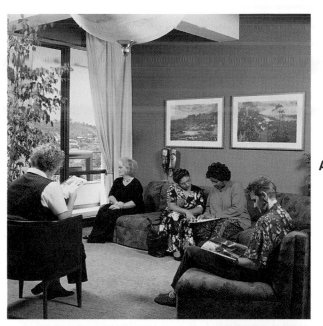

A

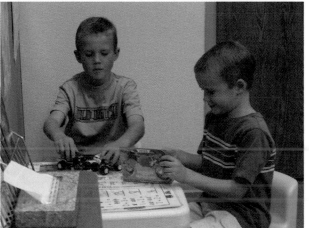

B

FIGURE 5-2

A reception area that creates a positive image. The room meets the needs of patients by offering a variety of reading material for older ones and activities for younger ones. (**A,** From Kinn ME, Woods M: The Medical Assistant: Administrative and Clinical, 8th ed, Philadelphia, Saunders, 1999.)

Final Decision Stage

The First Visit

Allow ample time for the dental healthcare team to meet the new patient. The appointment should never be rushed, and the patient should have the opportunity to get to know the dental healthcare team.

Financial policies should be explained to patients, and a written copy of these policies given to them for review when they get home. A consultation should take between 20 and 30 minutes.

Communication Skills

The skills of the staff and dentist are important elements in creating a positive first impression. Effectively communicating with patients to better understand their needs involves asking questions and transmitting the objectives of the dental healthcare team.

Attitude and Professionalism

Patients must leave the office after their first appointment honestly believing that the dental healthcare team cares about them as individuals, understands their needs, and is willing to work with them to improve their dental health. This will lead to mutual trust.

Managing Patient Expectations

When patients decide to make an appointment with a dentist, they have certain expectations. These expectations are formed during their initial investigation of the dental practice. During their investigation, they obtain information from several different sources: friends, advertisements or marketing campaigns, insurance companies, and professional referrals. Additionally, they often will call a dental office, ask questions, formulate an opinion, and, if satisfied, will make an appointment. It is at this point in the process that the expectations that patients have may not be fulfilled by the dental office staff. This discrepancy will occur if communications have been inadequate.

It is important to answer the question, "What can we, as a dental healthcare team, do to ensure that we are meeting the expectations of our patients?"

Create the image that you want your patients to see. This applies to everything from yellow page ads to the location of the office.

- Inform your patients about the vision and mission of the dental practice. Communicate this information. Include in letters, pamphlets, and brochures, and on Web pages information that clearly outlines the mission of the practice, office hours, types of insurance accepted, types of financial plans available, and types of patients seen (if

a specialty office), along with an introduction of the dental healthcare team. Include answers to often asked questions. List the procedure that will be followed at the first visit. Provide office hours and emergency telephone numbers.

- Provide all patients with a standard financial policy. Provide this for patients before they have to ask for the information.
- Clarify insurance information before dental treatment is begun. Ask patients to bring you a summary of their policy.
- Inform patients of the treatment process before treatment is begun, keep them informed of each step, and inform them as changes occur. Do not promise unrealistic results, and do find out (through feedback) what results the patient hopes to accomplish. If the expected results are not the same, then this must be worked out before treatment is begun. Patients often share this information with an assistant instead of the dentist. It is important that each member of the team understand the intended treatment and be able to communicate with the patient. Assistants should ask for clarification of any information that they do not understand before they speak with patients.
- Infection control or standard precautions are anticipated by all patients. Inform your patient of the process and steps you take in the office. Be prepared to answer questions about the procedures used in the office to protect patients and team members.
- Be prepared to interpret patients' messages by reading body language. What they are saying may not be what they actually mean.
- Patients want to be treated as special individuals. Keep notes about patient preferences, activities, special events, likes, and dislikes: "Mr. Perez, how did your granddaughter like the playhouse you built for her?" "Jennifer, I understand your wedding was picture perfect." Such statements send a message of caring for the patient as an individual. In addition, they open dialogue to help relieve anxiety about the pending dental treatment.

PROBLEM SOLVING

Good patient relations require that the dental healthcare team have effective problem-solving

REMEMBER

Patients whose expectations are realistic (created through effective communications) will be happy patients.

skills. Patients who choose not to follow instructions require special attention. The problem must first be identified, and then it must be solved. Some patients complain about everything. Some of their complaints will be justified, and others will not. Pressures inside and outside the dental practice will affect patients and how they cope. Dealing with angry patients requires skill and tact.

Noncompliance

Successful dental treatment requires the combined effort of the dental healthcare team and the patient. Frustration results when a patient chooses not to follow the dentist's instruction.

Identify the Problem

Each patient is an individual with different goals and ideals. As Maslow points out, motivation is not the same for each person, and we must discover what motivates our patients (see Figure 5-1).

Treatment that requires patients to change their habits, such as increasing the time spent brushing and flossing, may cause them to abandon these regimens. To solve this problem, it is necessary to make sure that before beginning treatment, patients understand what will be expected of them. When patients understand and accept a treatment, they will be more likely to follow the instructions. When noncompliance is discovered, explain to patients what will happen if they do not follow the recommended treatment:

John, I can understand your reluctance to stop jogging, but for a week after surgery, it is advised because of the possible complications, such as prolonged bleeding.

Ask open-ended questions (which require the patient to explain). Begin with "what," "why," "how," or "tell me":

Why do you feel that way?
Tell me why you don't think it is necessary.

Closed-ended questions require a simple answer—"yes" or "no"—and are used to confirm information:

Can you come next Tuesday?

Describe the outcome when the patient follows instructions:

Judy, I understand your teeth are sensitive and your gums bleed easily. If you brush and floss daily, within a few days, you will experience less sensitivity and bleeding.

Give positive instead of negative information:

Jeff, 85% of our patients have reported whiter teeth within the first week of treatment. Not *"It does not work in 15% of our patients."*

Take time to demonstrate techniques to patients. Show a patient correct brushing and flossing techniques, have them demonstrate back to you, and correct them when needed. Send patients home with instructions so that they can review the techniques at home. When patients understand how and why, they will be more likely to follow instructions.

A final technique is to ask the patient for help in solving the problem:

If we changed places, how would you help solve this problem?

REMEMBER

All detection of noncompliance must be entered into the patient's clinical record. State the problem, and document the action taken.

Complaints

When patients have a complaint, they will react in one of three ways: stop using the dental practice, voice their concern, or ignore the problem. Exiting the practice occurs when a patient chooses to leave instead of confronting the issue. Often, dental practices do not understand why a patient has left. This is unfortunate, because the underlying issue is not discovered or corrected. Some patients will choose to voice their opinion, which gives the dental practice the opportunity to identify and solve the problem. A few patients are "loyal" to the practice and therefore choose to ignore the problem instead of creating an unpleasant situation.

Angry Patients

Some patients bring with them outside issues that cause them to become angry easily. Some believe that the only way a problem will be solved is if they become angry. This gives them a feeling of power and control. Never assume that such a person is angry with you. If you look closely at the causes of their anger, you will discover that they are usually not angry with you personally. They are angry because of circumstances—most often, these are out of your control.

Dealing with angry patients requires a special talent to separate the issue from the person. Becoming personally involved and reacting negatively makes you the loser and gives control to the angry patient. Remaining professional is the key to successful resolution of the problem.

Steps in Identifying and Solving Complaints

1. Watch for changes in attitudes and nonverbal cues.
2. Consider both sides of the issue; the patient could be right.
3. Consider each complaint as an opportunity to improve patient services. "Thank you for bringing this to our attention, we will try to improve."
4. Listen to the full complaint without interruption before suggesting a solution to the problem.
5. Show empathy for the complainer by restating the issue in an empathetic tone of voice.
   "In other words, you are concerned with the way you will feel after the extraction."
   "You feel it is unfair that the insurance company will not cover sealants."
   "It sounds as though you might not have understood the extent of the treatment."
   "As you see it, it is upsetting when Dr. Edwards leaves you during treatment to see another patient."
6. Proceed only when the patient is in agreement that you understand the nature of the complaint.
7. Avoid phrases and words that put the complainer on the defensive:
   "You are the only person who has complained about . . ."
   "We have other patients who need our attention."
   "These are our rules; everyone has to follow them."
8. State what you will do next.
9. Assure the patient that you want him or her to continue using the services of the dental practice.

Steps to Consider When Dealing With an Angry Patient

1. Listen to the whole story. Do not interrupt the patient, even if the accusations seem ridiculous.
2. Do not pass judgment before you understand the reason for the anger.
3. Change the environment. Take the patient to another area, and offer water or a cup of coffee. Remove all barriers and sit down. (Sit at the same level—not behind a desk.)
4. Use humor, but be careful not to ridicule.
5. Do not involve others in the dispute. This will make it appear that you are "ganging up" on the patient. Listen to the full story, and then suggest involving another person to help solve the problem. (If you add others, which is sometimes advisable, ask permission first.)
6. Do not pass the patient off to another team member without explaining that the other person can help.
7. Do not become angry yourself. This will only increase the tension. Add a tone of empathy and understanding.
8. Try to find a positive aspect of the problem.
9. Ask the patient, "If you were in my shoes, how would you handle the situation?" or "How would you handle this situation?"
10. Above all else, *do not become defensive.* Always remain positive and professional.

PROVIDING OUTSTANDING CUSTOMER SERVICE

Some who are able to provide outstanding customer service have shared their successes with others. A composite of several different resources includes the following elements.

Team Strategies

- **Be available.** Adjust appointment hours to meet the needs of the patients you serve. Rotate the schedule to provide for both early morning and evening appointments. Provide for continued telephone coverage during lunch hours.
- **Have a unique image.** Develop an image that you want to be known for (you cannot be everything for everybody). Become the best at what you do well.
- **Show appreciation.** Show appreciation by thanking patients for their referrals. Become a kind and caring team, placing the needs of your patients above your own.
- **Personalize.** Keep in touch with patients; call them after treatment and inquire how they are doing. Personally call each patient to schedule recall appointments. Send birthday cards and holiday greetings.
- **Listen.** Develop listening skills. Be able to recognize concerns and address them. Identify individual patient needs.
- **Set goals.** Set practice goals. Measure your goals by industry standards and continually modify them to meet the needs of your patients.
- **Understand value.** Understand the value of a long-term patient, and constantly strive to provide quality care.

Personal Strategies for Providing Exceptional Patient Care

- Acknowledge patients when they arrive for an appointment. Greet them with a warm smile and a sincere "Hello."
- Answer the telephone within three rings, and greet the caller with a smile.
- Use the patient's name at least once during a conversation.
- Explain to the patient what will happen next.
- Identify verbal and nonverbal signals. Become aware of the warning signs that indicate that a patient is dissatisfied or concerned. Respond to the concern, and be willing to work with the patient until the problem is solved.
- Become an active listener.
- Observe confidentiality at all times. Safeguard the integrity of clinical records, and do not discuss patients with persons who are not team members.
- Do what you say you will do, when you say you will, 100% of the time.
- When patients leave, thank them for coming, bid them goodbye, wish them well, and tell them you are looking forward to seeing them the next time.

KEY POINTS

- **Good patient relations** include empathy, understanding, concern, and warmth for each patient.
- **Humanistic theory** is based on the works of Maslow and Rogers. Maslow identifies a hierarchy of needs. This hierarchy can be applied to a patient's motivation and desire to receive dental treatment. Rogers theorized that all healthy individuals believe in an ideal self and that they are constantly trying to achieve the ideal self as much as possible. Applying humanistic theories helps us to understand the needs of our patients and fellow team members.
- **A positive image** is necessary to attract and keep patients. Patients will go through several stages before they select a dentist:
  - Investigation stage
  - Initial contact stage
  - Confirmation of initial impression stage
  - Final decision stage
- **Managing patient expectations** is a process of communication. What image is being sent, and will the dental healthcare team live up to the expectations of the patient?
- **Problem solving** requires that the dental healthcare team develop skills that identify and solve problems of:
  - Noncompliance
  - Complaints
  - Anger
- **Providing outstanding patient care** requires a team strategy as well as personal characteristics:
  - Team strategies: availability, image, appreciation, personalization, goals, and values

- Personal characteristics: care for the patient as an individual, development of good listening and communications skills

Web Watch

Customer Service World

http://www.ecustomerserviceworld.com/earticlesstore.asp

Effective Complaint Handling

http://www.bbb.org/alerts/aticle.asp?ID=449

Tip Sheets: Quick Ideas to Consider for Everyday Challenges in Health Care

http://www.susanbaker.com/resources/tips/default.asp

 Log on to Evolve to access additional web links!

Critical Thinking Questions

1. On the basis of what you have learned in this chapter, explain how the humanistic theory applies to your acceptance of patients and their decisions about dental treatment.

2. A patient tells you he is upset with a fee that has been charged. He is standing at your desk with other patients nearby. You try to offer an answer, but the patient begins to raise his voice. What will you do?

3. A prospective patient passes through several stages of decision making before deciding to make an appointment with a dentist. List the stages, and give a brief description of what you can do as an administrative dental assistant to help project a positive image.

4. Describe the personal strategies that can help you provide outstanding patient care. Give examples.

Notes

OUTLINE

KEY TERMS AND CONCEPTS

Avoiding Style
Change
Compromising Style
Dominating Style
Electronic Noise
Filtering by Level
Formal Downward Channel
Horizontal Channel

Inappropriate Span of Control
Informal Channels
Integrating Style
Intergroup Conflict
Interorganizational Conflict
Interpersonal Conflict
Intragroup Conflict
Intraorganizational Conflict

Intrapersonal Conflict
Lack of Trust and Openness
Obliging Style
Rank and Status
Timing
Upward Channel
Work Overload

6

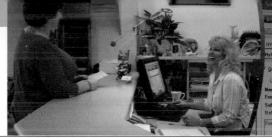

Dental Healthcare Team Communications

LEARNING OBJECTIVES

The students will:

1. Discuss the purpose of a dental practice procedural manual and identify the different elements of the manual.
2. Categorize the various channels of organizational communication and identify the types of communication that are used in each channel.
3. Identify and discuss barriers to organizational communications.
4. Describe different types of organizational conflict, and select the appropriate style for resolution.
5. Explain the purpose of staff meetings.

INTRODUCTION

A team can be described as a group of two or more persons who work toward a common goal. Similar to those on a sports team, all members must understand and practice established rules and have a common goal. An effective healthcare team requires a shared philosophy, excellent communication skills, the desire to grow and change, and the ability to be flexible while providing quality care for all patients.

DENTAL PRACTICE PROCEDURAL MANUAL

The dental practice procedural manual is a detailed manual that is used as a form of written communication. The objective of the manual is to provide a reference for all team members. This resource provides each team member with specific details on practice goals, personnel procedures, business office procedures, and clinical procedures. The manual should be developed as a team project, with each team member contributing in his or her specific area of expertise. As procedures change, it is the team members' responsibility to update the manual. The manual, to be effective, must be updated at regular intervals, and all team members be given updated manuals.

The key to developing a good procedural manual is to include as much information as possible without making the manual cumbersome. The idea is for the manual to be a resource for all team members. It will not be used on a daily basis by experienced team members, but it will be used to help train new team members and will serve as a guide for substitute team members or, when necessary, for the team member who fills in for another. The purposes of the manual are to provide written documentation of, and to eliminate inconsistency in, policies. Such inconsistencies are a common cause of conflict among members of the dental healthcare team.

The initial writing of the manual can be overwhelming if it is done without guidance. Several resources, including established manuals and workbooks, can be purchased through supply catalogues and consulting services.

Elements of a Procedural Manual

Practice Philosophy

- Mission Statement
- Vision Statement
- Goals and Objectives

General Instructions

- Mission Statement for the Manual (team mission statement)
- How to Use the Manual
- Responsibility for Updating and Revising

Personnel Procedures

- Hiring
- Work Schedules
- Job Descriptions
- Benefits
- Dress Codes
- Code of Conduct
- Grievance Procedures
- Reviews and Evaluations
- Termination Procedures

HIPAA (Health Insurance Portability and Accountability Act) Procedures

- Identify Who Manages HIPAA Compliance
- Establish a Plan for Compliance
- Identify the Components of HIPAA
- Describe the Roles and Responsibilities of Various Members of the Dental Healthcare Team

Business Office Procedures

- Specific Duties and Job Descriptions (detailed descriptions of each procedure and duty performed in the business office)
- Records Management Protocol (detailed information for each type of record)
- Ordering Information for All Supplies and Equipment

Clinical Area Procedures

- Specific Duties and Job Descriptions (detailed description of each procedure and duty performed in the clinical area, including identification of team member responsibilities)
- Description of the Inventory Procedure
- Description of the Hazardous Material Program
- Outline of Emergency Procedures

COMMUNICATIONS

Personal Communications

The basic rules of communication are outlined in Chapter 3. These rules and concepts apply to communication in general and can be used to enhance communication among members of the dental healthcare team.

Barriers to communication listed in Chapter 3 (semantics, jargon, credibility, preconceived ideas, emotions, stereotyping, noise, conflicting nonverbal communications) can be expanded and applied to communications among team members. It is an ongoing task to evaluate the communication skills of the team and to identify barriers that exist.

Organizational Communications

One of the most important elements of creating a dental healthcare team is the establishment and practice of effective communications. Similar to communications with patients, communications between team members must be effective. A team cannot perform at its highest potential if it has no communication skills. Communication includes the spoken word, the written word, and body language (see Chapter 3). Effective communication can be accomplished when there is a policy of open communication. This allows for identification of problems and provides a means for conflict resolution without the stress and anger that can occur with ineffective communications.

Channels

Information is transferred through a variety of different channels (directions): formal downward channels, horizontal channels, upward channels, and informal channels. The method or medium of communication is referred to as the *communication network*. Channels and networks are necessary means of facilitating organizational communication. Improper use of channels and networks is a characteristic of an ineffective dental healthcare team.

Formal Downward Channels

A **formal downward channel** of communication can best be described as communication that originates at the top of the organizational structure and moves downward. Several different types of organizational structure may be used (Figure 6-1). One common element within all structures is that one person or group is at the top of the structure. This can be the chief executive officer (CEO), the president, a board of directors, the manager, or the dentist.

Types of Communications Sent Through a Formal Downward Channel

- Policies
- Vision
- Goals
- Changes in rules and procedures
- Job designs
- Performance appraisals

Although several people or groups may participate in designing, writing, and implementing ideas and functions, ultimate responsibility rests at the top of the organization and is formally communicated downward to others (Figure 6-2).

Horizontal Channel

When communication goes across (horizontally) the organizational structure, it is transmitted between the members. The **horizontal channel** of communication is used primarily by members at the same level.

Types of Communications Sent Through a Horizontal Channel

- Goal setting
- Defining of goals and roles
- Improving methods of maintaining working relations
- Gathering and processing of information
- Sharing of day-to-day information

In a dental office, horizontal communications can and will include all members of the team and will affect how they relate to patients and how well they work together on a daily basis (Figure 6-3).

Upward Channel

For the dental healthcare team to work well together, there must be a means by which those at the lower level of the organizational structure can

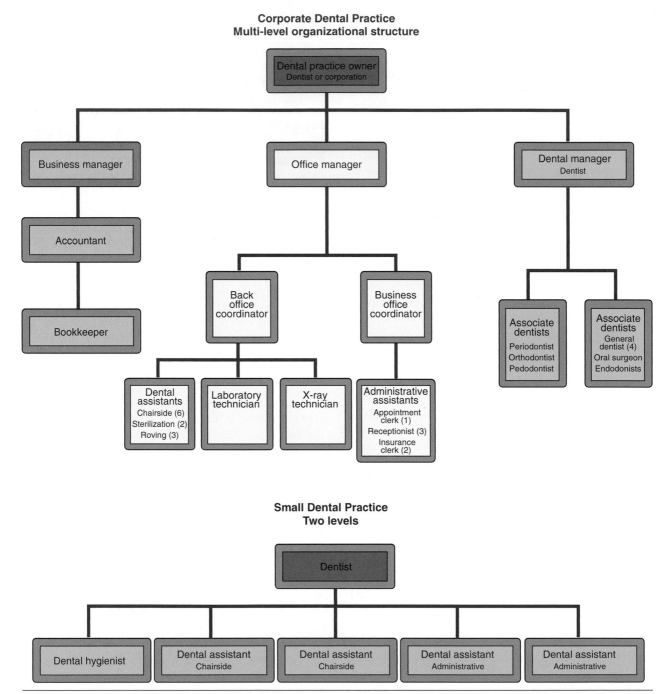

FIGURE 6-1

Top, Organizational chart of a business that is structured in several levels, typical of a large or corporate dental practice. *Bottom,* Organizational chart of a business consisting of two levels, typical of a small dental practice.

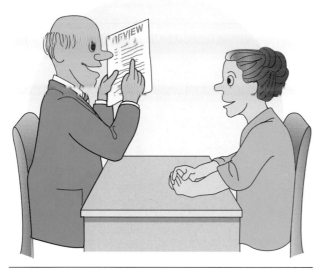

FIGURE 6-2
Example of a downward communications channel.

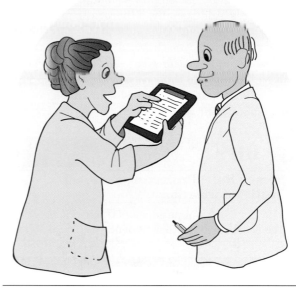

FIGURE 6-4
Example of an upward communications channel.

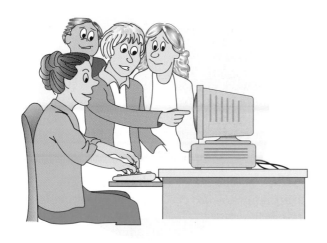

FIGURE 6-3
Example of a horizontal communications channel.

Types of Communications Sent Through an Upward Communication Channel

- Feedback
- Requests for assistance
- Problem solving
- Conflict resolution

A typical dental practice will have only two or three layers of organizational structure. It is vital for a successful team to be able to communicate in an upward direction, as well as downward and horizontally (Figure 6-4).

Informal Channel

Informal channels of communication are often referred to as "the grapevine." This type of communication takes place in an informal setting and does not include the official communications of the organization. Informal communications can be accurate or inaccurate. A good manager listens carefully to informal communications because they are a good indicator of the mood of staff members and reveal how they perceive formal communications. When questions are asked in an informal setting, this may

communicate with those at higher levels of the structure. An **upward channel** of communication is the flow of information from one level to a higher level. This can take place between two layers or can move upward through all layers. In most cases, this communication must move sequentially through all levels.

be an indication that the communication process is not effective and that employees do not understand the messages. Additionally, if there is an atmosphere of mistrust, informal communication may be the only way that employees have to state their position. Informal communications can be very destructive when employees use their time to repeat gossip and rumors about patients, fellow employees, or the management staff.

HIPAA

Privacy Rule: Protecting Personal Health Information

- Do not discuss a patient's PHI when it may be overheard by other patients

Types of Communications Sent Through an Informal Communication Channel

- Rumors
- Gossip
- Accurate information
- Inaccurate information
- Sharing and helping (informal)

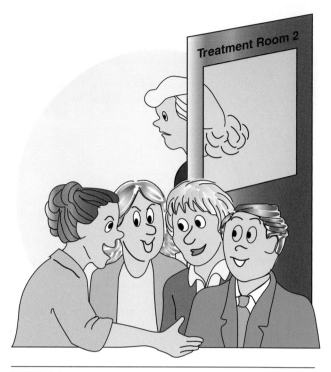

FIGURE 6-5
Example of an informal communications channel.

Members of the dental healthcare team must be very careful about how they use informal communications. Patients have the right of confidentiality, and this can be broken by gossip and rumors (in many cases, information is communicated without the knowledge of other team members). The layout of a dental practice is such that patients can overhear informal conversations between members of the dental healthcare team; therefore, it is vital that informal conversations be limited (Figure 6-5).

Organizational Barriers to Communication

Organizational barriers to communication create an undesirable environment for members of the dental healthcare team and the patients they serve. Stress due to poor communication is easily perceived by patients. Patients can feel the tension and may begin to question the motives of the dental healthcare team. Some communication barriers encountered in the dental office are the following:

- **Work overload:** Any amount or type of work that adds to daily stress. When employees feel the stress of work overload, they do not take the time to communicate effectively. In a dental practice, work overload can be caused by the volume of work, or by performing more than one job, filling in for an absent employee, accommodating emergency patients, constantly answering the telephone, and not managing time effectively.
- **Filtering by level:** Information sent is not received because it has been changed or stopped at some level. If, as an administrative dental assistant, you send a message or idea to the dentist and it is stopped or changed by the office manager, there is a breakdown in the upward flow of the message.
- **Timing:** A good idea not presented at the right time or in the right manner will not be accepted.
- **Lack of trust and openness:** When feedback is not accepted, it is very difficult to communicate effectively. This can occur at all levels of the organization and leads to conflict.
- **Inappropriate span of control:** This leads to lack of trust and fuels resentment. It may be the

result of poor communication, lack of direction, or poor or nonexistent policies and procedures.

- **Change:** When not accepted or understood, change places a barrier on communication. For some people, change is perceived as a negative. Good communication provides a means of discussing the need for change and how it will improve the organization.
- **Rank and status:** Some people use position (rank) as a form of power over others, which closes channels of communication.
- **Electronic noise:** In a dental office, it is common to encounter electronic noise from high-speed handpieces and other electronic equipment. This hinders communication of the full message (message sent is not heard, and feedback is incomplete).

ORGANIZATIONAL CONFLICTS

Not all conflict should be considered bad. Conflict is a common experience in any relationship. How we use conflict determines its benefit. If conflict is used as a weapon and is destructive, it is considered to be nonfunctional. If conflict is used as a means to identify a problem and improve a situation, it can be viewed as a valuable tool for change and improvement.

Constructive

Conflict can be constructive if:
- Team members improve their decision-making skills
- Different solutions to a problem are identified
- New solutions are developed
- Group solutions are devised for shared problems
- Team members find new ways to state their problems
- Team members are stimulated to become more creative, resulting in growth
- Individual and team performance is improved

Destructive

Conflict can be destructive if it:
- Causes unhealthy stress, leading to job burnout
- Reduces communications
- Produces an atmosphere of cynicism and mistrust
- Reduces job performance

- Increases resistance to change
- Affects quality of patient care

Classifying Conflict

Conflict has many different meanings and sources. Organizational conflict can be described as **intraorganizational conflict** (within the organization) and **interorganizational conflict** (between two or more organizations). Intraorganizational conflict can also be divided into levels between groups, departments, and individuals. There are four types of intraorganizational conflict:

- **Intrapersonal conflict:** Intrapersonal conflict (within oneself) occurs when an individual is expected to perform a task that does not meet his or her personal goals, values, beliefs, or expertise. For example, the dental hygienist who has to clean the darkroom may feel that this is not in her job description and is below her level of training.
- **Interpersonal conflict:** Interpersonal conflict (between two team members) occurs when members of the team at the same level (assistant and assistant) or different levels (hygienist and assistant) disagree about a given matter. This can occur between any two or more members of the dental healthcare team.
- **Intragroup conflict:** Intragroup conflict (within the group) occurs among members at the same level (assistant and assistant, dentist and dentist). This conflict usually occurs when there are differences in goals, tasks, and procedures.
- **Intergroup conflict:** Intergroup conflict (between two or more groups) occurs when members of one group are in disagreement with members of another group. For example, dental assistants may be in conflict with the management staff if the vacation schedule is set without personal consultation with each staff member. Conflict can also occur when dentists and hygienists do not agree with the Dental Practice Act.

Conflict-Handling Styles

The type of conflict, who is involved, and the amount of time that has elapsed before the problem is addressed determine which conflict style should be used to address the problem. There are appropriate and inappropriate situations for each style. Not every problem can be solved in the same manner, and the manner chosen may determine whether

---

Conflict-Handling Styles

Ways of handling conflict have been studied and identified by many researchers. Rahim describes the following styles:

- **Integrating style:** High concern for self and others (also known as *problem solving*). This style is collaborative because both parties work together in openness, exchanging information to achieve an equitable solution.
- **Obliging style:** Low concern for self and high concern for others (also known as *accommodating*). This style is one of self-sacrifice and giving to others.
- **Dominating style:** High concern for self and low concern for others (also known as *competing*). This type of person has a win–lose mentality and goes out to win with little regard for others. This person is usually very competitive.
- **Avoiding style:** Low concern for self and others (also known as *suppression*). This style is associated with sidestepping and buck passing. People who use this style avoid issues so as not to be in conflict with themselves and others and appear not to be aware of conflicts when they occur.
- **Compromising style:** Intermediate in concern for self and others. With this style, there is a give-and-take attitude; compromise is the key, and both parties are willing to give up something to arrive at a solution.

(Data from Rahim MA: Managing Conflict in Organizations, 2nd ed, Westport, CT, Praeger, 1992.)

---

resolution is successful. Conflict resolution is a complex process that takes time, knowledge, and understanding. Following are some suggestions for selecting the appropriate resolution style:

- **Integrating style:** This style works best when time is available to address the problem. Usually, problems are complex, and their resolution requires the expertise of more than one person. The problem must be identified, and then input from all members is needed for development of a solution. Once the solution is developed, the support of the full team is needed to implement the changes. Good communication is essential when this style is used. It is inappropriate to use this style when the problem is simple, when a decision is needed at once, or when other parties are unwilling to contribute, or they do not have the necessary problem-solving skills.
- **Obliging style:** This style is used when the issue is unimportant and someone is willing to defer to the other party to preserve a relationship. This style is sometimes used by people who are unsure about whether they are correct. It would be inappropriate to use this style if you believe that the other person is wrong or is behaving unethically.
- **Dominating style:** This style is used when a decision must be made quickly, and the results are trivial. It is also appropriate when an unpopular course of action is needed, when the decisions of others will be costly, or when an overly aggressive subordinate must be managed. This style is inappropriate when an issue is complex, when decisions do not have to be made quickly, or when both parties are equal in status or power.
- **Avoiding style:** This style is best used when an issue is trivial, when a cooling-off period is needed, or when the benefits do not go beyond the discord that the style will cause between the involved parties. It is inappropriate when the issue is important, when it is someone's responsibility to make a decision, or when a decision is needed quickly.
- **Compromising style:** This style is best used when both parties are equally powerful, when a consensus cannot be reached, when an integrating or dominating style is not successful, or when a temporary solution to a complex problem is needed. It is not appropriate when a problem is complex and requires problem-solving skills, or when one party is more powerful than the other.

STAFF MEETINGS

Staff meetings serve several different functions. They can be formal, informal, social, and so forth. Staff meetings should always be constructive and never destructive. They may serve as an effective tool for organizational communication and problem solving. The type and duration of the meeting depend on its purpose. Short meetings at the beginning of each day may be needed to prepare members

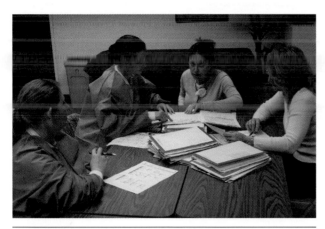

FIGURE 6-6
Morning team huddle technique to review charts and prepare for the day. (Courtesy of William C. Domb, DMD, Upland, CA.)

of the dental healthcare team for their day (Figure 6-6). Clinical charts are reviewed, and potentially difficult situations are identified. Longer staff meetings may include a week-long retreat to a resort. This type of meeting combines work and social interaction.

All types of meetings require a preset protocol. Setting of ground rules for a meeting helps to eliminate potential barriers when an unexpected gripe session evolves. Common guidelines for staff meetings are discussed in the following sections.

Before the Meeting

- Identify the type of meeting that will be held, that is, formal or informal. Describe the purpose of the meeting, that is, to share information (exchange of ideas or knowledge), to solve problems, or to set goals. Establish a protocol, and set the ground rules for various types of meetings.
- Set a date and time. Establish dates well in advance so that schedules can be set, and do not change the date, if at all possible. Regular meetings can be set a year in advance. When meetings are scheduled weekly, or even monthly, they will be viewed as normal. Try to avoid having meetings only when there is a problem.
- Develop an agenda. Appoint a team member to act as facilitator, note taker, and time keeper. Seek input from others on items they would like

included on the agenda. Agendas should include a review of minutes from the previous meeting, reports, old business, and new business. Post the agenda a few days in advance of the meeting.

During the Meeting

- Each member receives a copy of the agenda.
- The facilitator moves the meeting forward according to the agenda. It is easy for meetings to get out of hand if the protocol is not followed. The facilitator ensures that everyone follows the guidelines and keeps everyone focused.
- The note taker keeps notes. The notes are later typed; one copy is placed in a record book, and other copies are given to members present at the next meeting. Notes serve as documentation and serve as a method of recording what was discussed, who is responsible for implementing change or following through on actions decided upon, and what was decided. It is very important to keep records of meetings for future reference.
- Each team member is given an opportunity to voice opinions and to help in problem solving. It is also vital that one or two people should not be allowed to dominate the meeting. It is the duty of the facilitator to keep everything positive.
- The time keeper helps the facilitator move the meeting along. When there is much work to be accomplished in a short time, the responsibility of the time keeper is very important.

After the Meeting

- Minutes are typed and are properly distributed.
- Those who were assigned tasks must carry them out.

KEY POINTS

An effective dental healthcare team requires:
- Shared philosophy
- Excellent communication skills
- The desire to grow and change
- The ability to be flexible while providing quality care for all patients

A dental practice **procedural manual** is a form of written communication. It is a reference for all team members. This resource provides each team member with specific details about practice goals, personnel procedures, business office procedures, and clinical procedures.

Effective **organizational communications** are accomplished when the lines of communication are open. This allows for identification of problems and provides a means for conflict resolution without the stress and anger that can result from ineffective communication. The channels of organizational communications are as follows:

- Downward
- Horizontal
- Upward
- Informal

Barriers to organizational communications include the following:

- Work overload
- Filtering by level
- Timing
- Lack of trust and openness
- Inappropriate span of control
- Change
- Rank and status
- Electronic noise

Organizational conflict is common. How conflict is dealt with determines its benefit. If conflict is used as a weapon and is destructive, it is nonfunctional. If conflict is used as a means to identify a problem and improve the organization, it can be a valuable tool for change and improvement. Classifications of organizational conflict are listed here:

- Intrapersonal conflict
- Interpersonal conflict
- Intragroup conflict
- Intergroup conflict

Handling conflict can be done appropriately or inappropriately. Results depend on the style used to resolve the conflict. Conflict resolution can be accomplished with use of the following styles:

- Integrating style
- Obliging style
- Dominating style
- Avoiding style
- Compromising style

Staff meetings serve various functions. They can be formal, informal, or social. They should always be constructive and never destructive.

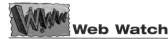

Web Watch

How to Resolve Conflicts—Without Killing Anyone

http://www.onlinewbc.gov/docs/manage/conflicts.html

How to Write a Policies and Procedures Manual

http://www.onlinewbc.gov/docs/manage/hrpolicy1.html

The Fine Art of Resolving Disputes

http://www.sba.gov/lubrary/successXIII/20-Resolving-Disputes.doc

 Log on to Evolve to access additional web links!

http://evolve.elsevier.com

 Critical Thinking Questions

1. With information in this chapter, in Chapter 1, and from outside resources, develop a code of conduct for a dental healthcare team. Work independently or in a small group. Support your code by referencing those of other organizations (e.g., the American Dental Association, the American Dental Assistants Association, school codes).

2. Select one of the four channels of organizational communications, and describe how communication flows. Give examples of the types of information communicated.

3. Amber is an office manager. She has worked her way up the dental assisting ladder (chairside assistant for 12 years, administrative assistant for 3 years, office manager for 1 year). James is a chairside assistant with 6 years of experience. He is very good with patients, and his assisting skills are excellent. Amber and James disagree about patient scheduling procedures. He is concerned because patients are squeezed into the schedule when needed and dental treatment is diagnosed during their recall appointments. Treatments take about 30 minutes for the dentist to complete. Amber wants patients seen on the days they request to be seen, to save them an extra trip, but most of all because this will boost daily production. James is concerned because when an extra patient is squeezed in, the following happens: Patients with scheduled appoint-

ments have to wait longer because of the addition to the schedule; when the schedule is running late, one of the assistants must stay during lunch or after work; and the dentist does not take a stand because Amber has been a loyal employee for 16 years.

- What are the problems that Amber, James, the dentist, and the patients have?
- What types of organizational conflict are involved?
- What style of conflict resolution would you use to solve this problem? Why?

OUTLINE

KEY TERMS AND CONCEPTS

Clinical Record
Consent Form
Correspondence Log
Dental History
Dental Radiograph
Diagnostic Model
Examination Form

Forensic Odontology
Individual Patient File Folder
Laboratory Form
Medical History
NSF
Objective Statement
Progress Notes

Registration Form
Risk Management
Subjective Statement
Treatment Plan
WNL

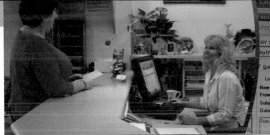

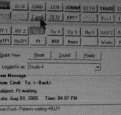

Patient Clinical Records

LEARNING OBJECTIVES

The student will:

1. List the functions of clinical records.
2. List key elements of record keeping and describe the significance of each element.
3. Define the two types of accessibility of clinical records.
4. Discuss methods used in the collection of information needed to complete clinical records.
5. Identify the components of a clinical record and describe the function of each component.
6. Discuss the function of risk management.
7. Identify situations that lead to patient dissatisfaction.

INTRODUCTION

The function of the **clinical record** (i.e., the patient's chart) is to provide the dental healthcare team with information. The objective of the dental healthcare team is to supply dental treatment that takes into consideration the needs of the patient. The whole picture cannot be correctly visualized if all the pieces are not present. The information collected during preparation of the clinical record, when complete, provides all of the necessary pieces.

The patient **registration form** introduces the patient to the dental practice and provides demographic and financial information that will be used to complete insurance forms and bill the patient. A comprehensive **medical history** alerts the dentist to drug allergies and medical conditions that may be affected by particular dental procedures. The **dental history** provides information about previous treatment; it also alerts the dental healthcare team to fears and apprehensions that the patient may have concerning dental treatment. The diagnostic information is used to formulate a **treatment plan.** Various other forms may also be used to aid the dental healthcare team.

When all of the pieces have been collected and placed together in an **individual patient file folder,** a total picture of the patient and the patient's needs can be visualized. Once the initial information is collected and a treatment plan is developed, the next section of the clinical record documents the dental treatment. At each visit, treatment is carefully and thoroughly recorded.

In addition, the clinical record serves as a legal document. This document can be used in defense of allegations of malpractice and can provide information for **forensic odontology** (dental conditions used for identification). Third party insurance carriers and managed care providers can mandate elements and organization of the clinical record.

The basic elements of all clinical records are the same, although formats and styles may vary from practice to practice. The format selected by the dentist may be determined by a specific organization, such as a professional organization, a managed care company, a corporation, an insurance company, or a practice management consultancy. The Dental Practice Act of each state may mandate required elements. Organizations may require specific forms

and a predetermined format to be used by all dental offices within that particular organization. Regardless of which system is used, the key elements to success are organization, consistency, and completeness.

Key Elements of Record Keeping
• Organization • Consistency • Completeness

It is the responsibility of the dental healthcare team to ensure that all aspects of the clinical record are accurate and easily accessible. In addition, the HIPAA (Health Insurance Portability and Accountability Act) Privacy Rule applies to the information contained in the patient's clinical record. The accessibility of clinical records is twofold. First, the dental healthcare team must know where the record is located at all times. Second, patients have the right to view the contents of their personal clinical records.

Each dental healthcare team member plays an important role in the collection, recording, and maintenance of clinical records. It is the responsibility of each member to ensure that the information contained within each clinical record is accurate, factual, and complete. The contents of the clinical record and all conversations with a patient are confidential and must be protected both ethically and as mandated in the HIPAA Privacy Rule (Figure 7-1).

COMPONENTS OF THE CLINICAL RECORD

Clinical records are a crucial part of the dental practice. Without accurate and well-organized clinical records, it would be impossible to determine the dental needs of each patient. The clinical record is the instrument used to communicate information on the health of the patient and the patient's dental needs, dental treatment, and financial responsibility.

The order in which these forms are used and placed in the clinical record is a personal preference

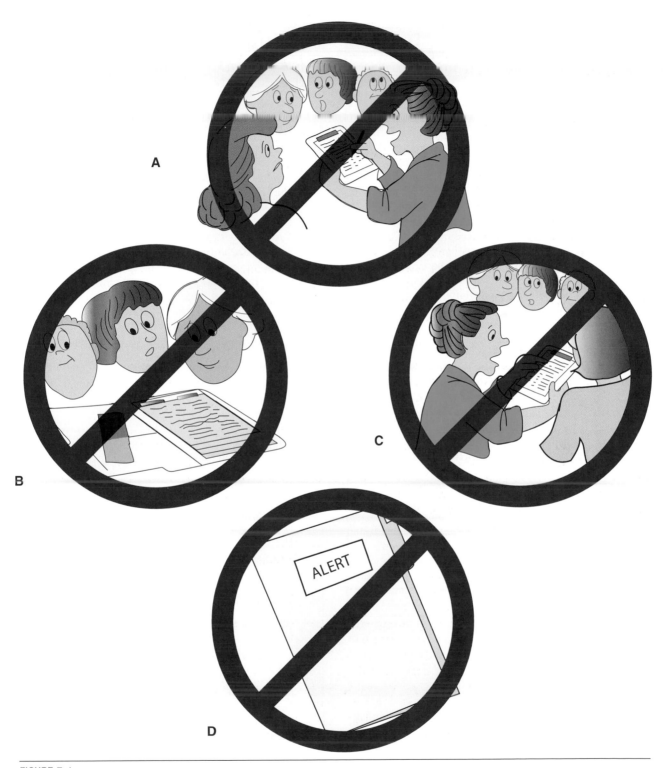

FIGURE 7-1
Safeguarding clinical records and complying with the HIPAA (Health Insurance Portability and Accountability Act) Privacy Rule. **A,** Do not ask patients questions in a place where others can hear the responses. **B,** Do not leave charts in places where others can read the content. **C,** Do not talk with staff members about patients where others can overhear the conversation. **D,** Do not place protected health information (PHI) on the outside of a clinical record.

HIPAA

Privacy Rules That Apply to Clinical Records

- **Access to Clinical Records:** Patients should be able to see the information in their clinical record. They may request to view the information or to obtain a copy. If errors are found, they may request that they be corrected. The dental office should provide access to the records or provide a copy within 30 days of the written request. A reasonable fee can be charged for copying the records.
- **Notice of Privacy Practices:** The dental office (or any covered entity) must provide patients with a copy of the notice while explaining how patients may use personal medical information and their rights under the HIPAA (see Figures 7-4 and 7-5).
- **Limits on Use of Personal Medical and Dental Information:** Private health information (PHI) contained in the clinical record can be shared only with other health professionals when the information is used for the care of the patient's health. PHI cannot be shared with others for purposes not related to their healthcare without written authorization from the patient.
- **Confidential Communications:** Healthcare professionals must take reasonable steps to ensure that their communications with patients are confidential. For example, when discussing PHI with a patient, do so in a private area, where it cannot be overheard by others. Patients may also request that you are not to contact them or leave a message at their home. The dental office must comply with such requests if they can be reasonably accommodated.

HIPAA

Roles and Responsibility of the Dental Healthcare Team

- **Written Privacy Procedures:** Written privacy procedures that identify which members of the staff will have access to private health information (PHI), how the information will be used, and when it may be disclosed. In addition, the policy must ensure that any business associates who may have access to the PHI will agree to follow the same procedures.
- **Employee Training and Privacy Officer:** The dental entity must provide adequate training and appoint a Privacy Officer. The plan should also state how policies will be monitored and what disciplinary actions will be taken if a policy is not followed by a staff member.
- **Public Responsibilities:** In limited circumstances, the Privacy Rule permits, but does not require, that covered entities continue certain existing disclosures of health information for specific public responsibilities, such as:
- Emergency circumstances
- Identification of the body of a deceased person or the need to determine the cause of death
- Research that involves limited data or that has been independently approved by an Institutional Review Board or privacy board
- Overall management of the healthcare system
- Judicial and administrative proceedings
- Limited law enforcement activities
- Activities related to national defense and security
- When no other law requires disclosures in these situations, covered entities may continue to use their professional judgment to decide whether to make such disclosures on the basis of their own polices and ethical principles.
- **Equivalent Requirements for Government:** Provisions of the privacy rule generally apply equally to private sector and public sector covered entities.

of the dental practice. Some forms may be consolidated to include more than one type of information. The key point is that all information must be located somewhere within the patient's clinical record. A "mock-up" of a typical clinical record is given on *pages* 123-140.

Steps for Collecting Information

1. **Call for first appointment.** Use a telephone information form to begin gathering information (*see page* 140).
2. **Before the scheduled appointment.** If time allows, forms for registration and dental and medical histories can be mailed to the patient before the first appointment. These forms can be part of a packet that also contains information about the dental practice and a welcome letter from the dentist. Forms can be completed at the patient's leisure. If forms are not completed before the appointment, the patient should be instructed to arrive 15 minutes early to complete them. To expedite form completion and prevent missing information, the patient should be informed of the types of information he or she will be required to provide, such as insurance information, types and dosages of medications being taken, and names and addresses of physicians and former dentists.
3. **Day of appointment.** When the patient arrives for the appointment, greet the patient and have all forms ready for completion (if not completed in advance). Give the patient a clipboard, a pen, and the paperwork that must be completed. Briefly explain to the patient how you would like the forms completed; this will help answer questions in advance. If the patient is a minor, it is necessary that a parent or guardian complete and sign the forms. Once the forms have been completed, they must be reviewed and checked for completeness (Figure 7-2). Another method that could be used is the interview technique. Patients are asked questions on the medical and dental history forms, and answers are recorded by the assistant. If this method is used, the interview must take place in a private area (Figure 7-3).
4. **Confirmation of information.** After the forms have been completed, a member of the dental healthcare team reviews the information with the patient. Notations should be made to clarify "yes" answers and incomplete answers. During the dentist's review of the forms, he or she may ask additional medical and dental questions according to available findings.
5. **Information collected during the examination.** Additional information is recorded on the proper form by the dental assistant, as directed by the dentist. The data entered must be neat, complete, and legible. Other such records include **dental radiographs, examination forms,** and **laboratory forms.**

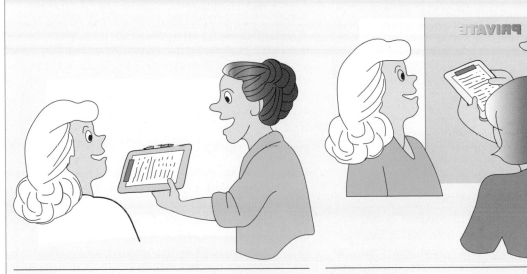

FIGURE 7-2
Administrative assistant and patient reviewing completed forms.

FIGURE 7-3
Patient and her mother being interviewed by an administrative assistant in a private location.

Components of the Patient Clinical Record

- Individual patient file folder*
- Dental radiographs*
- Acknowledgement of receipt of privacy practices notice*
- Registration form*
- Dental history form*
- Medical history form*
- Recall examination form
- Clinical examination form*
- Periodontal screening examination form
- Treatment plan form
- Problem priority list
- Progress notes form*
- Consent forms
- Signature on file form
- Financial arrangements form
- Correspondence log
- Telephone information form

*Necessary forms.

COLLECTING INFORMATION

To ensure consistency, a protocol for collection of information must be established and followed. A telephone information form (*see page* 135), a written script, and other methods will help the administrative dental assistant to collect all information needed to compile the clinical record.

REMEMBER

People outside the dental office may need to read the information contained within the clinical record. Therefore, use standard abbreviations and charting terminology.

Privacy Practices Notice

Three separate communication documents must be given to a patient to describe how health information may be used and disclosed, and how a patient can access his or her protected health information (PHI). The patient is first asked to read the *Notice of Privacy Practices* (Figure 7-4); he or she is then given *Instructions for Our Notice of Privacy Prac-*

tices (Figure 7-5), along with verification that the information was given to the patient *(Acknowledgment of Receipt of Privacy Practices Notice)* (*see page* 125).

Registration Forms

From a business perspective, the registration form contains information that will be used by the administrative assistant. The document includes demographic and insurance information needed to collect payment for dental services. It also includes key legal provisions that the patient agrees to by signing the form. There may also be separate **consent forms.** Study the Anatomy of a Dental Registration Form to understand all of the components of this important form (*page* 141).

Other Diagnostic Records

Several different types of diagnostic tools may be used in the evaluation and maintenance of a patient's dental health. The most common, radiographs (x-rays), digital radiographs, and periodontal evaluations, are easily stored in the patient's clinical record. Other types of diagnostic records include intraoral photography. With an intraoral imaging system, pictures can be used to visually record the condition of the patient's teeth and surrounding tissue. The system combines an intraoral camera with a computer to record and store images. A narrative and visual report can be stored in the computer or transferred to photographs, DVD, and videotapes. The narrative report is included in the clinical record, and a cross-referencing system is used to direct the reader to copies of the DVD, videotape, or computer record.

Diagnostic Models

Diagnostic models, or study models, are used as a tool in treatment planning. They are casts of the patient's mouth (Figure 7-6) and are not stored in the patient's clinical record; although they are part of the record, they are stored in a cabinet or box. To help locate models when needed, they should be stored alphabetically or numerically. Numeric filing works well for this purpose; the numbers are cross-referenced in the patient's clinical record and also in a master file.

Individual Patient File Folder

Components of the clinical record are organized and placed inside file folders; every patient has an individual file folder. Each file folder is identified with the patient's name in correct format for the filing system that is used by the individual dental practice. The style and size of the folder are determined by the filing system used. The standard folder size is 8½ by 11 inches. A fastening system is used to hold forms in place and to keep them from falling out. One or two pockets are attached to the inside of the folder to hold radiographs and other small items. Dividers can be placed inside the folder to organize the forms.

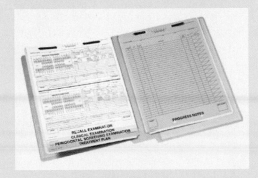

(Courtesy The Dental Record, Wisconsin Dental Associations, Milwaukee, WI.)

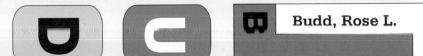

Budd, Rose L.

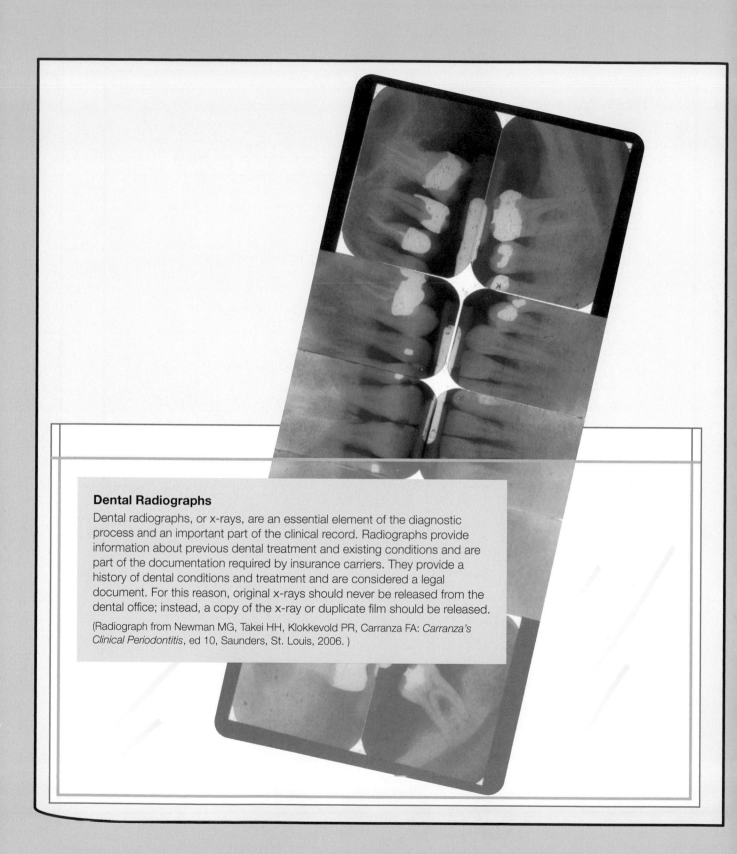

Dental Radiographs

Dental radiographs, or x-rays, are an essential element of the diagnostic process and an important part of the clinical record. Radiographs provide information about previous dental treatment and existing conditions and are part of the documentation required by insurance carriers. They provide a history of dental conditions and treatment and are considered a legal document. For this reason, original x-rays should never be released from the dental office; instead, a copy of the x-ray or duplicate film should be released.

(Radiograph from Newman MG, Takei HH, Klokkevold PR, Carranza FA: *Carranza's Clinical Periodontitis*, ed 10, Saunders, St. Louis, 2006.)

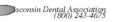
Canyon View Dental Associates
[Insert Name of Practice]

SECTION A: The Patient.

Name: _Rose L Budd_

Address: _1836 N Front Street_

Telephone: _555-1486_   E-mail: _RLBudd@townbank.com_

Patient Number: _326570_   Social Security Number: _123-45-6789_

SECTION B: Acknowledgement of Receipt of Privacy Practices Notice.

I, _Rose Budd_ , acknowledge that I have received a Notice of
Privacy Practices from the above-named practice.

Signature: _Rose Budd_   Date: _7/1/2006_
If a personal representative signs this authorization on behalf of the individual, complete the following:

Personal Representative's Name:

Relationship to Individual:

SECTION C: **Good Faith Effort**

Describe your good faith effort to

Describe the reason why the indiv

Acknowledgement of Receipt of Privacy Practices Notice

All patients or representatives of patients (parent, guardian, or personal representative) sign this form stating that they have received the Notice of Privacy Practices (Figure 7-4). **Section A** is the patient's information; **Section B** is signed by the patient or patient representative; **Section C** is completed by a member of the dental healthcare team only if the patient refuses to sign the form; **Signature** is provided by the authorized dental healthcare team member.

(Form courtesy The Dental Record, Wisconsin Dental Associations, Milwaukee, WI.)

SIGNATURE.
I attest that the above information is correct.

Signature: _Sharon Williams_   Date: _7/1/2006_

Print name: _Sharon Williams_   Title: _Privacy Officer_
Include this acknowledgement of receipt in the individual's records.

ACKNOWLEDGEMENT OF RECEIPT OF PRIVACY PRACTICES NOTICE

Form No. T303HA   © Michael Best & Friedrich, LLC

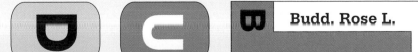

Budd, Rose L.

| 3 | 2 | 6 | 5 | 7 | 0 |

PATIENT NUMBER

welcome

Date __7/1/2006__

Patient's Name __Budd__ __Rose__ __L__ Date of Birth __7/17/52__ ☐ Male ☒ Female
Last   First   Initial

If Child: Parent's Name _____

How do you wish to be addressed __Rosie__
Single ☒ Married ☐ Separated ☐ Divorced ☐ Widowed ☐ Minor ☐

Residence - Street __1836 N Front Street__
City __Flora__ State __CA__ Zip __91711__
Business Address __123 S Business Way__
Telephone: Res. __555-4321__ Bus. __555-3210__

Fax _____ Cell Phone # _____

eMail __R.L.Budd@townbank.com__

Patient/Parent Employed By __Town Bank__

Present Position __N/A__

How Long Held __N/A__

Spouse/Parent Name __N/A__

Spouse Employed By __N/A__

Present Position __N/A__

How Long Held __N/A__

Who is Responsible for this account __Self__

Drivers License No. __M3205167__

Method of Payment: Insurance ☒ Cash ☐ Credit Card ☐

Purpose of Call __Check-up__

Other Family Members in this Practice __No__

Whom may we thank for this referral __Self__

Patient/parent Social Security No. __123-45-6789__

Spouse/Parent Social Security No. __N/A__

Someone to notify in case of emergency not living with you _____
__Evelyn Jones__

DENTAL INSURANCE 1ST COVERAGE

Employee Name __Rose Budd__ Date of Birth __7/17/52__
Employer Name __Town Bank__ Yrs. __12__
Name of Insurance Co. __Blue Cross__
Address __1116 Form St.__
__Los Angeles, CA 91110__
Telephone __310-555-6381__
Program or policy # __8476__
Social Security No. __123-45-6789__
Union Local or Group __N/A__

DENTAL INSURANCE 2ND COVERAGE

Employee Name _____ Date of Birth _____
Employer Name _____ Yrs. _____

Registration Form

Registration forms provide demographic and financial information about the patient and the person or persons financially responsible for payment of the dental fees. This form is divided into sections that help to organize the information (see p 141, Anatomy of a Dental Registration Form). Data collected on this form will be used to create a computerized database, complete insurance forms, and create a financial record. If the form is completed by the patient, make sure that all information is legible and complete.

(Form courtesy The Dental Record, Wisconsin Dental Associations, Milwaukee, WI.)

revoke all previous agreements to the contrary and agree to be responsible for payment of services not paid, by my dental care payor.
I attest to the accuracy of the information on this page.

PATIENT'S OR GUARDIAN'S SIGNATURE
__Rose Budd__

DATE __7/1/2006__

Form No. T110R

REGISTRATION

Form No. T150DH

DENTAL HISTORY

Form No. T140MH

MEDICAL HISTORY

PATIENT NUMBER `3 2 6 5 7 0`

welcome

Patient's Name **Budd** / **Rose** / **L** / **7/17/52**
Last / _First_ / _Initial_ / _Date of Birth_

1. Purpose of initial visit *Check up*
2. Are you aware of a problem? *yes*
3. How long since your last dental visit? *3 years*
4. What was done at that time? *cleaning*
5. Previous dentist's name *Frances Jones, DDS*
   Address: *Hong Kong* Tel.
6. When was the last time your teeth were cleaned? *3 years*

CIRCLE THE APPROPRIATE ANSWER. IF YOU DON'T KNOW THE CORRECT ANSWER, PLEASE WRITE "DON'T KNOW" ON THE LINE AFTER THE QUESTION.

7. Have you made regular visits? .... YES **(NO)**
   How often:
8. Were dental x-rays taken? .... **(YES)** NO
9. Have you lost any teeth or have any teeth been removed? .... YES **(NO)**
   Why?
10. Have they been replaced? .... YES NO
11. How have they been replaced?
    a. Fixed bridge _____ Age _____
    b. Removable bridge _____ Age _____
    c. Denture _____ Age _____
    d. Implant _____ Age _____
12. Are you unhappy with the replacement? .... YES NO
    If yes, explain
13. Would you like to know about permanent replacements? .... YES NO
14. Have you ever had any problems or complications with previous dental treatment? ... **(YES)** NO
    If yes, explain:
15. Do you clench or grind your teeth? .... **(YES)** NO
16. Does your jaw click or pop? .... YES **(NO)**
17. Have you experienced any pain or soreness in the muscles or your
    face or around your ear? .... **(YES)** NO
18. Do you have frequent headaches, neckaches or shoulder aches? .... **(YES)** NO
19. Does food get caught in your teeth? .... YES **(NO)**
20. Are any of your teeth sensitive to: ☐ Hot? ☒ Cold? ☐ Sweets? ☐ Pressure?
21. Do your gums bleed or hurt? .... **(YES)** NO
    When?
22. How often do you brush your teeth? *2/per day* When? *AM/PM*
23. Do you use dental floss? .... **(YES)** NO
    How often?
24. Are any of your teeth loose, tipped, shifted or chipped? .... YES **(NO)**
25. Are you unhappy with the appearance of your teeth? .... YES **(NO)**
26. How do you feel about your teeth in general?
27. Do you feel your breath is offensive at times? .... **(YES)** NO
28. Have you ever had gum treatment or surgery? *not sure* YES NO
    What?
    Where?
    When?
29. Have you had any orthodontic work?
30. Have you had any unpleasant dental experiences or is there anything about dentistry that you
    strongly dislike? *sometimes*
31. Do you have any questions or concerns? .... YES NO

I CERTIFY THAT THE ABOVE INFORMATION IS COMPLETE AND ACCURATE

PATIENT'S / GUARDIAN'S SIGNATURE *Rose Budd* DATE *7/1/2006*

DENTIST'S SIGNATURE _____ DATE _____

ANEST.

MED. ALERT
Penicillin
Codeine

DENTAL HISTORY

MEDICAL HISTORY

Form No. T150DH

Form No. T140MH

Dental History Form

The dental history form provides the dental healthcare team with information about the patient's previous dental treatment and concerns and identifies fears. The patient is requested to provide information about:

- Purpose of the visit
- Current dental problem
- Previous dentist
- Previous radiographs
- Brushing and flossing habits
- Previous orthodontic work
- Unpleasant dental experiences
- Questions or concerns

The patient is interviewed by the dentist, and notations are made. The patient and the dentist should sign the form. It is at this time that any adverse reactions to dentistry can be noted. This will assist the dental healthcare team in recognizing and calming fears.

(Form courtesy The Dental Record, Wisconsin Dental Associations, Milwaukee, WI.)

© 2004 Wisconsin Dental Association
(800) 243-4675

welcome

PATIENT NUMBER: 3 2 6 5 7 0

Patient's Name: Budd (Last) Rose (First) L (Initial) 7/17/52 (Date of Birth)

CIRCLE THE APPROPRIATE ANSWER, IF YOU DON'T KNOW THE CORRECT ANSWER PLEASE WRITE "DON'T KNOW" ON THE LINE AFTER THE QUESTION

COMMENTS

1. Physician's Name: _Robert Alexander_
   Address: _1346 Medical Way Suite B_ Tel:( )
2. Are you under a physician's care? .... **YES** NO
   Since when _3/95_ Why
3. When was your last complete physical exam? _2003_
4. Are you taking any medication or substances? .... **YES** NO
   (If yes, please list medications in comments section or on the back of this form.)
5. Do you routinely take health related substances? (Vitamins, herbal supplements, natural products) .. YES NO
6. Are you allergic to any medications or substances? (please list) .... **YES** NO
7. Do you have any other allergies or hives? .... YES **NO**
8. Do you have any problems with penicillin, antibiotics, anesthetics or other medications? .... **YES** NO
9. Are you sensitive to any metals or latex? .... YES **NO**
10. Are you pregnant or suspect you may be? .... YES **NO**
11. Do you use any birth control medications? .... YES **NO**
12. Have you ever been treated for or been told you might have heart disease? .... YES **NO**
13. Do you have a pacemaker, an artificial heart valve implant, or been diagnosed with mitral valve prolapse? .... YES **NO**
14. Have you ever had rheumatic fever? .... YES **NO**
15. Are you aware of any heart murmurs? .... YES **NO**
16. Do you have (high) or low blood pressure? (please circle) .... **YES** NO
17. Have you ever had a serious illness or major surgery? .... YES NO
    If so, explain

estrogen
penicillin/codeine

infant
high 192/67

18. Have you ever h...
    growth or other ...
19. Do you have infl...
20. Do you have any...
21. Do you have any...
22. Have you ever b...
23. Do you have any...
24. Do you have any...
25. Do you have any...
26. Are you diabetic...
27. Do you have fai...
28. Do you have ast...
29. Do you have epi...
30. Do you or have y...
31. Have you tested...
32. Do you have AID...
33. Have you had or...
34. Do you or have y...
35. Do you smoke, ...
36. Do you regularly...
37. Do you habitually...
38. Have you had ps...
39. Have you taken ...
    phentermine (fer...
40. Do you have any...

Medical History Form

A comprehensive medical history is necessary to ensure that the medical needs as well as the dental needs of the patient are being met. Careful review of the medical history will alert the dentist to possible interactions between dental treatment and medical treatment. The medical history will provide information that may require a consultation between the physician and the dentist. Cooperation between the professions allows the dental healthcare team to recommend treatment that takes into consideration the well-being of the total patient. It is at this time that allergies and other conditions that require special consideration are noted in the patient's clinical record. A sticker, colored pens, stamps, or preprinted boxes may be used to identify such special conditions. The goal is to alert all members of the dental healthcare team; such items should be used in a manner that is consistent and that results in easy visualization of the identifier. To protect the confidentiality of the patient, alerts should not be placed on the outside of the folders, where they may be read by other patients.

(Form courtesy The Dental Record, Wisconsin Dental Associations, Milwaukee, WI.)

41. Is there anything else we should know about your health that we have not covered in this form? _None_
42. Would you like to speak to the Doctor privately about any problem? .... YES NO

I CERTIFY THAT THE ABOVE INFORMATION IS COMPLETE AND ACCURATE

PATIENT'S / GUARDIAN'S SIGNATURE _Rose Budd_ DATE _7/1/2006_
DENTIST'S SIGNATURE _Mary A. Edwards_ DATE _7/1/2006_

ANEST.

MED. ALERT
Penicillin
Codeine

Form No. T140MH

MEDICAL HISTORY

PATIENT'S NAME ___Budd___ ___Rose___ ___L___ ___7/17/52___
Last   First   Initial   Date of Birth

PRESENT CONDITIONS

B
L
RIGHT   LEFT
L
B

1 2 3 4 5 6 7 8 9 10 11 12 13 14 15 16
A B C D E F G H I J
T S R Q P O N M L K
32 31 30 29 28 27 26 25 24 23 22 21 20 19 18 17

Date 1-12-2007   Hygienist ___   Dr ___
X-Rays None BW None PAN None FMX N/A PA N/A

Regional Exam	Soft Tissue	HYG INS
☐ Head & Neck	☑ Lips ☑ Pharynx	TBI ✓
☐ Skin	☑ Cheeks ☑ Floor	Floss
☐ TMJ WNL	☑ Palate ☑ Tongue	Hyg aids Floss THREADER FL No

BP		Plaque	Calculus	Bleeding
110/68	DISEASE CONTROL PROGRESS			
Pulse 78				

NO.	PROBLEMS
21	Occlusal Canies

COMMENTS: _____   Treatment Schedule ☐

IS THERE ANY CHANGE IN MEDICAL HISTORY OR MEDICATION? YES ☐ NO ☐ (Enter below or on the Medical History Update Form)

CONDITION	MEDICATION	DOSAGE	DATE
No changes at this time			

ANEST.	I certify that the above information is complete and accurate. PATIENT'S OR GUARDIAN'S SIGNATURE *Rose Budd* DATE 1/12/2007	MED. ALERT Penicillin Codeine

---

PATIENT'S NAME _____
Last   First   Initial   Date of Birth

Date ___ Hygienist ___ Dr. ___
X-Rays ___ BW ___ PAN ___ FMX ___ PA ___

Regional Exam	Soft Tissue	HYG INS

PRESENT CONDITIONS

B
L
RIGHT
B

1 2 3 4 5 6 7 8 9 10 11 12 13 14 15 16
32 31 30 29

COMMENTS: _____   Treatment Schedule ☐

IS THERE ANY CHANGE

			DATE

ANEST.	I certify that the above information is complete and accurate. PATIENT'S OR GUARDIAN'S SIGNATURE ___ DATE ___	MED. ALERT Penicillin Codeine

Recall Examination Form

After the initial medical history is collected, it is vital that the history be updated on a regular schedule. Patients who have series histories should be asked at each visit whether there has been a change in their medical status. Some forms provide space that can be used to record any changes in medical history or in medications. After the form has been updated, it is signed by both the patient and the dental healthcare team member.

(Form courtesy The Dental Record, Wisconsin Dental Associations, Milwaukee, WI.)

Form No. T161RE
RECALL EXAMINATION
Form No. T170CE
CLINICAL EXAMINATION
Form No. T181PS
PERIODONTAL SCREENING EXAMINATION
Form No. T201TP
TREATMENT PLAN

Budd, Rose L.

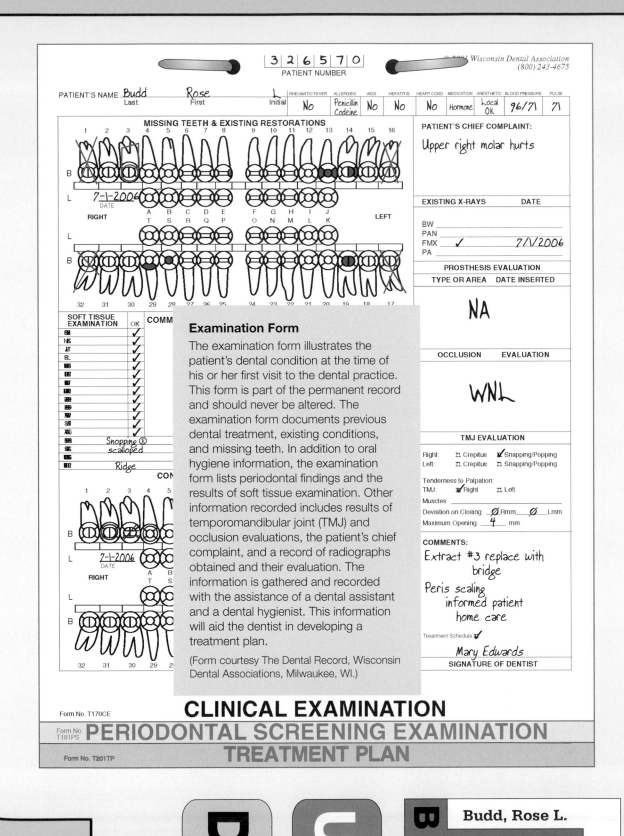

PATIENT NUMBER: 3 2 6 5 7 0
© 2001 Wisconsin Dental Association
(800) 243-4675

PATIENT'S NAME: Budd (Last) Rose (First) L (Initial)

RHEUMATIC FEVER	ALLERGIES	AIDS	HEPATITIS	HEART COND.	MEDICATION	ANESTHETIC	BLOOD PRESSURE	PULSE
No	Penicillin Codeine	No	No	No	Hormone	Local Ok	96/71	71

MISSING TEETH & EXISTING RESTORATIONS

1 2 3 4 5 6 7 8 9 10 11 12 13 14 15 16

B
L
7-1-2006 DATE

RIGHT
A B C D E F G H I J
T S R Q P O N M L K
LEFT

L
B

32 31 30 29 28 27 26 25 24 23 22 21 20 19 18 17

SOFT TISSUE EXAMINATION — OK

(checkmarks listed)

Snapping ® scalloped
Ridge

1 2 3 4 5
B
L
7-1-2006 DATE
RIGHT
A B
T S
L
B
32 31 30 29

PATIENT'S CHIEF COMPLAINT:
Upper right molar hurts

EXISTING X-RAYS   DATE
BW _____
PAN _____
FMX ✓   7/1/2006
PA _____

PROSTHESIS EVALUATION
TYPE OR AREA   DATE INSERTED
NA

OCCLUSION   EVALUATION
WNL

TMJ EVALUATION
Right: ⊓ Crepitus   ✓ Snapping/Popping
Left: ⊓ Crepitus   ⊓ Snapping/Popping

Tenderness to Palpation:
TMJ: ✓ Right   ⊓ Left
Muscles: _____
Deviation on Closing: Ø Rmm   Ø Lmm
Maximum Opening: 4 mm

COMMENTS:
Extract #3 replace with bridge
Peris scaling
informed patient
home care

Treatment Schedule ✓

Mary Edwards
SIGNATURE OF DENTIST

Form No. T170CE
CLINICAL EXAMINATION

Form No. T181PS
PERIODONTAL SCREENING EXAMINATION

Form No. T201TP
TREATMENT PLAN

Examination Form

The examination form illustrates the patient's dental condition at the time of his or her first visit to the dental practice. This form is part of the permanent record and should never be altered. The examination form documents previous dental treatment, existing conditions, and missing teeth. In addition to oral hygiene information, the examination form lists periodontal findings and the results of soft tissue examination. Other information recorded includes results of temporomandibular joint (TMJ) and occlusion evaluations, the patient's chief complaint, and a record of radiographs obtained and their evaluation. The information is gathered and recorded with the assistance of a dental assistant and a dental hygienist. This information will aid the dentist in developing a treatment plan.

(Form courtesy The Dental Record, Wisconsin Dental Associations, Milwaukee, WI.)

Budd, Rose L.

PATIENT'S NAME: Budd (Last) Rose (First) L (Initial)

326570

Wisconsin Dental Association
(800) 243-4675

Date of Birth: 7/17/52

DATE: 7-1-2006 THERAPIST: Sue Greavy

PROBING – Place probe as close to the contact point as possible, directed along the long axis of the tooth. Take the mesial, mid and distal measurements from the buccal aspect. Repeat for lingual aspect. Record only those measurements over 3mm.
BLEEDING – After probing each quadrant, note whether or not bleeding has occurred. Indicate the bleeding area by circling the pocket in red.
MOBILITY – Move each tooth between two instrument handles in a bucco-lingual direction and attempt to depress each tooth in its socket. Grade each tooth accordingly: 0 - Movement of less than 0.5mm; 1 - 0.5mm to 1.0mm; 2 - 1.0mm to 2.0mm; 3 - Movement of more that 2.0mm or depressible.
FURCATION – Probe from the buccal and lingual. Record accordingly: 0 - Normal; 1 - Slight; 2 - Moderate; 3 - Through and through.
RECESSION – Measure the exposed surface from the cemental enamel junction (CEJ) to the gingival crest. Enter the distance in millimeters (mm).

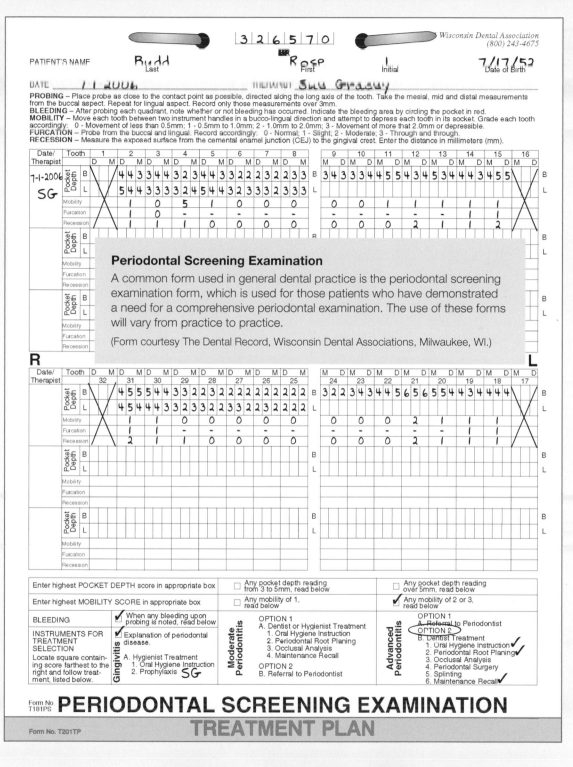

Periodontal Screening Examination

A common form used in general dental practice is the periodontal screening examination form, which is used for those patients who have demonstrated a need for a comprehensive periodontal examination. The use of these forms will vary from practice to practice.

(Form courtesy The Dental Record, Wisconsin Dental Associations, Milwaukee, WI.)

R   L

Enter highest POCKET DEPTH score in appropriate box	☐ Any pocket depth reading from 3 to 5mm, read below / ☐ Any pocket depth reading over 5mm, read below
Enter highest MOBILITY SCORE in appropriate box	☐ Any mobility of 1, read below / ✔ Any mobility of 2 or 3, read below

BLEEDING — ✔ When any bleeding upon probing is noted, read below

INSTRUMENTS FOR TREATMENT SELECTION — ✔ Explanation of periodontal disease.
Locate square containing score farthest to the right and follow treatment, listed below.

Gingivitis
A. Hygienist Treatment
1. Oral Hygiene Instruction
2. Prophylaxis SG

Moderate Periodontitis
OPTION 1
A. Dentist or Hygienist Treatment
1. Oral Hygiene Instruction
2. Periodontal Root Planing
3. Occlusal Analysis
4. Maintenance Recall

OPTION 2
B. Referral to Periodontist

Advanced Periodontitis
OPTION 1
A. Referral to Periodontist
OPTION 2
B. Dentist Treatment
1. Oral Hygiene Instruction ✔
2. Periodontal Root Planing ✔
3. Occlusal Analysis
4. Periodontal Surgery
5. Splinting
6. Maintenance Recall ✔

Form No. T181PS
PERIODONTAL SCREENING EXAMINATION
TREATMENT PLAN
Form No. T201TP

Budd, Rose L.

PATIENT NUMBER 3 2 6 5 7 0

PATIENT'S NAME __Budd__ __Rose__ __L__ __7/1/2006__
Last / First / Initial / Date

DATE	TREATMENT PLAN	FEE	ALTERNATE TREATMENT	FEE	PROB # ASGN
7/1/2006	#3 Extraction	83⁻			2
7/1/2006	#2-4 3 unit Fix Br	2160	PUD	745⁻	3
7/1/2006	UR quad perio scaling	100⁻			4
7/1/2006	UL quad perio scaling	100⁻			4
7/1/2006	LL quad perio scaling	100⁻			4
7/1/2006	LR quad perio scaling	100⁻			4
7/1/2006	Prophy + polish	65⁻			5
7/1/2006	Patient selected Fix Br				
	Total	2708⁰⁰			

Treatment Plan Form

The treatment plan is derived from information collected in the clinical record. The dentist reviews the medical history, previous dental history, and results of the diagnostic examination and determines what work is needed to ensure that the best interests of the patient are protected. This is done with no insurance coverage or managed care contract. Each patient is treated in the same way, regardless of socioeconomic factors or insurance coverage. The patient is presented the full case and then may decide on alternative treatment that will meet insurance company mandates or financial need. This allows the patient to make an informed decision about needed dental treatment.

Once the treatment plan has been presented and the course of treatment has been decided, a financial plan can be prepared.

(Form courtesy The Dental Record, Wisconsin Dental Associations, Milwaukee, WI.)

RELEASE

I accept the above treatment plan. I understand that because of unexpected circumstances, the treatment, the fees for treatment and/or the materials required as explained to me at this time, may require some changes after actual care has begun.

PATIENT'S/GUARDIAN'S SIGNATURE __Rose Budd__ DATE __7/1/2006__

ANEST.

MED. ALERT
Penicillin
Codeine

TREATMENT PLAN

Form No. T201TP

Budd, Rose L.

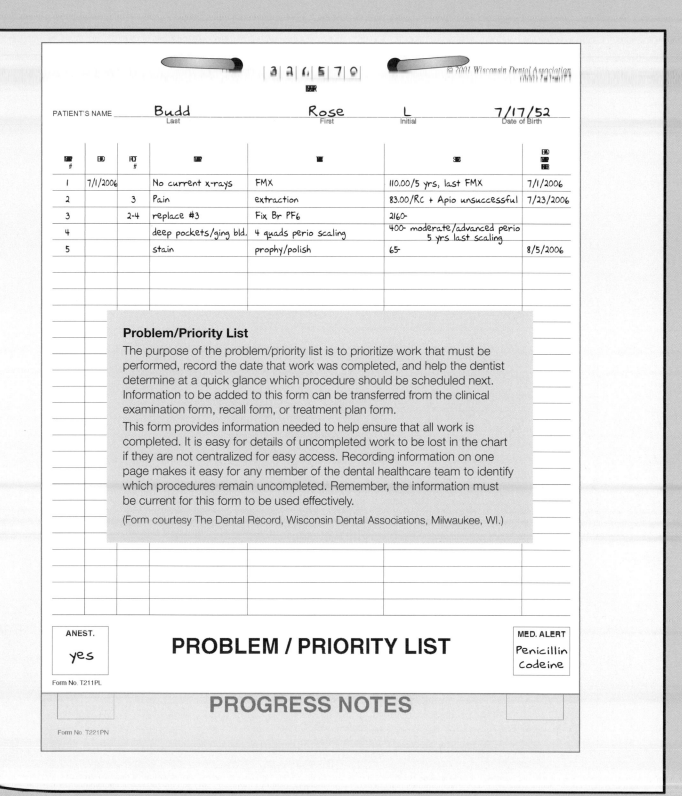

PATIENT'S NAME   Budd   Rose   L   7/17/52
                   Last   First   Initial   Date of Birth

#		#				
1	7/1/2006		No current x-rays	FMX	110.00/5 yrs, last FMX	7/1/2006
2		3	Pain	extraction	83.00/RC + Apio unsuccessful	7/23/2006
3		2-4	replace #3	Fix Br PF6	2160-	
4			deep pockets/ging bld.	4 quads perio scaling	400- moderate/advanced perio 5 yrs last scaling	
5			stain	prophy/polish	65-	8/5/2006

Problem/Priority List

The purpose of the problem/priority list is to prioritize work that must be performed, record the date that work was completed, and help the dentist determine at a quick glance which procedure should be scheduled next. Information to be added to this form can be transferred from the clinical examination form, recall form, or treatment plan form.

This form provides information needed to help ensure that all work is completed. It is easy for details of uncompleted work to be lost in the chart if they are not centralized for easy access. Recording information on one page makes it easy for any member of the dental healthcare team to identify which procedures remain uncompleted. Remember, the information must be current for this form to be used effectively.

(Form courtesy The Dental Record, Wisconsin Dental Associations, Milwaukee, WI.)

ANEST.
yes

PROBLEM / PRIORITY LIST

MED. ALERT
Penicillin
Codeine

Form No. T211PL

PROGRESS NOTES

Form No. T221PN

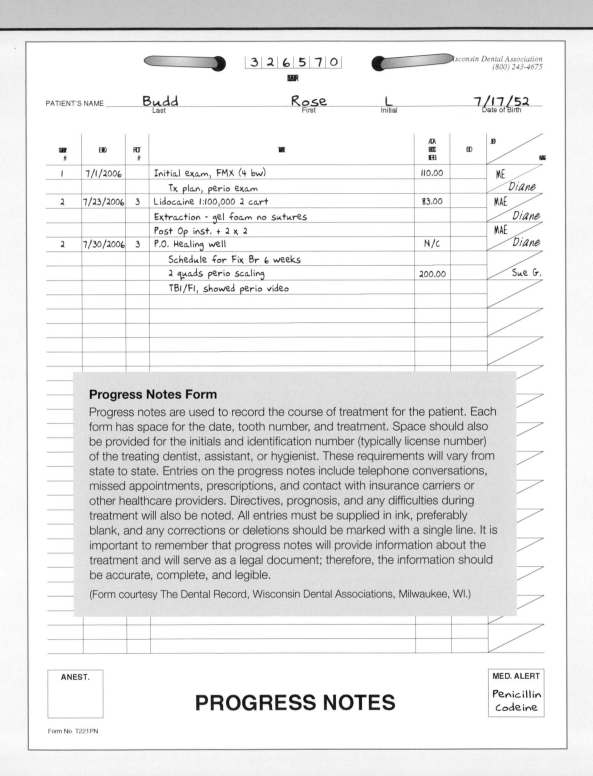

326570

Wisconsin Dental Association
(800) 243-4675

PATIENT'S NAME **Budd** **Rose** **L** **7/17/52**
Last   First   Initial   Date of Birth

#	DATE	TOOTH #	TREATMENT	ADA CODE FEE	PD	INIT NOS
1	7/1/2006		Initial exam, FMX (4 bw)	110.00		ME
			Tx plan, perio exam			Diane
2	7/23/2006	3	Lidocaine 1:100,000 2 cart	83.00		MAE
			Extraction - gel foam no sutures			Diane
			Post Op inst. + 2 x 2			MAE
2	7/30/2006	3	P.O. Healing well	N/C		Diane
			Schedule for Fix Br 6 weeks			
			2 quads perio scaling	200.00		Sue G.
			TBI/FI, showed perio video			

Progress Notes Form

Progress notes are used to record the course of treatment for the patient. Each form has space for the date, tooth number, and treatment. Space should also be provided for the initials and identification number (typically license number) of the treating dentist, assistant, or hygienist. These requirements will vary from state to state. Entries on the progress notes include telephone conversations, missed appointments, prescriptions, and contact with insurance carriers or other healthcare providers. Directives, prognosis, and any difficulties during treatment will also be noted. All entries must be supplied in ink, preferably blank, and any corrections or deletions should be marked with a single line. It is important to remember that progress notes will provide information about the treatment and will serve as a legal document; therefore, the information should be accurate, complete, and legible.

(Form courtesy The Dental Record, Wisconsin Dental Associations, Milwaukee, WI.)

ANEST.

PROGRESS NOTES

MED. ALERT
Penicillin
Codeine

Form No. T221PN

PATIENT NUMBER: 3 2 6 5 7 0

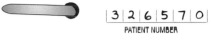

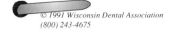
© 1991 Wisconsin Dental Association
(800) 243-4675

PATIENT'S NAME: **Budd** (Last) **Rose** (First) **L** (Initial) **7/17/52** (Date of Birth)

I hereby authorize **Mary A. Edwards, DDS**
DOCTOR'S NAME

and whomever he/she may designate as his/her assistants, to perform upon me the following operation and/or procedures:

Extraction-#3
Fixed PFM Bridge-#2-#4
Four quadrants of perio scaling

I request and authorize him/her to do whatever he/she deems advisable if any unforeseen condition arises in the course of these designated operations and/or procedures calling, in their judgment, for procedures in addition to or different from those now contemplated.

I consent to the abo[...]
treatments and the cons[...]

I consent to the abo[...]
and the known material [...]

I further consent to [...]
drugs that may be deeme[...]
the administration of any[...]
cardiac arrest, and aspira[...]
injury to blood vessels a[...]

I am informed and fu[...]
In oral surgery, the most [...]
discomfort, stiff jaws, los[...]
loss or injury to adjacent t[...]
fractures, sinus exposure [...]
ing in the jaw which mig[...]

I realize that in spite [...]
sary and desired by me [...]
acknowledge that no guarantees have been made to me concerning the results of the operation or procedure.

Consent Form

This form outlines the work that will be done, describes reasonable results, and alerts the patient to complications that could result from treatment. It also explains the responsibility the patient assumes in assuring that treatment will be successful. The use of consent forms allows the patient to ask questions about the treatment and helps establish a partnership between the patient and the dental healthcare team. It is believed that these forms and the signatures of patients should help to reduce the number of malpractice suits. These forms should be designed with the assistance of an attorney, who will check the form for legal content.

(Form courtesy The Dental Record, Wisconsin Dental Associations, Milwaukee, WI.)

I have provided as accurate and complete a medical and personal history as possible including those antibiotics, drugs, medications and foods to which I am allergic. I will follow any and all instructions as explained and directed to me and permit prescribed diagnostic procedures.

I have had the opportunity to ask questions and receive answers to and responsive explanations for, all questions about my medical condition, contemplated and alternative treatment and procedures, and the risk and potential complications of the contemplated and alternative treatments and procedures, prior to signing this form.

Patient or Guardian's Signature **Rose Budd**   Date **7/1/2006**
Dentist's Signature **M. Edwards**   Date **7/1/2006**
Witness's Signature **Diane Feller**   Date **7/1/2006**

CONSENT FORM

Form No. 243CF

Form 250SF — **SIGNATURE ON FILE**

Form 260FA — **FINANCIAL ARRANGEMENTS**

Form No. T231CL — **CORRESPONDENCE LOG**

   Budd, Rose L.

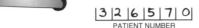

PATIENT NUMBER

© 1991 Wisconsin Dental Association
(800) 243-4675

PATIENT'S NAME   *Budd*   *Rose*   *L*
                   Last   First   Initial

I hereby authorize payment directly to _____ *Mary*
of the dental benefits otherwise payable to me.   DEN

_____ *Rose L. B*
SIGNATURE (INSURED P

7/1/2006
DATE

Signature is valid for two years from the above date, u

_____

_____

Mary A. Edwar
ATTENDING D.D.S. N

is authorized to provide any insurance company(s), claim adminis
information concerning health care advice, treatment or supplie
purpose of evaluating and administrating claims for benefits.

This authorization is valid for the term of coverage of the policy or
which ever is shorter.

I know I have a right to receive a copy of this authorization upo
this authorization is as valid as the original.

_____ *Rose Budd*   *7/1/2006*
PATIENT OR AUTHORIZED PERSON'S SIGNATURE   DATE

Signature on File Form

The purpose of the signature on file form is to provide a process that allows the dental practice to submit insurance claim forms without the patient's signature. With the use of computer-generated insurance forms and electronic submissions, it is not possible to have patients sign each form with an original signature. Therefore, patients are asked to sign a form that authorizes the dentist to submit claims without the signature.

The form provides two types of authorization. The first authorizes the dentist to submit claims and request direct reimbursement (authorization to issue the check in the name of the dentist). The second authorization states that the patient will release any information in his/her clinical record that will be needed by the insurance company. *Remember, all information contained in the patient's clinical record is confidential and cannot be released to anyone without the written permission of the patient.*

(Form courtesy The Dental Record, Wisconsin Dental Associations, Milwaukee, WI.)

Form 250SF

SIGNATURE ON FILE

Form 260FA

FINANCIAL ARRANGEMENTS
CORRESPONDENCE LOG

Form No. T231CL

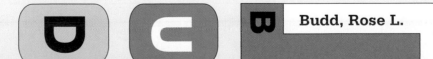

Budd, Rose L.

PATIENT'S NAME   _Budd_   _Rose_   _L_
                     Last   First   Initial

I   _Rose_   have had my treatment plan and options explained to me and hereby authorize this treatment to be performed by Dr. _Mary Edwards_

Patient's Signature   _Rose Budd_   Date _7/23/2006_
(Parent or Guardian MUST sign if patient is a minor)

I also understand that the cost of this treatment is as follows and that the method of paying for the same will be:

Total (Partial) estimate of treatment	$	_2708.00_
Less:		
Initial Payment	−	_1000.00_
Insurance Estimate if Applicable	−	_1000.00_
Other _____	−	_0_
Balance of Estimate Due	$	_708.00_

Terms: Monthly Payment $ _236.00_ over a _3_ month period.

PLEASE CONTACT THE BUSINESS OFFICE IF YOU ARE UNABLE TO MEET YOUR FINANCIAL OBLIGATION

The truth in lending Law enacted in 1969 serves to inform the borrowers and installment p... amounts financed. This law applies to this office whenever the office extends the courtesy o... finance charge is made.

The signature below indicate a mutual understanding of the ESTIMATE ... ule of payment as noted.

Today's Date _7/23/2006_   _Rose Budd_
                                        Signature of Responsible Party

                       Sharon Williams
                             Financial Advisor

Note: THIS IS AN ESTIMATE ONLY, if treatment plan should change please request an a... This estimate is valid for 90 days from the date above IF treatment has not begun within that makes this agreement invalid.

Financial Arrangements Form

The use of the financial arrangements form places in writing the total estimated cost of the proposed dental treatment, when payments are expected, and the amount. It meets regulations by providing a "truth in lending" statement and gives instructions on what should be done if a payment cannot be made. By signing the form, patients state that they understand what is going to be done, agree to the estimated fee, and accept the payment schedule.

(Form courtesy The Dental Record, Wisconsin Dental Associations, Milwaukee, WI.)

Form 260FA

FINANCIAL ARRANGEMENTS

CORRESPONDENCE LOG

Form No. T231CL

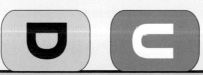

Budd, Rose L.

324 Wisconsin Dental Association
(800) 243-4675

3 2 6 5 7 0
PATIENT NUMBER

PATIENT'S NAME ___Budd_____Rose_____L_____
                        Last   First   Initial

NO.	DATE RECEIVED	DATE SENT	CORRESPONDENCE TO / FROM	INS.	SPEC. REF.	RX	REASON
							OTHER / COMMENTS
1.		7/7/2006	Blue Cross				Pre-Auth
2.	7/14/2006		Blue Cross				Auth Received
3.	7/15/2006		Rose B				Financial Agreement
4.							
5.							
6.							
7.							
8.							
9.							
10.							
11.							
12.							
13.							
14.							
15.							
16.							
17.							
18.							
19.							
20.							
21.							
22.							
23.							
24.							
25.							
26.							

Correspondence Log

Any correspondence related to the patient's care should be logged in on this form, with copies placed in the patient's clinical record. This includes letters of referral to specialists, communications to insurance carriers, and correspondence that records financial matters.

(Form courtesy The Dental Record, Wisconsin Dental Associations, Milwaukee, WI.)

REFERRAL, INSURANCE, PRESCRIPTION
CORRESPONDENCE LOG

Form No. T231CL

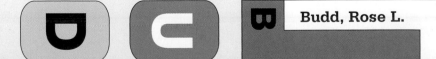

Budd, Rose L.

THAYER DENTAL LABORATORY, INC.

131 OLD SCHOOLHOUSE LANE, P.O. BOX 1204
MECHANICSBURG, PA 17055
717-697-6324 / 800-382-1240 / FAX: 717-697-1412
"YOUR PARTNER IN MASTERING NEW TECHNOLOGIES"

DR. _Mary Edwards_   RETURN DATE: _10/18/2006_
PATIENT: _Rose Budd_   DATE SENT: _10/10/2006_

MALE ☐   FEMALE ☒   AGE: _54_   FACIAL SHAPE: _Sq. oval_

STUMPF SHADE: _____

SHADE DESIRED: _____

MOULD: _____

SURFACE:		OCCLUSAL STAIN:	
SMOOTH	☐	NONE	☐
MODERATE	☐	LIGHT	☐
HEAVY	☐	MEDIUM	☐
		DARK	☐

DEGREE OF TRANSLUCENCY: MINIMUM ☐   MODERATE ☐   MAXIMUM ☐

RETURN: METAL ☐ BISQUE ☐ FINISHED ☐ INDIVIDUAL ☐ SPLINTED ☐

COPING DESIGN (PLEASE CIRCLE ONE):

FULL PORCELAIN COVERAGE | LINGUAL METAL COLLAR | FULL METAL COLLAR | BUCCAL CUSP (PORCELAIN/ METAL OCCLUSAL) | FULL METAL OCCLUSAL (VENEER) | FULL PORCELAIN COVERAGE | FULL COVERAGE LINGUAL | 2/3 COVERAGE LINGUAL

PONTIC DESIGN (PLEASE CIRCLE ONE):

SANITARY | FULL RIDGE | MODIFIED | BULLET | OVATE

MARGIN DESIGN: NO METAL TO SHOW ☐
HAIRLINE METAL MARGIN ☐   PORCELAIN BUTT ☐

IF NO OCCLUSAL CLEARANCE:
METAL
REDUC

INSTRU

UPPER — RIGHT / LEFT — LOWER

Laboratory Forms

Laboratory forms are used to communicate instructions to dental laboratory staff in the fabrication of a dental prosthesis. This form or prescription is required in most states to prevent the illegal practice of dentistry. This form contains specific information that communicates to the laboratory what needs to be done. It is important to keep a copy of this form in the patient's chart for reference. The laboratory prescription includes the patient's name or identification number, along with date, instructions, signature, and license number of the prescribing dentist.

(Form courtesy Thayer Dental Laboratory, Inc., Mechanicsburg, PA.)

SIGNATURE: _Mary Edwards_   LICENSE: _____
ADDRESS: _4546 Avery Way_
CITY: _Canyon View_   STATE: _CA_   ZIP: _91783_
WE NEED: BOXES ☐   RX PADS ☐   FED-X AIRBILLS ☐   MAILING LABELS ☐
(SEE REVERSE SIDE FOR TERMS & CONDITIONS)

3 2 6 5 7 0
PATIENT NUMBER

N.P. # ____ _yes_ ____

NAME _Budd, Rose L_

IF CHILD:
PARENT'S NAME _____

ADDRESS _1836 N Front Street Flora, CA 91711_

TELEPHONE: HOME _555-1486_   BUSINESS _555-3210_   CELL _____

DENTAL INSURANCE _Blue Cross_   MEDICAL ASSISTANCE _N/A_

DATE OF LAST DENTAL VISIT _5 yrs_   ARE X-RAYS AVAILABLE? Yes ☐ No ☒

NAME OF FORMER DENTIST _F. Jones_

ADDRESS _Hong Kong_

TELEPHONE _____

PAIN ☐ ✓   WHERE

TOOTHACHE _Sometimes_

LOST FILLING ☐

OTHER SYMPTOMS _Had a_
area has never fel

PREMEDICATION REQUIRED BECAU

PROSTHETIC JOINTS _____

MITRAL VALVE PROLAPSE _____

PURPOSE OF VISIT:

RELIEF OF PAIN ☐ ✓

EXAMINATION ☐ ✓   PR

PATIENT WISHES TO SEE: DR.

ATTITUDE:

FRIGHTENED ☐   HOSTILE

REMARKS: _____

APPOINTMENT ON: _7/1 10 am_

X-RAYS SENT OR CALLED FOR: YES ☐   NO ☐   DATE: _____

WHOM MAY WE THANK FOR THIS REFERRAL: _____

INFORMATION TAKEN BY: _Sharon W_   DATE: _6/28/2006_

TELEPHONE INFORMATION

Form No. T320TI

Telephone Information Form

The process of collecting information used in the clinical record begins when the patient first contacts the dental practice, which typically involves a telephone call. Data collection can begin immediately with a telephone information form. This form guides the receptionist through a series of questions and provides space for recording the answer. This form provides spaces in which the patient's name, address, and home and work telephone numbers can be recorded. The receptionist is able to discern the reason why the patient is calling for an appointment, insurance information, last visit to a dentist, and the name and address of the previous dentist. When a patient calls with a dental emergency, subjective information can be recorded. Subjective information includes the chief complaint, the presence of swelling, the area of the problem, and whether the patient is experiencing other symptoms. Medical questions may be asked to determine whether the patient requires medication before dental treatment. In addition to patient information, this form provides space in which other information may be recorded, such as scheduled appointments, requests for radiographs from a previous dentist, the name of the person who referred the patient, and when a thank you letter for the referral was sent.

This form serves two purposes. First, the information is arranged in an organized manner, providing consistency and logic to the questions being asked in a format that can be followed by any team member who answers the telephone. Second, the form ensures that all of the necessary information is collected.

(Form courtesy The Dental Record, Wisconsin Dental Associations, Milwaukee, WI.)

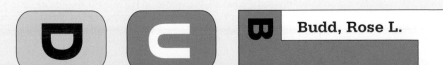

Budd, Rose L.

ANATOMY OF A DENTAL REGISTRATION FORM

(1) PATIENT INFORMATION SECTION

This includes demographic data that will be used in preparing financial and insurance statements.

(2) INSURANCE INFORMATION

This includes all of the informatin needed to complete and process dental insurance claim forms. This information is also used to detemine the eligibility for and the dental insurance coverage of the patient.

(3) RESPONSIBLE PARTY SECTION

This relates to the person or persons who are financially responsible for the payment of the dental account. This is not to be confused with insurance companies or others who will act as third party in the payment of the patient's dental fees. This concept is confusing and often misinterpreted by patients.

Adult patients are responsible for their own account, and when married they are jointly responsible (in most states) along with their spouse. Minor children's accounts are the responsiblity of their parents. In the case of divorced parents, the court assigns responsiblity to one or both parents. Determining financial responsiblity is confusing for both the dental assistant and the patient. The bottom line is that the patient or parents are responsible for payment. Insurance companies do not guarantee payment and therefore cannot be held responsible.

(4) NECESSARY TREATMENT STATEMENT

This statement, when signed by the patient, serves as a consent to treatment.

(5) RELEASE OF INFORMATION

Before any information can be released concerning the treatment of a patient, a statement must be signed by the patient authorizing the release. A similar statement and signature will be required when information is released to another dentist, medical doctor, or to any the authorized agency.

(6) CONFIRMATION THAT THE PATIENT IS RESPONSIBLE FOR ALL DENTAL COSTS

This statement helps eliminate the confusion of who is ultimately responsible for all the dental costs. By informing the patient of the fees and coordinating a payment plan between the patient and the insurance carrier, the dentist or assistant ensures that the patient is fully aware of all financial responsibility prior to the beginning of dental treatment.

(7) CERTIFICATION THAT THE INFORMATION PRESENTED IS ACCURATE

This is signed by the patient or parent.

Form

© 2003 Wisconsin Dental Association
(800) 243-4675

0 0 0 1 3 8
PATIENT NUMBER

welcome

Date _____

(1) Patient's Name _____ Date of Birth _____ ❑ Male ❑ Female
Last   First   Initial

If Child: Parent's Name _____

How do you wish to be addressed _____
Single ❑ Married ❑ Separated ❑ Divorced ❑ Widowed ❑ Minor ❑

Residence - Street _____

City _____ State ____ Zip _____

Business Address _____

Telephone: Res. _____ Bus. _____

Fax _____ Cell Phone # _____

eMail _____

Patient/Parent Employed By _____

Present Position _____

How Long Held _____

Spouse/Parent Name _____

Spouse Employed By _____

Present Position _____

How Long Held _____

Who is Responsible for this account _____

(3) Drivers License No. _____

Method of Payment: Insurance ❑ Cash ❑ Credit Card ❑

Purpose of Call _____

Other Family Members in this Practice _____

Whom may we thank for this referral _____

Patient/parent Social Security No. _____

Spouse/Parent Social Security No. _____

Someone to notify in case of emergency not living with you _____

DENTAL INSURANCE 1ST COVERAGE

(2) Employee Name _____ Date of Birth _____
Employer Name _____ Yrs. _____
Name of Insurance Co. _____
Address _____

Telephone _____
Program or policy # _____
Social Security No. _____
Union Local or Group _____

DENTAL INSURANCE 2ND COVERAGE

Employee Name _____ Date of Birth _____
Employer Name _____ Yrs. _____
Name of Insurance Co. _____
Address _____

Telephone _____
Program or policy # _____
Social Security No. _____
Union Local or Group _____

(4) **CONSENT:**
I consent to the diagnostic procedures and treatment by the dentist necessary for proper dental care.

(5) I consent to the dentist's use and disclosure of my records (or my child's records) to carry out treatment, to obtain payment, and for those activities and health care operations that are related to treatment or payment.
I consent to the disclosure of my records (or my child's records) to the following persons who are involved in my care (or my child's care) or payment for that care.

(6) My consent to disclosure of records shall be effective until I revoke it in writing.
I authorize payment directly to the dentist or dental group of insurance benefits otherwise payable to me. I understand that my dental care insurance carrier or payor of my dental benefits may pay less than the actual bill for services, and that I am financially responsible for payment in full of all accounts. By signing this statement, I revoke all previous agreements to the contrary and agree to be responsible for payment of services not paid, by my dental care payor.
I attest to the accuracy of the information on this page.

(7) PATIENT'S OR GUARDIAN'S SIGNATURE _____

DATE _____

Form No. T110R

REGISTRATION

(Form courtesy of The Dental Record, Wisconsin Dental Association, Milwaukee, WI.)

(Form courtesy The Dental Record, Wisconsin Dental Association, Milwaukee, WI.)

Canyon View Dental Associates   © 2002 Wisconsin Dental Association
(800) 243-4675

[Insert Name of Practice]

NOTICE OF PRIVACY PRACTICES

THIS NOTICE DESCRIBES HOW HEALTH INFORMATION ABOUT YOU MAY BE USED AND DISCLOSED AND HOW YOU CAN GET ACCESS TO THIS INFORMATION.

PLEASE REVIEW IT CAREFULLY. THE PRIVACY OF YOUR HEALTH INFORMATION IS IMPORTANT TO US.

OUR LEGAL DUTY

Federal and state law requires us to maintain the privacy of your health information. That law also requires us to give you this notice about our privacy practices, our legal duties, and your rights concerning your health information. We must follow the privacy practices we describe in this notice while it is in effect. This notice takes effect April 14, 2003, and will remain in effect until we replace it.

We reserve the right to change our privacy practices and the terms of this notice at any time, provided such applicable law permits the changes. We reserve the right to make the changes in our privacy practices and the new terms of our notice effective for all health information tha t we maintain, including health information we created or received before we made the changes. Before we make a significant change in our privacy practices, we will change this notice and make the new notice available upon request.

You may request a copy of our notice at any time. For more information about our privacy practices, or for additional copies of this notice, please contact us using the information listed at the end of this notice.

USES AND DISCLOSURES OF HEALTH INFORMATION

We use and disclose health information about you for treatment, payment, and health care operations. For example:
Treatment: We may use your health information for treatment or disclose it to a dentist, physician or other health care provider providing treatment to you.

Payment: We may use and disclose your health information to obtain payment for services we provide to you. We may also disclose your health information to another health care provider or entity that is subject to the federal Privacy Rules for its payment activities.

Health Care Operations: We may use and disclose your health information for our health care operations. Health care operations include quality assessment and improvement activities, reviewing the competence or qualifications of health care professionals, evaluating practitioner and provider performance, conducting training programs, accreditation, certification, licensing or credentialing activities. We may disclose your health information to another health care provider or organization that is subject to the federal privacy rules and that has a relationship with you to support some of their health care operations. We may disclose your information to help these organizations conduct quality assessment and improvement activities, review the competence or qualifications of health care professionals, or detect or prevent health care fraud and abuse.

On Your Authorization: You may give us written authorization to use your health information or to disclose it to anyone for any purpose. If you give us an authorization, you may revoke it in writing at any time. Your revocation will not affect any uses or disclosures permitted by your authorization while it was in effect. Unless you give us a written authorization, we cannot use or disclose your health information for any reason except those described in this notice.

To Your Family and Friends: We may disclose your health information to a family member, friend or other person to the extent necessary to help with your health care or with payment for your health care. Before we disclose your health information to these people, we will provide you with an opportunity to object to our use or disclosure. If you are not present, or in the event of your incapacity or an emergency, we will disclose your medical information based on our professional judgment of whether the disclosure would be in your best interest. We may use our professional judgment and our experience with common practice to make reasonable inferences of your best interest in allowing a person to pick up filled prescriptions, medical supplies, x-rays, or other similar forms of health information. We may use or disclose information about you to notify or assist in notifying a person involved in your care, of your location and general condition.

Appointment Reminders: We may use or disclose your health information to provide you with appointment reminders (such as voicemail messages, postcards, or letters.)

Disaster Relief: We may use or disclose your health information to a public or private entity authorized by law or by its charter to assist in disaster relief efforts.

Public Benefit: We may use or disclose your medical information as authorized by law for the following purposes deemed to be in the public interest or benefit:
- as required by law;
- for public health activities, including disease and vital statistic reporting, child abuse reporting, FDA oversight, and to employers regarding work-related illness or injury;
- to report adult abuse, neglect, or domestic violence·

Form No. T302HN   © Michael Best & Friedrich, LLC

FIGURE 7-4

Notice of Privacy Practices forms are given to all patients and outline the various HIPAA mandates. (Courtesy The Dental Record, Wisconsin Dental Association, Milwaukee, WI.)

- to health oversight agencies;
- in response to court and administrative orders and other lawful processes;
- to law enforcement officials pursuant to subpoenas and other lawful processes, concerning crime victims, suspicious deaths, crimes on our premises, reporting crimes in emergencies, and for purposes of identifying or locating a suspect or other person;
- to coroners, medical examiners, and funeral directors;
- to an organ procurement organizations;
- to avert a serious threat to health or safety;
- in connection with certain research activities;
- to the military and to federal officials for lawful intelligence, counterintelligence, and national security activities;
- to correctional institutions regarding inmates; and
- as authorized by state worker's compensation laws.

PATIENT RIGHTS

Access: You have the right to look at or get copies of your health information, with limited exceptions. You may request that we provide copies in a format other than photocopies. We will use the format you request unless we cannot practicably do so. You must make a request in writing to obtain access to your health information. You may request access by sending us a letter to the address at the end of this notice. If you request copies, we will charge you a reasonable cost-based fee that may include labor, copying costs, and postage. If you request an alternative format, we will charge a cost-based fee for providing your health information in that format. If you prefer, we may—but are not required to—prepare a summary or an explanation of your health information for a fee. Contact us using the information listed at the end of this notice for more information about fees.

Disclosure Accounting: You have the right to receive a list of instances in which we or our business associates disclosed your health information over the last 6 years (but not before April 14, 2003). That list will not include disclosures for treatment, payment, health care operations, as authorized by you, and for certain other activities. If you request this accounting more than once in a 12-month period, we may charge you a reasonable, cost-based fee for responding to these additional requests. Contact us using the information listed at the end of this notice for more information about fees.

Restriction: You have the right to request that we place additional restrictions on our use or disclosure of your health information. We are not required to agree to these additional restrictions, but if we do, we will abide by our agreement (except in an emergency). Any agreement we may make to a request for additional restrictions must be in writing signed by a person authorized to make such an agreement on our behalf. Your request is not binding unless our agreement is in writing.

Alternative Communication: You have the right to request that we communicate with you about your health information by alternative means or to alternative locations. You must make your request in writing. You must specify in your request the alternative means or location, and provide satisfactory explanation how you will handle payment under the alternative means or location you request.

Amendment: You have the right to request that we amend your health information. Your request must be in writing, and it must explain why we should amend the information. We may deny your request under certain circumstances.

QUESTIONS AND COMPLAINTS

If you want more information about our privacy practices or have questions or concerns, please contact us using the information listed at the end of this notice.

If you believe that:

- we may have violated your privacy rights,
- we made a decision about access to your health information incorrectly,
- our response to a request you made to amend or restrict the use or disclosure of your health information was incorrect, or
- we should communicate with you by alternative means or at alternative locations,

you may contact us using the information listed below. You also may submit a written complaint to the U.S. Department of Health and Human Services. We will provide you with the address to file your complaint with the U.S. Department of Health and Human Services upon request.

We support your right to the privacy of your health information. We will not retaliate in any way if you choose to file a complaint with us or with the U.S. Department of Health and Human Services.

Provider Contact Office: Canyon View Dental Associates

Telephone: 555-0101   Fax: 555-0202

E-Mail: medwards@cuda.com

Address: 4546 North Auery Way Canyon View, CA 91783

Form No. T302HN   © Michael Best & Friedrich, LLC

FIGURE 7-4, cont'd

For legend see opposite page.

Canyon View Dental Associates
[Insert Name of Practice]

INSTRUCTIONS FOR OUR
NOTICE OF PRIVACY PRACTICES

Purpose: This Notice of Privacy Practices presents the information that the HIPAA Privacy Rules require us to give our patients regarding our privacy practices.

We must provide this Notice to each patient no later than the date of our first service delivery to the patient, after April 14, 2003. We must also have the Notice available at the office for patients to request to take with them. We must post the Notice in our office in a clear and prominent location where it is reasonable to expect any patients seeking service from us to be able to read the Notice. Whenever we revise the Notice, we must make the Notice available upon request on or after the effective date of the revision in a manner consistent with the above instructions. Thereafter, we must distribute the Notice to each new patient at the time of service delivery and to any person requesting a Notice. We must also post the revised notice in our office as discussed above.

We must make a good faith effort to obtain a written acknowledgement of receipt of this Notice from each individual with whom we have a direct treatment relationship and to whom we provide this Notice, except in emergency situations. If we do not obtain the acknowledgement, we must document our efforts and the reason we did not obtain the acknowledgement. The last page of the Notice is a written acknowledgement that each patient should sign. We should keep the acknowledgement in the patient's medical record.

This Notice is copyrighted by Michael Best & Friedrich, LLC and licensed to WDA Professional Services, Inc. Any duplication or distribution of this form by other parties requires the prior written approval of Michael Best & Friedrich, LLC and WDA Professional Services, Inc.

[This Notice does not constitute legal advice. This Notice is based on federal law. Requirements reflected in this Notice are subject to change based on changes in federal law or subsequent interpretative guidance. This Notice should be modified to reflect state law that is more stringent than the federal law or other state law exceptions that apply.]

© Michael Best & Friedrich, LLC
Form No. T301HI

FIGURE 7-5

Instructions for Our Notice of Privacy Practices: Required to be given to all patients. The notice identifies the necessary patient documentation that the HIPAA Privacy Rules require. (Courtesy The Dental Record, Wisconsin Dental Association, Milwaukee, WI.)

CLINICAL RECORDS RISK MANAGEMENT

Risk management is a process that identifies conditions that may lead to alleged malpractice or procedures that are not in compliance with mandated regulations. Through a process of identifying and correcting possible conditions or violations, the dental healthcare team can lessen the risk of malpractice suits and deliver quality care to all patients.

Major issues that may cause the patient to question the quality of dental treatment include poor communications, poor dental healthcare team relationships, and poor record keeping. These problems can reduce the level of confidence between the patient and the dental healthcare team. During risk management evaluations, these areas should be identified and corrected before they create a need to defend in an alleged malpractice case.

A second area that can lead to legal actions or sanctions is noncompliance with statutes and regulations established by federal law, identified in the state Dental Practice Act, proscribed in professional organizations' codes of conduct, or outlined in con-

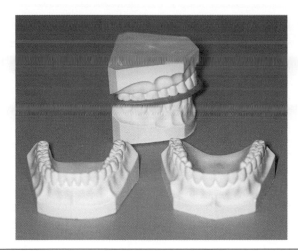

FIGURE 7-6
Diagnostic model. (From Bird D, Robinson D: Torres and Ehrlich Modern Dental Assisting. 8th edition. St. Louis, WB Saunders, 2005, p 775.)

tracts between the dental practice and third party insurance carriers. Noncompliance can lead to fines, revocation of licenses, cancellation of contracts, and lawsuits. It is the duty of the dental healthcare team to be informed of statutes, regulations, and mandates and to follow them to the best of their ability. The American Dental Association, state dental associations, third party insurance carriers, managed care providers, and other professional organizations have spent a great deal of time researching and developing action plans to alert the dental healthcare team to problem situations. These organizations conduct seminars and workshops to help the dental healthcare team identify problems and improve quality of care.

Maintaining Clinical Records

Experts in risk management have identified poor record keeping as a major justification for cases that are decided in favor of the patient. Poor records are sloppy, disorganized, and, in most cases, illegible. The primary reasons for keeping adequate files are to support the need for dental treatment and to justify the actions of the dentist. If the clinical record is incomplete and cannot support the need for treatment, legal cases are decided in the patient's favor. It is impossible to recount all the details of each patient's treatment when you are asked ques-

tions in the future unless good records are available that you can refer to.

The administrative dental assistant plays a key role in protecting the dental practice from such lawsuits. The process begins and ends with the administrative assistant. It is the administrative dental assistant who collects the initial data when a patient first enters the dental practice and initiates the clinical record process. After a patient has received treatment, the clinical record is returned to the business office. It is the responsibility of the administrative assistant to check each chart to make sure all necessary forms have been completed and that the entries meet mandated criteria. Through a checks-and-balances routine, the entire dental healthcare team takes part in the assurance that information is organized, complete, and legible. Regulations and mandates of record keeping vary from state to state and from organization to organization. It is therefore necessary for you to become familiar with the requirements of each state and each organization in which you work.

Procedures for Specific Tasks

Entries

All entries must be legible and must be entered in nonerasable ink. The entry must be signed and dated, and, in some states, must include an identification number (such as a license or social security number). If a correction is made, the error should be crossed out with a single line that is dated and initialed (Figure 7-7). Abbreviations should be used consistently, and a copy of definitions should be kept on file. *Rationale:* An illegible entry or the presence of whiteout can imply that something has been hidden. If abbreviations are not understood, they will confuse the reader, members of the court, or other health professionals and can lead to an incorrect interpretation.

Patient Identification

The patient's name or number should be placed on all pages of the clinical record (as illustrated in Rose Budd's clinical record) and on all radiographs, cast models, laboratory prescriptions, and correspondence. *Rationale:* If records become separated, it may be very difficult to locate the master file,

INCORRECT WAY TO MAKE A CHANGE

PROBLEM #	DATE	TOOTH #	TREATMENT	ADA CODE OR FEE	DISC.	DR. ASST./HYG.
1	7/1/98		Initial Exam, FMX (4 bw)	110.00		ME
			Tx plan, perio exam			Diane
2	7/23/98	3	Lidocaine 1:100,000 2 cart	83.00		MAE
			Extraction - gel foam no sutures			Diane
			~~quads perio scaling~~			
			Post Op inst. + 2×2			
	7/30/98	3	P.O. Healing well			MAE
					N/C	Diane

CORRECT WAY TO MAKE A CHANGE

PROBLEM #	DATE	TOOTH #	TREATMENT	ADA CODE OR FEE	DISC.	DR. ASST./HYG.
1	7/1/98		Initial Exam, FMX (4 bw)	110.00		ME
			Tx plan, perio exam			Diane
2	7/23/98	3	Lidocaine 1:100,000 2 cart	83.00		
			Extraction - gel foam no sutures			Diane
			~~2 quads perio scaling~~ 7/28 MAE			
			Post Op inst. + 2×2			
	7/30/98	3	P.O. Healing well			MAE
					N/C	Diane

FIGURE 7-7
Incorrect way to make a change and correct way to make a change.

and vital information may become permanently lost.

Statements

Statements about patients must be truthful, factual, and objective. Guesses about how patients feel or why they did something can lead to problems if the records leave the dental practice. It is best to report only documented findings (objective findings). *Rationale:* Records can be read by patients and released to others. In a legal proceeding, they will be read by members of the court.

An example of a subjective statement is as follows:

Mary has a real attitude today.

This statement does not provide information. It is only an interpretation of an observation. Mary could have an "attitude" because of a nondental problem, or this could be Mary's normal personality.

An example of an **objective statement** is this:

Mary said that she is upset because she had to wait for 20 minutes.

This statement is based on factual information given by Mary.

Progress Notes

Notations should include the diagnosis, treatment, and amount and type of anesthetic, as well as the

INCORRECT SPACING OF ENTRIES

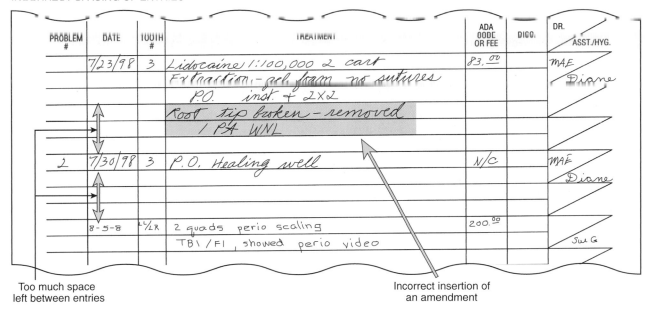

Too much space
left between entries

Incorrect insertion of
an amendment

CORRECT SPACING OF ENTRIES

Correct way to
amend an entry

FIGURE 7-8
Incorrect spacing of entries and correct spacing of entries.

brand names of materials used. Postoperative instructions or unusual occurrences should also be noted. Spacing between entries should be consistent and limited to one or two lines (Figure 7-8). *Rationale:* If spacing is inconsistent, it may appear that information was added at a later date. If it is necessary to add additional information, you are advised to date the entry and state that you are amending the original entry. In addition to recording treatment information, it is suggested, for good risk management, that information on correspondence, telephone conversations, missed appointment noncompliance, and prescriptions also be recorded in the progress notes.

Correspondence

Correspondence includes letters between professionals concerning the dental health of the patient, referral letters, letters between the dentist and the patient concerning dental treatment, insurance inquiries, and letters of dismissal. In addition, all correspondence received should be noted in the progress notes and a copy placed in the clinical record. If a **correspondence log** is used, information can be entered there and cross-referenced to the clinical records.

Telephone Conversations

All telephone conversations with other professionals, pharmacies, insurance carriers, and patients should be recorded and a brief description given stating the significance for any patient's dental care.

Missed Appointments

Documentation of missed and broken appointments establishes the intent of the dentist to complete work in a timely manner and to provide postoperative care. Missed appointments should be followed up with a letter to the patient explaining the importance of continued treatment and outlining the consequences if additional appointments are missed. Place a copy of such letters in the patient's clinical record.

Failure to Follow Instructions

Documenting postoperative or other instructions establishes that the information was given to the patient. Likewise, documenting failure of the patient to follow instructions establishes the patient's noncompliance. The consequences of noncompliance must be explained to the patient, in writing; one copy is given to the patient, and another copy is placed in the patient's clinical record.

Prescriptions

Records must be kept of all prescription and nonprescription drugs given to the patient. The name of the drug, quantity and dosage, and date given must be recorded in the progress notes. Other recommendations or prescriptions, such as for radiographs, laboratory tests, physical therapy, or a dental prosthesis, must be noted also, and a copy of the prescription must be placed in the patient's clinical record.

REMEMBER

Information left out of records is assumed, in a court of law, to have never existed.

Rationale

Consider what would happen if, during an examination, a patient showed no signs of an abnormal condition, and therefore, no mention of the examination was added to the clinical record. An outside professional or an attorney who later reads the record may conclude that the examination did not take place. Even if no significant condition was found, a notation still needs to be made. The use of abbreviations such as **WNL** (within normal limits) and **NSF** (no significant findings) can simplify the process yet still provide documentation that an examination did in fact take place.

Other forms and documentation may be required or recommended by risk management experts. It is important to remember that all of these tools are designed to help the dental healthcare team meet the needs of the patient. By keeping good records, being organized, communicating efficiently, and establishing a partnership with patients, the dental healthcare team helps protect the practice from alleged malpractice cases.

COMPUTERIZED MANAGEMENT OF CLINICAL RECORDS

In the past, a dental practice may have used a computer only to maintain accounting information. Now, computers are used to organize and maintain complex business and clinical records. It is no longer a luxury to have a computer system; it is a necessity. The types of records that are maintained in a computer system include patient clinical and financial information, insurance tracking, recall systems, and appointment scheduling. In addition, computers are now being used to record clinical findings, to access online services, to electronically transfer insurance information, and to communicate with patients, referring dentists, and other professional organizations. The use of computers in the dental practice is discussed in Chapter 17.

HIPAA

Security Standards That Apply to Electronic Clinical Records

- Administrative safeguards:
  - Identification of who will supervise compliance with HIPAA (Health Insurance Portability and Accountability Act) Security Standards
  - Staff clearance procedure that identifies which members of the staff will have access to electronic protected health information (EPHI)
  - Termination procedure
  - Security incident procedures
  - Contingency plan, including data backup plan, disaster recovery plan, and emergency mode operation plan
- Physical safeguards:
  - Protection of electronic systems, equipment, and data that contain EPHI from environmental hazards and unauthorized intrusion
  - Retention of off-site computer backups
- Technical safeguards:
  - Access control, including unique user identification (password and biometric systems)
  - Emergency access procedures
  - Audit controls

Clinical Records

The role of computer-generated clinical records in the dental practice is limitless. The dream of a totally paperless dental practice may soon become a reality. Software is being designed that will ensure the authenticity of clinical records. Digital and scanned radiographs, progress notes, periodontal charting, clinical charting, and so forth can be stored within a computer system. The advantages of a computerized clinical record include reduced storage space and less time required for shuffling papers. Charts will be permanently stored on disk, and information can be transferred elsewhere without removal of the original document from the storage area.

The ability to easily read computer-generated progress notes takes the guesswork out of trying to interpret handwriting. Entries are stamped with the code of the person making the entry (computer signature). Computer software can be designed with safeguards that ensure that all needed information is entered before the program can be closed. This procedure helps to create documents that include all of the necessary elements of good record keeping: organization, consistency, and completeness.

KEY POINTS

- The function of the clinical record is to provide the dental healthcare team with information. The **registration form** provides demographic and financial information needed to complete insurance forms and bill the patient. The **medical history** and **dental history** provide the dentist with information needed to diagnose the patient's condition. **Treatment plans** and clinical charts document necessary treatment. **Progress notes** document treatment that is performed. A variety of other forms help to organize and maintain a complete record for each patient.
- It is the responsibility of the administrative dental assistant to maintain organized clinical records. The administrative dental assistant collects information, organizes the clinical record, checks for completeness, and safeguards the integrity of the record.
- **Risk management** is a process that identifies conditions that can lead to alleged malpractice or to procedures that are not in compliance with mandated regulations. Through the process of identifying and correcting possible conditions or violations, the dental healthcare team can limit the number of alleged malpractice suits and deliver quality care to all patients. The primary reasons for keeping adequate files are to support the patient's need for dental treatment and to justify the dentist's actions.

Web Watch

    Log on to Evolve to access additional
http://evolve.elsevier.com   web links!

Critical Thinking Questions

1. Role play. Use the telephone information form as a guide, and with another student, simulate a telephone conversation according to the following scenario: A new patient calls the dental office to schedule an appointment to have a tooth checked. The tooth has been hurting for about 3 weeks.

2. Mary Smith has an appointment for her first visit to the dental practice. The reception area is crowded when she arrives. Jim, the administrative dental assistant, greets Mrs. Smith.
   - How should Jim complete the information collection process?
   - What forms are included in the process?
   - Form a small team, and discuss situations that may arise that will require an approach that is different from than the one selected by Jim. Write an action plan for each of the following situations, including statements of the problem and the solution: The patient is a minor; the patient is physically challenged; the patient has specific medical problems.

3. Obtain a copy of your state's Dental Practice Act. List the mandates for clinical record keeping.

4. The administrative dental assistant plays a key role in protecting the dental practice from legal actions. Describe the role, and outline the duties that are the responsibility of the administrative dental assistant that pertain to the clinical records.

Notes

OUTLINE

KEY TERMS AND CONCEPTS

Accounts Payable
Accounts Receivable
Aging Labels
Alphabetic Filing
Bank Statements
Business Records
Business Reports
Card Files
Chronological Filing
College Degrees
Color Coding
Confidential Personnel Records
Cross-Referencing
File Folders
File Labels

Filing Segment
Filing Unit
Financial Reports
Geographic Filing
Guides
Hyphenated Names
Indexing
Inspecting
Insurance Records
Lateral File Folders
Lateral Files
Numeric Filing
Out-Guides
Patient Information
Payroll Records

Periodic Method
Perpetual Method
Personnel Records
Professional Correspondence
Retention
Royal and Religious Titles
Simplified Filing Standard Rules
  for Personal Names
Sorting
Subject Filing
Tax Records
Titles and Suffixes
Transfer Methods
Vertical File Folders
Vertical Files

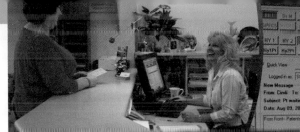

8

Information Management

LEARNING OBJECTIVES

The student will:

1. List and describe the five filing methods outlined in this chapter.
2. Classify personal names according to ARMA (the Association for Information Management) Simplified Filing Standard Rules by correctly indexing names as they will appear on filing labels.
3. List the type of filing methods used for filing accounts payable, accounts receivable, bank statements, and financial reports, as well as personnel records.
4. Describe methods that can be used for filing patient information.
5. Prepare a new patient's clinical record for filing.
6. Prepare a business document for filing.

INTRODUCTION

The responsibilities of the administrative dental assistant in the management of information and records are multifaceted. In today's dental practice, the storage of information may involve both paper files and electronic files. Although methods of documentation may vary, the principles of a records management program will always be the same. According to the International Organization for Standardization (ISO), in *Information and Documentation—Records Management,* a general policy should involve ". . . the creation and management of authentic, reliable and useable records, capable of supporting business function and activities for as long as they are required." The importance of collecting the correct information and preparation of a dental record were discussed in Chapter 7. This chapter discusses basic methods used in a systematic approach to the storage and retrieval of information (filing).

Once it has been created, a record (paper and electronic) should remain accessible, usable, reliable, and authentic. Systems for electronic records should also ensure that these criteria will be maintained through any type of system change for the entire period of retention of this information, including any change in software or in the practice management system.

HIPAA

Security Rule: Protecting Electronic Personal Health Information (ePHI)

- **Confidentiality:** Only authorized individuals may access electronic health information
- **Integrity:** The information does not change except when changed by an authorized person
- **Availability:** Authorized persons can always retrieve ePHI regardless of circumstances

The purposes of following a systematic approach to information management are to simplify the retrieval process and to ensure the precise location of documents and records. In a paper environment, a storage system will include a filing system that contains metal filing cabinets and methods for organizing documents and records. In an electronic environment, the storage system includes hard drives (located on individual PCs and network servers) and portable devices (CDs, tapes, and portable mega storage devices).

Filing systems are used in almost all areas of daily life. Think of a supermarket. Products are divided into categories—produce, dairy, meat, frozen foods, canned goods, and so forth. Once you locate a product category, you will find that it has been subdivided into other areas. For example, when you are shopping for a can of cream of mushroom soup, you first have to locate the general area where "soup" is shelved. You locate the aisle by reading the overhead signs. Once in the correct aisle, you find the soup section; it will be subdivided by brands. You locate the brand of soup you are shopping for, and then you discover that the different types of soup are shelved alphabetically. This system helps you find the can of cream of mushroom soup quickly and efficiently.

Filing in the dental office follows the same principles. First, you locate the file cabinet that contains the information you want to retrieve. Second, you identify the location within the cabinet that contains the subject area. Subjects may be subdivided alphabetically. This eases the retrieval process and ensures that documents are available when needed.

FILING METHODS

A filing system provides a method for placing files in a prescribed order so that they can be located and retrieved by any member of the dental healthcare team. It is the responsibility of the dental professional to safeguard the integrity and confidentiality of all documents. This cannot be guaranteed if records are misplaced or are not returned to their proper locations. It is advisable to follow one of the standardized methods for filing information. Brief descriptions of five of the basic filing systems are provided.

Alphabetic

Alphabetic filing follows strict rules. These rules have been standardized by ARMA (the Association for Information Management) and are recognized as an American National Standard by the American National Standards Institute (ANSI). The purpose of standardization is to establish consistent methods of filing.

Standards must be applied to each and every document, patient record, or other medium that is to be stored. This is not a haphazard process; it must be followed exactly by each person who indexes, codes, and files. When these steps are followed, the integrity and safety of all records can be maintained.

All basic filing methods, with the exception of the chronological system, require alphabetic arrangement. Most of the filing within the dental practice is done alphabetically. Sometimes, a numeric filing system is used (e.g., for clinical records).

The arrangement of a name, subject, or number is referred to as **indexing** and constitutes a filing segment. Before a personal name, business name, or organizational name is indexed, it must be arranged in the correct order. A name, subject, or word is broken down into units. ARMA has defined a unit and filing segments as follows:

> A *filing unit* may be a number, a letter, a word, or any combination of these as stated. . . .

One or more filing units are a *filing segment* (i.e., the total name, subject, or number that is being used for filing purposes).

Following is a description of what makes up each unit and the order in which units are placed, with personal names and business or organizational names used as examples.

- **Unit 1:** *Personal name rule:* Last name (*surname;* also known as the *family name*). *Business / organizational name rule:* First name of the business or organization (business and organizational names are filed as written).
- **Unit 2:** *Personal name rule:* First name (given name); can also be the initial of the first name. *Business / organizational name rule:* Second name as written.
- **Unit 3:** *Personal name rule:* Middle name or initial. *Business / organizational name rule:* Third name as written.
- **Unit 4:** *Personal name rule:* Titles, appendages, and degrees (e.g., Prince, Sr., DDS). *Business / organizational name rule:* Fourth name as written.

NAME AS WRITTEN	NAME AS FILED			
	Unit 1	Unit 2	Unit 3	Unit 4
Robert A. Weingart, DDS (personal name rule)	Weingart	Robert	A.	DDS
Robert A. Weingart, DDS (Business name rule)	Robert	A.	Weingart	DDS

Chart Label (Personal Name)

Weingart, Robert A., DDS (comma is placed between the last name and the first)

File Label (Business Name)

Robert A. Weingart, DDS

The following are examples based on the ARMA **Simplified Filing Standard Rules** for personal names.

Names with prefixes. When a surname has a prefix, such as De, La, Mac, Mc, O', or Van, the prefix is indexed and filed as one unit with the surname.

Business and organizational names follow the same rules as personal names.

Personal and professional titles and suffixes. Titles and suffixes are not used as a filing unit except when they are needed to distinguish between two or more identical names. When used, titles and suffixes are placed in the last filing unit and are filed as written. (Punctuation is ignored.) Specific filing guidelines specify that suffixes are filed in numeric sequence when needed for identification.

When **college degrees** are used, they are placed in the last unit and are used for indexing only, to distinguish between two identical names.

NAME AS WRITTEN	NAME AS FILED			
	Unit 1	Unit 2	Unit 3	Unit 4
Allen	Allen			
A. C. Allen	Allen	A.	C.	
A. C. Allendale	Allendale	A.	C.	
Alice Allendale	Allendale	Alice		
Charles Allendale	Allendale	Charles		
Charlotte Allendale	Allendale	Charlotte		

NAME AS WRITTEN	NAME AS FILED			
	Unit 1	Unit 2	Unit 3	Unit 4
Mark De Anza	De Anza	Mark		
Josie De La Cruz	De La Cruz	Josie		
James M. El Camino	El Camino	James	M.	

NAME AS WRITTEN	NAME AS FILED			
	Unit 1	Unit 2	Unit 3	Unit 4
James Hall	Hall	James		
James C. Hall	Hall	James	C.	
James C. Hall, Sr.	Hall	James	C.	Sr.
James C. Hall, Jr.	Hall	James	C.	Jr.
James C. Hall, III [third]	Hall	James	C.	III [third]
James C. Hall, V [fifth]	Hall	James	C.	V [fifth]

NAME AS WRITTEN	NAME AS FILED			
	Unit 1	Unit 2	Unit 3	Unit 4
Judith L. Green	Green	Judith	L.	
Judith L. Green, DDS	Green	Judith	L.	DDS
Judith L. Green, DMD	Green	Judith	L.	DMD
Julia J. Green	Green	Julia	J.	
Julia J. Green, Ed.D	Green	Julia	J.	Ed.D

NAME AS WRITTEN	NAME AS FILED			
	Unit 1	Unit 2	Unit 3	Unit 4
Lynn Marie Jones	Jones	Lynn	Marie	
Mary Ann Jones-Scott	Jones-Scott	Mary	Ann	
Mary Kelly	Kelly	Mary		
Sandra Kelly-Jones	Kelly-Jones	Sandra		

NAME AS WRITTEN	NAME AS FILED			
	Unit 1	Unit 2	Unit 3	Unit 4
Duchess of York	Duchess (of)	York		
Father O'Malley	Father	O'Malley		
Madame Curie	Madame	Curie		
Pastor Ralph	Pastor	Ralph		
Sister Mary Frances	Sister	Mary	Frances	

Hyphenated names. Hyphenated surnames are treated as one unit.

Royal and religious titles. When titles are followed by a single name, they are filed as written.

Rarely are titles such as Mr., Mrs., Ms., and Miss or military titles used in indexing, unless they are required to distinguish between two identical names. When they are used, these are indexed in the last unit and are alphabetized in the abbreviated form.

When filing records with properly indexed names, one should follow these basic rules:

- The first *letter* that is different in *any unit* determines the alphabetical order.
- Single names are filed before the same name followed by an initial or name.
- Initials are filed before the spelled out name.
- Abbreviations are filed as if they were spelled out. Example: St. becomes Saint, 3rd becomes Third.
- Nicknames are treated as first (given) names.
- Business and organizational names are filed as written, with the business letterhead used as a guide.

Numeric

Numeric filing is used for very large numbers of records. In this system, records are filed according to the number assigned. A key component to this system is cross-referencing. **Cross-referencing** is a method that identifies what other name (or number) a record may be filed under. In numeric filing, an alphabetic listing of all records is used to match names with numbers. Most practice management computer software programs use a numeric system. When a new patient name is entered into the system, the computer assigns the patient a number. The computer can locate patient records by entering a number or an alphabetic configuration (name).

In the numeric system, the order in which the number falls determines its place in the filing system. This is much like counting: 100, 101, 102. Groups of numbers may be assigned to letters of the alphabet that correspond with surnames (last names)—for example, 100 to 999 may be assigned to surnames beginning with *A;* 1,000 to 1,999 may be assigned to surnames beginning with *B;* and so forth. File guides are used in the filing cabinet to identify specific numeric sections.

A computer system works well with this method because it can assign numbers and provide cross-referencing.

Geographic

Geographic filing categorizes records according to a geographic location, such as city, ZIP code, area code, state, or country. Each document is coded and filed according to the selected geographic locator.

Subject

The purpose of **subject filing** is that it allows the retrieval of information according to subject. In this system, files are arranged alphabetically by subject and then within each subject by subgroup (e.g., company name). This system works well for business records (Figure 8-1).

Chronological

Chronological filing allows one to locate documents according to date, month, or year (Figure 8-2). Files are first sorted alphabetically by subject and then within each subject by chronology.

TYPES OF INFORMATION

Information that is stored can be divided into two broad categories: business and patient information. Within each of the two categories, subjects are divided into more specific topics.

Business Records

Business records consist of all documents that pertain to the operation of the dental practice. Business records are divided into several different topics, and a variety of methods exist for their retrieval and storage.

Accounts Payable

Accounts payable records track and store information about the money the practice pays to others for services and supplies (see Chapter 15). Records are divided and categorized by subject and then by vendor, according to the filing system selected. For example, an office may divide accounts according to general headings, such as dental supplies, laboratory, office supplies, and utilities. Once major headings have been developed, it is necessary to subdivide by vendor (see Figure 8-1).

Accounts Receivable

Accounts receivable records track money that is owed to the dental practice (see Chapter 14). Accounts receivable records are stored in a different location or file from accounts payable. When a computerized system is used, these records are stored within the computer under the heading of "Patient Accounts." If a peg board or manual system is used, ledger cards are filed alphabetically in a small metal file box (see Chapter 14).

Bank Statements and Financial Reports

Bank statements and **financial reports** are financial records that are filed according to subject, and then subdivided chronologically (see Figure 8-2).

Personnel Records

Personnel records relate to matters that pertain to the employees of the dental practice. These records include **payroll records,** which document financial information about each employee. The records are filed by subject (payroll) and then subdivided alphabetically by employee name. Each employee file is subdivided chronologically (by payroll period).

Confidential personnel records contain information about the employee's work record. These files contain employment contracts, performance reviews, and documentation of noncompliance. They must be secured and cannot be made available to nonauthorized people.

Tax Records

Tax records are filed by subject, and then subdivided into types of reports or records. These records usually cover a specified period of time, and therefore are subfiled chronologically. Tax reports include payroll, business, and corporate tax reports.

Business Reports

Business reports include profit and loss statements, practice production, and other specified reports that categorize a subject area. Reports are filed by subject, and then subdivided chronologically.

Insurance Records

Insurance records include contracts with third party carriers (insurance companies) and insurance

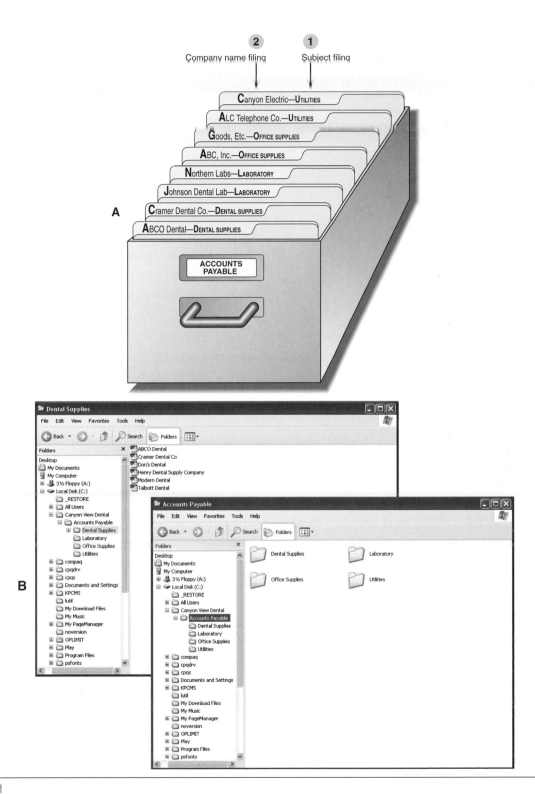

FIGURE 8-1
Subject filing: **A,** Traditional subject filing: Accounts payable, with general headings and subheadings. **B,** Computerized subject filing: Accounts payable, with general headings and subheadings.

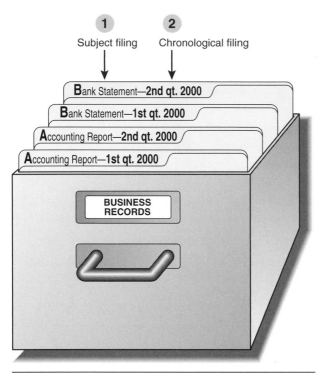

① Subject filing   ② Chronological filing

Bank Statement—2nd qt. 2000
Bank Statement—1st qt. 2000
Accounting Report—2nd qt. 2000
Accounting Report—1st qt. 2000

BUSINESS
RECORDS

FIGURE 8-2

Chronological filing: Financial reports, with general headings (subject filing) and subheadings (chronological filing).

policies that cover areas of the dental practice. These contracts and policies are filed according to subject.

Professional Correspondence

Professional correspondence includes correspondence between individuals and professional organizations. Files are organized by subject (e.g., Dental Specialty), and then are divided into specific subject areas (Endodontics). Specific subjects are then subdivided according to individual or organization (Figure 8-3).

Patient and Insurance Information

Patient Information

Patient information is stored within the clinical record (see Chapter 7). Information contained within the record deals strictly with treatment of the patient. The record does not include financial accounts or insurance forms. Clinical records are filed alphabetically or numerically in a variety of different storage cabinets.

Insurance Records

Insurance records are stored separately from patients' clinical records. Insurance forms are filed in a manner that is specified by each dental practice (see Chapter 11). Forms can be filed by insurance company, and then subdivided by patient. Chronological filing categorizes the forms according to the date the work was completed or the date the claim was filed. Once a claim has been paid, it is pulled from the original file and is refiled in the Paid Claims file.

FILING EQUIPMENT

Storage of information is achieved by putting documents into the correct file folder and placing the folder into the filing unit. The purposes of the filing unit are to store documents safely and to provide a system for easy retrieval. Most dental offices use more than one type of system. Business information may be stored in vertical files while patients' clinical records are placed into a lateral filing unit. Patient ledger cards are stored in small metal boxes, and recall cards may be filed in an index box. Sizes and configurations of filing cabinets vary according to the needs of the dental practice.

Vertical Files

Vertical files are cabinets that consist of one to five drawers that are arranged one on top of another. When these cabinets are used for storage of business records, a frame can be inserted into each drawer to accommodate hanging files. Hanging files can be labeled, and then individual files can be organized within each hanging file (see Figure 8-1).

Lateral Files

Lateral files, or open files, are very popular with dental professionals. They can take the form of modular units or built-in shelving systems. They take up less floor space and blend with the current trend in office design (Figure 8-4). File folders used in this system have side tabs.

Card Files

Card files, or Rolodex files, are designed for quick reference of telephone numbers and addresses and

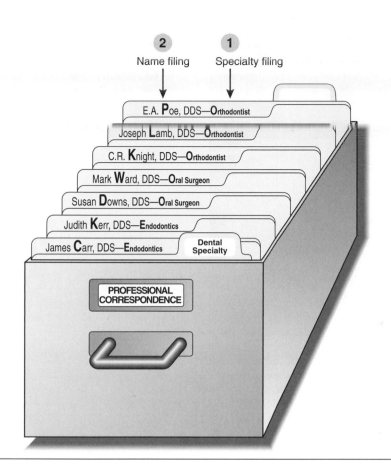

FIGURE 8-3
Professional correspondence filing: Organized by subject, subdivided into specific areas, and then subdivided by individual or organization.

can be used in a recall system. Their small size allows them to be set on a desk or countertop.

FILING SUPPLIES

Once a filing method and appropriate filing equipment have been selected, supplies are needed to complete the system.

File Folders

File folders come in a variety of formats. They are usually made of heavy stock paper, which adds durability. File folders are used to store documents, patient record forms, and business reports.

Vertical File Folders

Vertical file folders are used with vertical filing systems and have tabs located at the top of the file

(see Figure 8-2). Labels are placed on the tab to identify the contents of the folder. The location of the tab varies from folder to folder; this provides a means to look at more than one tab at a time. Folders that have a series of three tabs, far left, center, and far right, are referred to as $^1/_3$ cut. Folders with a series of five tabs are referred to as $^1/_5$ cut.

Organization of the filing cabinet can involve a hanging file system. This system uses a frame from which files hang. Hanging files can hold several file folders, can provide tabs for indexing, and can be moved easily to accommodate rearranging of files. Hanging files work well in systems in which files must hold more than one file folder.

Lateral File Folders

Lateral file folders are used for clinical records and come in a variety of formats and designs. Tabs

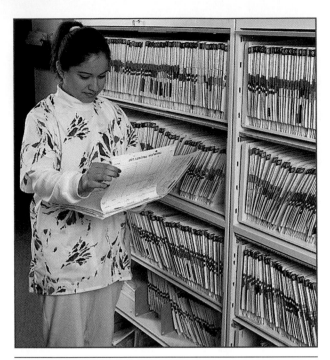

FIGURE 8-4
Lateral filing system. (Courtesy The Dental Record, Madison, WI.)

are located on the sides of the folders. Indexed labels and color-coded labels are placed on the tabs (Figure 8-5). Each folder consists of one or two fasteners designed to keep patient record forms in place (see Chapter 7). Each also has one or two pockets in which radiographs and loose papers can be kept. Some file folders have dividers that help organize forms within the clinical record.

Guides

Guides are used to divide filing systems into small sections. The guide is typically made of heavy stock paper and may be laminated for durability. In the alphabetic system, each letter of the alphabet has a guide. When files are large, additional guides or dividers can be used to subdivide the sections. Smaller sections have less chance of being misfiled.

Out-Guides

Out-guides are used to fill the space occupied by a file that has been removed from the system. The out-guide can simply denote that a record has been removed, or it may contain information stating the location of the record, who removed it, and when it

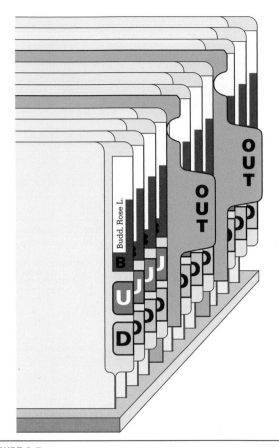

FIGURE 8-5
Lateral file with out-guides showing where records have been removed.

will be returned. The primary purpose of the out-guide is to signify that a record has been removed from the system (see Figure 8-5).

File Labels

The style and location of **file labels** are based on the filing system and must be used consistently. You must be careful to select the correct label for the file folder and to index it according to the selected method. Labels can be typed or computer generated.

Color Coding

The purpose of **color coding** in a filing system is to provide visual identification. Charts are marked with color tabs. If the charts are filed properly, a uniform pattern will be visible. When a chart is filed incorrectly, the colored pattern will be broken, alerting you of the error. Typically, a color coding system uses a different color for the first 13 letters of the alphabet and then repeats the color with a mark, such as a wide band, for the second half of the alphabet. Systems may use from one to three colors per file. Color coding can be used in vertical and lateral systems, but it is more effective when used within a lateral filing system.

Aging Labels

The use of **aging labels** allows for quick and easy visual identification of when a patient was last seen in the dental practice. This type of identification allows the transfer of charts from active to inactive files. A label is put on a new patient's chart to indicate the year the patient was first seen. The next year that the patient is seen, a new label is placed over the old. At designated intervals, charts are removed from the active files and are placed in the inactive files. Time lapse varies from practice to practice.

Aging labels can also be used to track patient treatments. When a treatment is completed, the chart is flagged with the appropriately colored label. If a patient does not complete a treatment, the chart can be easily identified and the proper steps can be taken to reschedule the patient. By adding a month label, the chart can be flagged for recall. The use of colored labels can also distinguish the primary dentist and the type of insurance. The most important element of a successful coding system is that it is kept simple. Every member of the dental health-care team should be able to use the system.

PREPARING THE CLINICAL RECORD

When a patient visits the office for the first time, the administrative dental assistant, in addition to collecting the correct data each time a patient visits the

ANATOMY OF AN INDEXED FILE FOLDER

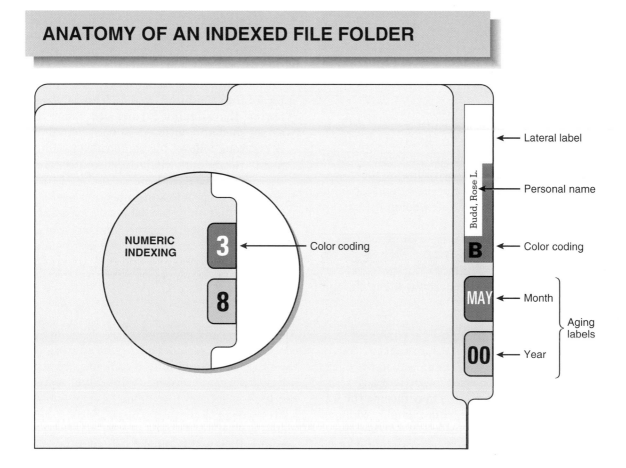

office, is responsible for placing all forms in a file folder and correctly labeling the folder.

General Guidelines

1. Check each form for the necessary information.
2. Make sure each form within the clinical record can be identified by the patient's name or account number. This provides a way of identifying forms if they should become separated from the folder.
3. Fasten forms in the correct order.

Preparing the Label

1. Determine the indexing method to be used (i.e., alphabetic or numeric).
2. Type the name or number on a label. (Become familiar with the different rules of indexing. It is very important to follow the same rules and to be concise in their application.)
3. Place the label on the file folder.

Coding the File Folder

1. Place corresponding color tabs according to the guidelines of the selected color coding system.
2. Place other coding labels according to preset guidelines (e.g., aging, year, month).

Cross-Referencing (Numeric Indexing)

Record the patient's name and chart number on your cross-reference list.

A computer system can aid in the preparation of file folders by printing labels according to the guidelines of the indexing system, assigning account numbers, and creating cross-referencing lists.

PREPARING BUSINESS DOCUMENTS

Business documents are prepared for filing through the following steps.

Inspecting

Check the document and make sure that it is ready to file. You will need to develop a method by which you can indicate that the document is ready to be placed in the filing system. This may include the initials of the dentist or other team member who has been working with the document, a simple checkmark, or a stamp.

Indexing

Once the document has been released for filing, the next step is to determine where the document should be filed and what method of indexing is required. A file folder will have to be prepared for a document that is to be filed for the first time (see Figures 8-1 and 8-2).

Coding

If you are using a subject method of filing, you may want to write the subject in the upper right-hand corner of the document. If the subject appears in the heading of the document, you can simply underline or highlight it. Subheadings can also be identified and coded.

Filing Procedures

Filing is more than putting away documents. You must follow the steps below to ensure that files are *concise, consistent,* and *convenient.*

- The first step is to be *concise* when preparing clinical records for filing. This includes labeling the clinical record according to the indexing rules for the selected method of filing.
- The second step is to be *consistent* in placing the record into the filing system. This is done by following the simplified rules for filing that are established and outlined for each dental practice. If everyone follows the same rules in filing documents, documents will be consistently returned to the same place each time.
- The third step is to store files in *convenient* locations so that they can be easily accessed. When files are indexed concisely and are consistently placed in the correct order in a convenient place, documents are easy to find and are safeguarded against loss or damage.

Sorting

After records and documents have been indexed and coded, they are sorted. During the **sorting** phase of the process, records and documents are separated into categories according to the filing method and the location of the files. This is a systematic step that will save time during filing. Records and documents are separated and placed in the same order in which they will be filed.

Sorting speeds up the filing process because you will not have to move back and forth from one end of the filing system to the other, opening and closing file drawers. Instead, you will work in order from one end of the system to the other, saving time and steps. Many accessories, such as a basket with file guides, can aid you in the sorting process. The key is to select a method that works well for you.

Putting Records and Documents into Their Final Place

The final step in the filing process is putting away records. Most people dread this process because they find it time consuming, boring, and unfulfilling. If you approach this part of filing with a positive attitude and are well organized, you will move quickly through the task.

How to Safeguard Records

Clinical, business, and tax records, as previously stated, are important elements of the dental practice. If they are lost, damaged, or poorly maintained, they can serve no useful purpose. It is your responsibility to safeguard each and every document and to maintain the integrity of the contents.

HIPAA

The HIPAA Privacy Rule covers the protection of all PHI in paper form, and the HIPAA Security Rule applies to all electronic protected health information (ePHI).

Know where records are at all times. Records should never be removed from the office. Copies of records can be made when the information is needed for work outside the office.

Records should be returned to the file cabinet at the end of each day. The chance of losing or destroying them is reduced when records are kept in the file cabinet. Vertical files offer some protection from fire and water damage if files are tightly compressed and drawers are locked. Those lateral files that are in cabinets provide the best protection; drawers should be closed and locked. Ledger cards and other file cards that are usually set out during the day should be placed at night in a file drawer for storage and protection.

A computerized system should be backed up on a regular basis and the backup files stored off site. It is costly, time consuming, and almost impossible to recapture information that is lost in a computer system.

HIPAA

Security Rule

• Ensure the integrity and confidentiality of ePHI.
• Protect against any reasonable anticipated threats or hazards to the security or integrity of the ePHI.
• Protect against unauthorized uses or disclosures of the ePHI.

Retention and Transfer of Records

The quantity of records in storage can become large and cumbersome. A policy must be established for the systematic removal of records. Most records must be retained for a particular length of time; however, inactive records do not have to be stored in active files. Active files should be located to provide easy access for business office staff. When files become inactive, they should be moved to a less convenient area, such as the bottom filing drawers or a cabinet located away from the business office.

Retention

Which records must be retained and for how long vary from state to state, according to the type of record. **Retention** of patient records also depends on the extent of treatment, whether radiographs have been taken, and regulations established by third party insurance carriers. It is advisable to keep records of patients who have received extensive dental treatment and to retain full mouth radiographic surveys indefinitely because of their significance in forensic dentistry.

Federal regulations and state statutes of limitations determine the retention of business records. Each state establishes periods during which records can be used in legal proceedings; this is referred to as the *statute of limitations*. After the statute of limitations expires, records can no longer be used in legal matters. Records that fall into this category are contracts, open accounts, and accident reports.

The federal government has assembled a set of regulations that determine the length of time records that deal with federal issues must be kept. These records include payroll reports, tax reports, receipts and bank statements, and other documentation used in the preparation of reports.

It is the responsibility of the administrative dental assistant to become familiar with regulations and statutes that govern the place of employment. Before you destroy any files, you should seek the advice of an accountant or an attorney. You should destroy records and files only under the direct order of your employer. Once files have been released for destruction, care should be taken to destroy them appropriately. Services are available that destroy records, or you can do so by yourself. A cross-reference list should be kept to denote the types of documents being destroyed, the time period that the documents represented, and the method used for destruction. It is essential that records be destroyed appropriately, so that they can never be used for fraud.

Transfer Methods

A filing system works best when the storage area is accessible and the files are not overcrowded. Therefore, this space should be used only for active files. To provide space for active files, a routine must be developed for the systematic removal of inactive files. Two types of **transfer methods** have been developed for the systematic removal of inactive files.

The **perpetual method** uses a system that identifies files and records that have been inactive for a predetermined length of time or that are no longer required for quick reference. As soon as a file or record reaches this interval, it is removed from the active filing system and placed in the inactive filing system. For example, if you are using aging labels, you will be able to visually identify records that are ready to be removed from the active filing system. You have predetermined that all charts will be placed in the inactive file if a patient has not been seen in the practice for a period of 3 years. Monthly, you quickly scan the files and pull all charts of patients who have not been seen for the past 3 years. This method will ensure that you do not overcrowd

your filing space. Computer systems can also generate monthly reports that list all records that should be removed from the active file.

The **periodic method** works well for business records. At a determined time, usually the end of the year, all files are transferred to the inactive file, and the same types of files in the inactive file are transferred to storage boxes. For example, all financial reports, payroll records, and other monthly reports are transferred to the inactive file to make room for the new year's reports and records. The previous year's reports are removed from the inactive file and boxed for storage. Boxes that go into storage can be marked with the year that they can be legally destroyed. When new boxes go into storage, old boxes marked for destruction can be removed and destroyed. Once again, a well-organized cross-referencing system is needed to track boxes and their content.

Active and inactive files must be kept in the dental practice for easy access. The chance that records will need to be accessed drops significantly with the passing of each year, but they still must be retained. Storage of countless boxes of files becomes expensive and serves no useful purpose unless they are properly cross-referenced. A solution to this problem is imaging.

This process places images of the contents of files and records on storage disks, microfilm, or magnetic tape. Scanners and other imaging equipment transfer images via computer to storage disks. Microfilming takes pictures of documents and reduces the size of the image, resulting in the ability to store several hundred documents on a reel of film. Disks, tapes, and reels, which have the capability to hold thousands of records, take up a fraction of the space that is required to store the original records. When an imaging system is used, it also cross-references the contents, which makes it possible to search documents quickly and easily, even 30 years later. Storage of original documents and radiographs may or may not be necessary, depending on the type of document. Each dental practice must establish a protocol that describes its policies on document storage.

KEY POINTS

The purposes of developing a systematic approach to filing are to simplify the retrieval process and to ensure the precise locations of documents. Guaranteeing integrity and safeguarding all documents are primarily the responsibilities of the administrative dental assistant.

Within the dental practice, more than one type of filing system may be used. The filing system will be determined by the type of information that must be filed. Information can be divided into two broad categories: (1) business documents and patient-related documents, and (2) clinical records and patient insurance forms. The five basic filing methods are as follows:

- Alphabetic
- Geographic
- Numeric
- Subject
- Chronological

Personal names and business or organizational names are indexed according to ARMA Simplified Filing Standard Rules. The arrangement of a name, subject, or number is referred to as indexing. Names are broken down into units; a group of units is a segment. When filing documents with properly indexed names, follow these basic rules:

- The first letter that is different in any unit determines the alphabetic order.
- Single names are filed before the same name followed by an initial or name.
- Initials are filed before the name spelled out.
- Abbreviations are filed as if they were spelled out.
- Nicknames are treated as first names.
- Business and organizational names are filed as written.

Effective storage of information is achieved by matching the type of document with the correct file folder and placing it within the filing unit. Documents can be stored in vertical files, which have one to five drawers. Vertical files require the use of file folders with tabs located at the top. Lateral file units make up a shelving system that uses side tab folders. The lateral unit is popular for the storage of clinical records because several different coding methods can be applied.

Documents must be stored for a specified length of time, depending on the type of document and the legal requirements. A policy must be developed that systematically identifies documents that should be moved from the active to the inactive files.

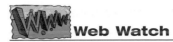 **Web Watch**

American Health Information Management Association

http://www.ahima.org

 Log on to Evolve to access additional web links!

Critical Thinking Questions

1. Apply what you have learned in this chapter to create a filing system for the following business documents. Describe how you would arrange the documents, and identify the method you would use. Write file labels, and arrange them in the correct sequence for the chosen method.

   Monthly bank statements from ABC National Bank (January to December 2000)

   Quarterly bank statements from RBB from the same period (January to December 2000)

   Monthly business reports; practice production reports, practice collection reports, hygiene production reports, associate dentist's production reports, primary dentist's production reports

2. Correctly index the following names and write them as you would on a filing label. Arrange the indexed names in alphabetical order:
   - W.P. Hazelton
   - Victor J. Carlucci, Jr.
   - Sung Kim
   - Robert James McCarty
   - R. Davison
   - Mary Anne Lucchesi
   - Mark Sandwell
   - Liz Famillian
   - James Lloyd
   - Damian Carmona
   - Brook M. Calloway
   - Ben DeFrank

3. Using the above names, develop a numbering system:
   - Assign each patient a different six-digit number.
   - Index the numbers (each number is a different unit).
   - Create a cross-reference list.
   - Place the numbers in sequence.

OUTLINE

Introduction

Mechanics of Scheduling

- Selecting the Appointment Book (manual and electronic)
- The Art of Scheduling
- Scenarios for Scheduling
- Results of Poor Scheduling

Making Appointments

Time-Saving Techniques

- Develop Call Lists
- Maintain Daily Schedule Sheets
- Establish a Daily Routine

KEY TERMS AND CONCEPTS

Appointment Book
Appointment Cards
Art of Scheduling
Bookmarks
Call Lists
Columns
Daily Schedule Sheets
Electronic Scheduler
Hardbound Books
Loose Leaf Appointment Books
Matrixing
Mechanics of Scheduling
Month Tab
Predated Appointment Pages
Productivity
Undated Appointment Pages
Units
Week at a Glance
Wirebound Appointment Books

9

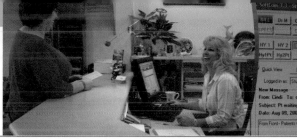
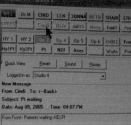

Dental Patient Scheduling

LEARNING OBJECTIVES

The student will:

1. Describe the mechanics of scheduling.
2. Identify criteria required for matrixing an appointment book. Apply the criteria selected, and properly matrix an appointment book.
3. Discuss different methods used to identify when specific procedures should be scheduled.
4. List the criteria for making an appointment book entry.
5. Discuss the seven different scenarios of appointment scheduling, and formulate an action plan to solve the problems presented.
6. List the steps to be followed in making an appointment.
7. Fill out an appointment card and a daily schedule.
8. Describe the use of a call list.
9. List the steps to be followed in performing the daily routine associated with the appointment schedule.

INTRODUCTION

Developing and implementing an organized, functional schedule for a dental practice requires time, experience, and the cooperation of the entire dental healthcare team. The process of scheduling appointments involves more than entering names in a book or keying into a computer. Scheduling is a complex process that has two main elements. The first is the **mechanics of scheduling,** which includes selecting the appointment book (manual or electronic), outlining or **matrixing,** and entering information.

The second is the **"art" of scheduling.** The first step in the art of scheduling is to work with the dental healthcare team and answer a few questions. These questions (such as how much time is required to complete a procedure [i.e., total time from patient to patient]) help identify when the dental healthcare team is the most productive. The second step is to develop a process for monitoring and adjusting the schedule to meet the goals set by the dental healthcare team.

Scheduling can be done by anyone, but effective scheduling is a skill that must be developed. Traditionally, scheduling was assigned to a single individual with little input from other members of the staff. In today's dental practice, the mechanics and the art of scheduling should be combined for efficient scheduling, which takes into consideration the needs of both the patient and the dental healthcare team.

MECHANICS OF SCHEDULING

Selecting the Appointment Book (manual and electronic)

The **appointment book** in today's dental practices can be either manual or electronic and is a tool that, when used efficiently, helps organize the daily schedule of the dental practice. The book identifies who will be performing which tasks, on what date, and at what time. The book outlines which treatment rooms are available and at what times. It identifies who is going to be seen, the treatment that will be performed, and the amount of time required to complete the treatment.

The size of the manual book is determined by the style and the function that it will serve. Appoint-

HIPPA

Privacy Rule: Protect the Confidentiality of Patient Treatment

Appointment books contain protected health information (PHI) and must be kept out of sight. Ensure that an open appointment book or computer screen cannot be seen by patients when you are scheduling appointments.

ment books come in several different styles. The most common style is the **week at a glance.** When the book is open, this style allows the assistant to view the full week, Monday through Saturday. When fully opened, books range in size from $9 \times 22^{7}/_{8}$ inches to as large as $11 \times 35^{1}/_{4}$ inches. When selecting a style, you must consider the number of practitioners you are scheduling for and the amount of desk space that is available for the opened book. In a large practice with several practitioners, it may be necessary to have an individual book for each practitioner.

REMEMBER

Appointment books are considered legal documents and can be a valuable tool in the defense of alleged malpractice; therefore, they must be kept in storage for the prescribed length of time.

Binding

In addition to the size of the book, the type of binding must be considered. Bindings are routinely available in three styles: hardbound, loose leaf, and wirebound.

Hardbound books should be used only in very small practices. Because they do not hold up well when opened frequently, their use should be limited.

Loose leaf appointment books offer several advantages. Pages can be removed and placed in permanent storage as they are filled, providing for a less bulky appointment book. It is easy to insert new pages as needed, and at the end of the year, pages for the new year can be added to provide for a smooth transition from year to year.

Wirebound appointment books provide flexibility in the space they need. When opened, they lie flat, which makes it easier to make entries near the binding. When more desk space is needed, they can be folded back on themselves to provide extra space. They store easily, and their use avoids the loss or removal of pages.

Columns

Pages of the appointment book are divided into **columns.** The function of the column is to organize the schedule and identify who is performing the treatment, who the patient is, why the patient is being seen, and what will be done. Columns can be assigned to an individual practitioner or treatment room or can be used to record additional information about the patient. The number and size of the columns in an appointment book depend on the style selected by the dental practice—for example, Canyon View Dental Associates employs two dentists, Dr. Edwards and Dr. Bradley, and two dental hygienists, Vivian and Diane. These employees work at different times. Because more than two practitioners are never in the office at one time, the practice can use a two-column appointment book. If the practice expands its hours or wants to include more information in the appointment book, a new appointment book style with additional columns would be needed.

Another way to schedule is to assign each treatment room a column in the appointment book. This means that the number of columns would equal the number of treatment rooms. (This form of scheduling requires advanced techniques and should not be attempted without a full understanding of the principles.)

Units

Each column is divided into time segments. Each segment represents a unit (**units** are either 10- or 15-minute intervals).

There are *four units per hour* when scheduling 15-minute intervals (Figure 9-1) and *six units per hour* when scheduling 10-minute intervals (Figure 9-2). The dental healthcare team will usually refer to the number of units needed for a procedure instead of the amount of time. For example, three units may be requested for a procedure. If a 15-minute unit is being used, a 45-minute block of time is needed to complete the procedure (30 minutes for a 10-minute unit). Consistency is very important; everyone needs to speak the same language.

Food for Thought

The dentist has just told you that he needs four units to complete a procedure. Is that 1 hour or 40 minutes?

Additional Appointment Book Features

The color of the appointment book can be selected to coordinate with the office decor. If more than one appointment book is used, the colors of the covers can be used to distinguish one book from another at a quick glance.

Bookmarks, colored tabs, and other accessories are easy ways to divide the appointment book according to month or week. For example, a **month tab** makes it easy to turn to a given month. This is especially handy when you are scheduling a few months in advance. **Bookmarks** are used to identify the current week so it can be turned to quickly.

Appointment books and pages for appointment books can be ordered with or without dates. **Pre-dated appointment book pages** are convenient and are used when schedules stay consistent. **Undated appointment book pages** are used when flexibility is needed. For example, flexibility is needed when a practitioner works only a few days a week at a given location. With undated pages, the administrative dental assistant can customize the design of the appointment book. Loose leaf appointment books accommodate undated pages well because they can be added easily.

Codes can be customized to fit the needs of any dental practice, but they are useful only if they are understood by each member of the dental healthcare team. Be careful not to use too many codes or other information that may clutter the entry and make it very difficult to read.

REMEMBER

Identify the patient and the procedure, and indicate the time the patient will be in the dental treatment room. When listing additional information, carefully use the space provided to ensure that the entry remains legible and easy to read.

ANATOMY OF AN APPOINTMENT BOOK PAGE

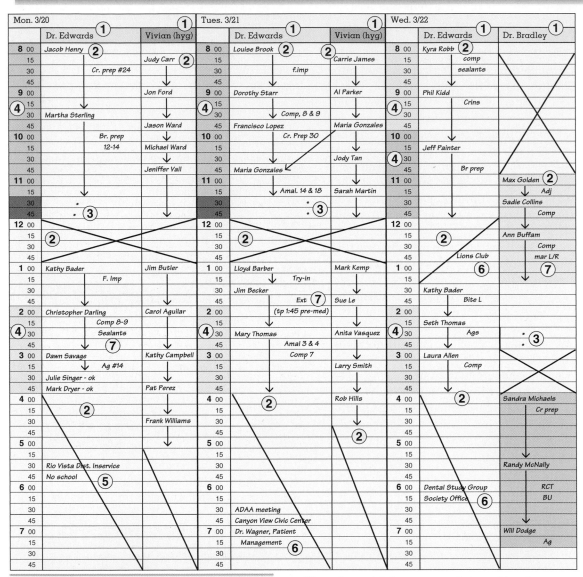

Appointment Book Matrix

Once the style of the appointment book is selected, the next step in the organization of the appointment book is to custom configure the pages. This is referred to as the **appointment book matrix**. The purpose of the matrix is to configure or outline the pages. Electronic schedulers are matrixed during the initial computer set-up function. The program will customize the appointment book following the specifications of the dental practice. (See Fig. 9-2)

Steps in matrixing an appointment book

1 Assign each practitioner a column for the day and clearly identify. If you are scheduling by treatment room, identify the treatment room assigned to each column.

2 Mark the columns so it can be easily determined by anyone looking at the appointment book what time the first procedure begins, when lunch or dinner will be scheduled, and when the last procedure ends.

③ During the course of the day it may be necessary to schedule emergency patients. The appointment book can be matrixed to identify a specific block of time each day in anticipation of an emergency. Dovetailing is another method used for short appointments and emergencies. For example, the dentist will need to wait 10 to 20 minutes after giving anesthetic before proceeding with the procedure, allowing time to check another patient.

④ With careful planning and attention to detail, the appointment book can be matrixed to identify when and where specific procedures should be scheduled. Colored highlighters, small colored sticky notes or colored book tabs (sticky notes and book tabs can be reused) will help identify blocks of time and procedures to be scheduled. When using a computerized scheduler, this type of function can be programmed into the system.

⑤ Identify when the local schools are on break or have days off. This is useful because teachers and children will be available for appointments without missing school.

⑥ Information other than patient appointments can be placed in the appointment book, which will help organize the function of the office. Items included are: professional meetings for the dentist and auxiliary, such as dental society meetings, dental assistant and dental hygienist society meetings; study clubs and continuing education courses; vacations; and important deadline dates, such as quarterly taxes, payroll deposits, or other dates important to the dental office.

⑦ When making entries in the appointment book, care should be taken to write legibly and in pencil. Entries include the patient's name (both the first and last name), the amount of time needed for the procedure (indicated by an arrow), and a code for the procedure. It may also be advisable to include a telephone number for confirmation (especially for a new patient), a code to indicate if lab work is needed for the procedure, and if the lab work has returned from the lab. It may be necessary to indicate if the patient requires premedication, or any other information that is vital to the case.

Some common codes are:

- C – appointment needs confirmation
- ₵ – confirmed
- cr – crown
- ag – amalgam
- comp – composite
- ext – extraction
- prophy – prophylaxis
- RP – root planing
- rc – root canal (rct)
- fl – fluoride treatment
- p.o. – post operative appointment
- br – bridge
- prep – preparation (crown, bridge, inlay, or onlay)
- ins – insertion (placement of crown, bridge, inlay, or onlay)
- tp – told patient
- L – lab work
- ○ – lab work returned from the lab

The **electronic scheduler** or computerized system incorporates many of the same features as those described above for the manual appointment book. During the system set-up, a series of questions will be asked that are designed to customize the scheduler to the individual practice, including the number of practitioners or treatment rooms, time blocks for specific procedures, operating hours of the dental practice, days of the week, and production goals. Once the system is programmed, it may operate in a number of modes, such as manual selection, wherein the assistant selects the appointment day and time, and automatic mode, in which the assistant enters the procedures and the computer selects the day and time for the appointment. In addition, the electronic scheduler will track missed appointments, provide up-to-date call lists at a push of a key, and search the database for incomplete treatment plans and unscheduled recalls. The primary difference between the manual appointment book and the electronic scheduler is the method in which data are entered and the ability with the electronic scheduler to do a variety of specialized tasks quickly and efficiently (see Chapter 17 for additional information).

The Art of Scheduling

The art of scheduling is important when the rules are established and maintained. The key to the art of scheduling is to determine when the dental healthcare team is the most productive and how, through effective scheduling, the goals and philosophy of the dental practice can be met. This is not a simple one-step procedure. It takes time and the cooperation of all members of the team. The process is ongoing, allowing for adjustments when needed to meet the goals of the dental practice.

Productivity

Productivity in dentistry is a complex concept. There are two types of **productivity.** The first is determined by the amount of dental treatment that is completed, and the second is determined by the amount of money collected. The amount of treatment that is provided can be increased by efficient scheduling, and the amount of money collected can be increased by effective collection methods. Maintaining efficiency in both areas is a function of the administrative assistant. In this chapter, ways to

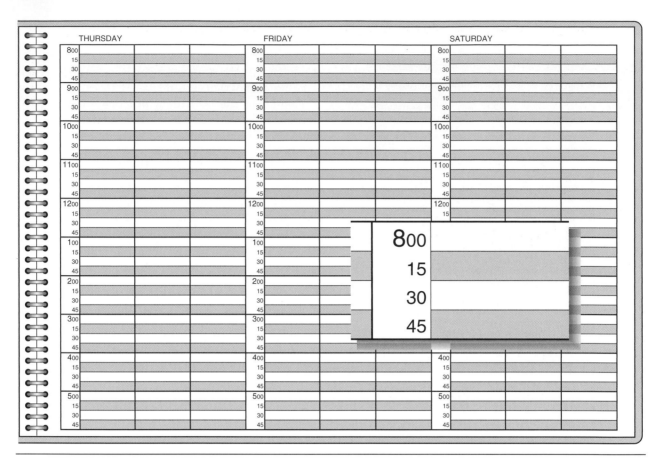

FIGURE 9-1

Appointment book, 15-minute units. (Courtesy of Colwell, a Division of Patterson Dental Companies, Champaign, IL.)

increase productivity through efficient scheduling are discussed. (See Chapter 13 for a discussion of collection productivity.)

The answers to four key questions will help you maximize scheduling efficiency:

1. *At what time of day does the dental healthcare team work smarter and faster?* This can be determined by selecting the time of day that the dentist performs best. Some dentists are "morning people." They wake up early and are eager to start work. Because this type of person is most productive in the early morning, difficult and challenging work should be scheduled then. The dentist will be able to remain focused on the task and will complete the procedure without becoming overly stressed or fatigued. As the day

passes and the dentist's ability to remain focused decreases, the type of procedure scheduled should be changed. This is an appropriate time for shorter appointments and less challenging work. For the dentist who wakes up later and is less focused in the mornings (also known as the "I don't do mornings" person), schedule the easier tasks first. Increase the difficulty of the procedure according to the dentist's internal clock to enhance productivity and reduce stress. Synchronization of work schedules with team members' internal work clocks will help increase productivity and meet the needs of patients.

2. *How much time is needed to complete a procedure?* This question is not easy to answer. Theoretically, the same procedure should consistently

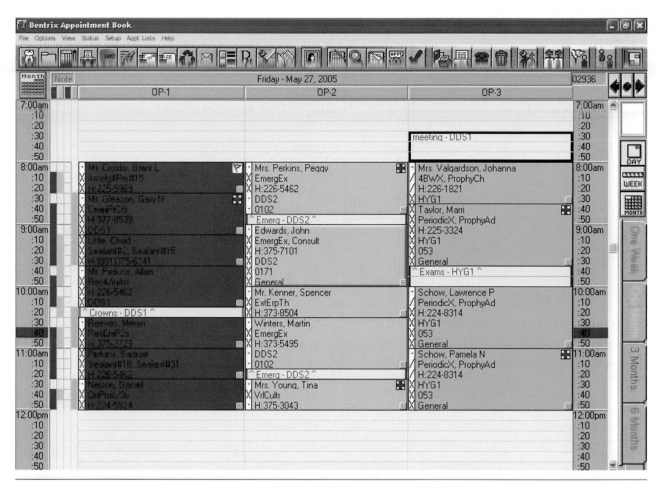

FIGURE 9-2

Electronic appointment book, 10-minute units. (Courtesy Dentrix Dental Systems, American Fork, UT.)

take the same amount of time. All patients are different, however, and what takes 3 units of time for one patient may take 4 units for another. To determine procedure times, you must average the times over several different patients. Once the average procedure time is determined, a list can be made to identify the amounts of time to allot for specific treatments. This process requires constant monitoring and adjusting. In addition to the amount of time it takes to complete the procedure, the amount of time it takes to properly clean and ready the room for the next patient must be considered. This time varies by procedure (minimum, 10 minutes). More complex procedures require longer clean-up times to ensure that proper infection control protocol is followed.

3. *Which procedures may require the assistance of an extended function dental assistant?* Depending on the duties dental assistants are allowed to perform (these are outlined in the Dental Practice Act of each state), the assistance of an extended function dental assistant may be needed. When extended function dental assistants are used, the amounts of time they will spend with patients must be considered when procedures in which they will assist are scheduled. For example, for a procedure that requires 4 units of chair time, the dentist may spend 3 units with the patient and the assistant may spend 1 unit. The dentist is then available for 1 unit with another patient. (This unit would be a good time for procedures such as examinations,

postoperative check-ups, and appointment adjustments.)

4. *Who will do the scheduling?* The scheduling process requires the cooperation of the entire dental healthcare team through constant monitoring and adjustment of procedural times. The physical entering of information into the appointment book can be assigned to one or two persons. It will be their responsibility to matrix the appointment book and to schedule as efficiently as possible according to the guidelines developed by the dental healthcare team. When more than one person schedules appointments, it may be better to use an electronic scheduler. More advanced software programs can matrix the electronic scheduler and outline the times of day when certain procedures should be performed (discussed in Chapter 17).

Scenarios for Scheduling

Scheduling would be easy if every patient and every procedure could be treated in exactly the same way, but this is not the case. Dental healthcare teams are continually faced with complex problems that require well-established guidelines that are also flexible. The scheduler must maintain control of the appointment book and must be creative in meeting the needs of both the dental healthcare team and the patient. At times, it is very difficult to accommodate everyone.

Scenario One: The Emergency Patient

Dorothy Star calls the office and informs you that she has a "pounding toothache" and has to see the dentist today.

With the help of a telephone information form, questions can be asked to determine where the pain is located, how long the pain has been present, if there is swelling, and whether there are other symptoms that will help determine if the patient must be seen "today." If the appointment book has been matrixed to allow for emergency patients, the patient can be informed of the appointment time. It is advisable to tell emergency patients that the dentist can see them for the immediate problem and relieve the discomfort. If more extensive work is needed, another appointment must be made.

If emergency time has not been worked into the daily schedule, a time will need to be selected. Find

a scheduled procedure that will allow the dentist to leave this patient momentarily to attend to the emergency patient without interfering with the amount of time scheduled for the first patient (this type of scheduling requires experience).

REMEMBER

"Dentists shall be obliged to make reasonable arrangements for the emergency care of their patients of record."—ADA Principles of Ethics and Code of Professional Conduct, January 2005, Chicago, IL.

Sometimes, patients cannot come in during a period when you can work them in. If these patients can wait, they can be scheduled for another day. The dental healthcare team, however, may have to be flexible and schedule the patient at a different time, such as during someone's lunch hour or at the end of the day. This type of scheduling should be avoided and done only after all other options have been explored. (Caution: Other patients should not be inconvenienced because of the poor planning or lack of flexibility of another patient. You may help one patient but lose others in the process.)

Scenario Two: The "Afternoon Only" Patient

Francisco Lopez must have extensive dental work performed, and he is concerned about the amount of time he will lose from work. Mr. Lopez is a production manager and is in charge of the production line from 8:00 AM to 12 NOON. He expresses an interest in scheduling his appointments in the afternoon.

A treatment plan must be prepared for each patient, and the steps in the treatment must be prioritized (see Chapter 7, Priority List). When scheduling appointments, the assistant can clearly identify from the priority list the order in which treatment steps must be performed and can determine the types of procedures that have to be scheduled.

The assistant can explain to the patient that the more extensive work, the crown and bridge, must be scheduled in the morning because this is when the dentist performs more extensive procedures. The less extensive work can be scheduled in the afternoon. By explaining the scheduling process to the patient and showing a willingness to divide the work so that part of it can be completed in the afternoon, the assistant demonstrates concern for the patient while maintaining control of the appointment book.

Scenario Three: The Chronically Late Patient

Julie Singer is a very busy professional woman. If you schedule her for a 2:00 PM appointment, she will rush into the office at 2:08.

Several factors enter into scheduling chronically late patients. First, the patient who is late even by as short a time as 8 minutes can and will affect the schedule. Second, patients who rush have racing pulses. Their higher-than-normal blood pressures may cause other problems if they are given local anesthetic before their vital signs return to normal.

The one thing that you can do with patients who you know will be late is to schedule them 15 minutes early for their appointment. Inform the patient who is scheduled to see the dentist at 2:00 that the appointment is at 1:45. This will allow time for the patient to arrive late and rest before he or she is seen by the dentist.

REMEMBER

This technique can backfire if patients discover you are scheduling them early. The entire dental healthcare team must know when you have done this in case a patient should call and ask the time of the appointment. Place a notation in the appointment book that clearly identifies the time the patient was told ("tp 1:45" to indicate "told patient 1:45").

When patients are always late for their appointments, dental healthcare team members should ask themselves why. In some cases, the dental office is the cause for late arrivals. Patients who consistently must wait to be seen by the dentist may develop the attitude that it does not make any difference if they arrive late; after all, they always wait for the dentist. It is very important to set the example. If we expect our patients to be on time, then we must be on time for them. Occasions will arise when it is impossible to see a patient within 10 minutes of arrival. When this occurs, the patient should be informed of the delay and given an approximate time that the dentist will be available. It may be necessary to give the patient the option of rescheduling the appointment.

Scenario Four: The Canceled Appointment

Al Parker often cancels his appointment at the last minute because he cannot leave work.

When patients cancel appointments often, look beyond the reasons they give. Fear is frequently the reason appointments are canceled. When this occurs, steps can be taken to relieve the fear through an established patient management protocol. These steps should be outlined by the dentist and may include premedication to relieve anxiety. Other reasons for cancellation include inability to pay for the visit, a lack of understanding of the importance of keeping appointments, and a lack of understanding of the consequences that may occur when prescribed dental treatments are not received. Once the reasons for constant cancellations have been determined, steps can be taken to help patients keep their appointments.

REMEMBER

For legal reasons, document all missed, broken, and rescheduled appointments.

Scenario Five: The Student Who Cannot Miss School

Kyra Robb is a student, and her mother wants her scheduled for appointments after 3:00 in the afternoon.

Most patients, if given a choice, would schedule their appointments when it is the most convenient for them. Peak appointment times usually occur in the later afternoon, early evening, and holidays when the dental office is open. Controlling these time slots is difficult.

REMEMBER

The dental assistant must maintain control of the appointment book while meeting the needs of patients. Peak time slots should be given only to those who cannot possibly come at any other time. If the appointment book has been matrixed, it is essential that the types of procedures scheduled in particular time slots are the types that the slots are designed for. Again, when patients understand the reasons why they need to be scheduled at less than ideal times (because it is in their best interest), they are usually willing to compromise.

Historically, dental practices have scheduled patients between the hours of 8:00 AM and 5:00 PM. In today's society, many patients are unwilling to change their schedules to meet the needs of dental practices. In addition, the number of dental practices is increasing. The need to attract and keep patients has resulted in the establishment of extended hours. It is not uncommon to find dental practices that are open evenings and weekends to meet the needs of dental patients.

Scenario Six: The Patient Who Arrives on the Wrong Day

Jeff Painter arrives for his appointment. When you check the schedule, you discover that he is due on Wednesday at 10:00 AM, not on Tuesday.

It is always a delicate situation when a patient arrives on the wrong day or at the wrong time; this must be treated with tact and diplomacy (no matter who is at fault). First, inform unexpected patients that you have them on the schedule at a different time and ask if they have their appointment card with them. (It is crucial to give all patients an appointment card.) Check the appointment card and determine who is at fault. If it is the patient, politely point out the error and offer your condolences. If it is a short procedure that you can work into the schedule without inconveniencing other patients, offer to do so. If the error was made by a member of the dental healthcare team, again, offer your condolences and try to work the patient into the schedule. (Flexibility in the schedule may be needed at this time.)

Scenario Seven: Unscheduled Appointments

Mrs. Sarah Martin is an older patient with lots of free time. She will drop by the dental office wishing to see the dentist for a "quick appointment" to adjust her partial. It is very difficult to say no to Mrs. Martin.

Patients who drop in and request service can create a very difficult situation. If they have a true emergency and cannot wait until another time, they will have to be accommodated. It works best if you agree to have the dentist see them and tell them when the dentist will be available for an emergency situation and explain that they will have to wait until that time.

Patients who can very easily be seen on a different day must be informed that it is not office policy to see drop-in patients for nonemergency appointments because it takes away from the patients who are scheduled, and that it is the dentist's philosophy to give all patients full attention during treatment. This is a very delicate situation and must be explained to the patient without causing an angry reaction.

In addition to unscheduled patients, unscheduled procedures can cause problems. For example, a patient who is scheduled for a recall appointment is discovered to need a couple of simple restorations. Instead of having the patient return another day, the dentist may wish to squeeze the patient into the schedule. This technique works only if the dentist has enough time to properly attend to the patient. This practice generally does more harm than good. The only person who appreciates this addition to the schedule is the patient. The dental healthcare team will be stressed by the added procedure, and other patients will be inconvenienced by having to wait.

During the day, the dentist's schedule can be interrupted for a variety of reasons, for example, by telephone calls, visits from sales representatives, and friends who "just stop by." All of these situations, if not controlled, add stress to the day for the dental healthcare team and for patients. When interruptions get out of control, the situation must be addressed. Identify the problem, and work out a solution.

Other Patients Who Require Flexibility

Children. Schedule short appointments for children in the morning. Once children are comfortable and trust the dental healthcare team, the length of the appointment can be increased. Cranky children are not easy for the dentist to treat; try to schedule them when they are at their best.

Difficult patients. Any patient who requires extra time and energy is a difficult patient. Some patients question everything the dentist does, and thus, the dentist will need additional time to answer all of their questions. Some patients cannot sit still, some constantly complain, some are fearful and need extra reassurance, and some will not stop talking (even when their mouths are full of dental materials).

Results of Poor Scheduling

Problem: Patients have to wait longer than 10 minutes before they are seen by the dentist.

Results:

1. Patients will arrive late because they always have to wait for the dentist.
2. Patients are offended when the dentist does not consider their time valuable.
3. Patients feel the stress of the dental healthcare team.
4. Patients will look for another dentist who will respect their time and is less stressed.

Problem: There is not enough time to complete the scheduled treatment.

Results:

1. Patients begin to question the quality of the work the dentist is performing.
2. Patients have to make more trips to the dentist than needed because their treatment was not scheduled efficiently.
3. Care is not taken to provide quality work.
4. Members of the dental healthcare team become stressed and overworked.
5. Patients will look for another dentist who will provide quality care.
6. Members of the dental healthcare team will look for another employer who will respect their time and develop a true team spirit in the delivery of dental care.

REMEMBER

Effective scheduling is a powerful practice builder. Patients want service. When the schedule serves the needs of only a few, the system of scheduling must be reevaluated and adjusted.

MAKING APPOINTMENTS

Appointments are made in one of three ways: (1) The patient calls or is called for an appointment. (2) The patient is present in the dental office and needs follow-up work in the near future. (3) The patient preschedules an appointment at the conclusion of a recall appointment. Each of these situations requires a slightly different approach.

1. *Patient calls for an appointment.* With the use of the telephone information form, the assistant can quickly identify the nature of the patient's call and ask the necessary questions in a logical manner to determine what type of appointment should be scheduled and to record the necessary information for follow-up. Once the appointment has been made and recorded in the appointment book or electronic scheduler, the assistant should repeat the information and the time of the appointment: "Mrs. Thomas, I have scheduled you for an appointment on Tuesday, July 3rd, at 2:30 PM. You are scheduled with Dr. Edwards. At that time, she will be replacing your old restorations, and you can plan on spending about one and one-half hours with us. Are there any other questions I can answer for you? Thank you for calling, and we will see you on July 3rd." It is important to record all relevant information on the telephone information form, enter the name and procedure in the appointment book or electronic scheduler, and repeat the information back to the patient before the call is ended. It is easy to become distracted by another phone call or patient, and it is very embarrassing to have a patient show up for an appointment that was not entered into the appointment book.

2. *Patient schedules follow-up appointment.* The patient has completed treatment for the day and is checking out at the front desk. The assistant records all necessary information into the appointment book or electronic scheduler, completes the appointment card, and hands it to the patient. As the assistant then repeats the information (date, day of the week, time, and procedure), the patient reads the appointment card and confirms that the information is correct.

3. *Patient preschedules a routine check-up appointment at the conclusion of a recall appointment.* When patients schedule an appointment 4 to 6 months in advance of the date, you handle it the same way as the previous situations. You schedule the appointment, inform the patient, give him or her an appointment card, and verify that the information on the card is correct. In addition, you explain the recall

procedure and tell the patient that he or she will receive a card in the mail a few weeks before the appointment. You may want to remind the patient of the importance of keeping the appointment and notifying the dental office if there is a need to change it. This type of an appointment must be confirmed.

REMEMBER

Scheduling recall appointments in advance will require careful monitoring and special consideration. Caution: Do not fill the schedule to capacity 6 months out; you will not be able to accommodate new patients or reschedule appointments in a timely manner.

Appointment cards are written reminders to patients of their next appointment. The design and style of the card vary widely from practice to practice. The card is usually the size of a business card and is printed on medium-weight paper. Information that should be included on the card is shown in Figure 9-3.

In addition to the traditional appointment card, many innovative ideas have been developed to help patients remember their appointments. Appointment cards may have a sticky patch on the back so that patients can place them on a calendar. Refrigerator magnets are another popular form of appointment card. They come in many colors and styles, but

---

Canyon View Dental Associates
Mary A. Edwards, DDS
200-555-3467

M _____

has an appointment

_____
day   month   date   time

We have reserved this time for you. If you are unable to keep this appointment please call the office at least 24 hours in advance.

FIGURE 9-3
An appointment card.

---

the purpose is still the same: to remind patients of the day, date, and time of their appointment.

TIME-SAVING TECHNIQUES

Develop Call Lists

Call lists are an important tool with which you can keep the schedule full when there is a sudden appointment change. Patients who are in need of dental treatment and are willing to come in on short notice are placed on the list. Patients who have a flexible schedule can also be placed on the list. Another method for filling openings in the appointment schedule is to identify patients who are scheduled who may need extended treatment. Instead of doing just one quadrant of amalgams, it may be possible to do two. If this method is used, the administrative assistant will need to:

1. Identify those patients who may need additional treatment by placing a notation in the appointment book.
2. Notify patients in advance that the dentist will be able to complete additional procedures (saving them a future trip to the office), and obtain their approval.

Maintain Daily Schedule Sheets

Daily schedule sheets contain information transferred from the appointment book or electronic scheduler and are used in treatment rooms, doctors' private offices, laboratories, and other work areas. These sheets contain patients' names, scheduled procedures, and amounts of time needed. Any other reminders for the day may be included (Figure 9-4). If changes or additions to the schedule are made during the day, the assistant simply revises each schedule sheet.

HIPAA

Privacy Rule: Protect the Confidentiality of Patient Treatment

Schedule sheets contain PHI and must be kept out of sight.

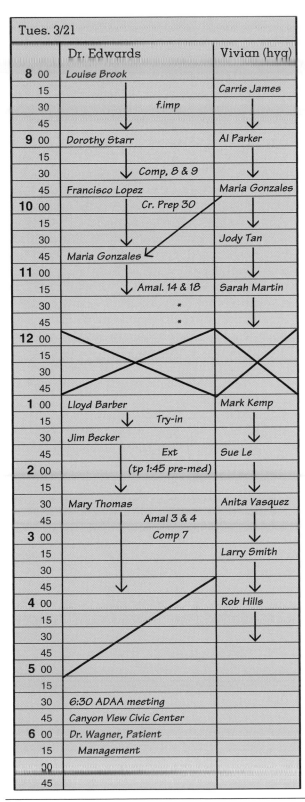

Tues. 3/21

	Dr. Edwards	Vivian (hyg)
8 00	Louise Brook	
15		Carrie James
30	f.imp	
45		
9 00	Dorothy Starr	Al Parker
15		
30	Comp, 8 & 9	
45	Francisco Lopez	Maria Gonzales
10 00	Cr. Prep 30	
15		
30		Jody Tan
45	Maria Gonzales	
11 00		
15	Amal. 14 & 18	Sarah Martin
30	*	
45	*	
12 00		
15		
30		
45		
1 00	Lloyd Barber	Mark Kemp
15	Try-in	
30	Jim Becker	
45	Ext	Sue Le
2 00	(tp 1:45 pre-med)	
15		
30	Mary Thomas	Anita Vasquez
45	Amal 3 & 4	
3 00	Comp 7	
15		Larry Smith
30		
45		
4 00		Rob Hills
15		
30		
45		
5 00		
15		
30	6:30 ADAA meeting	
45	Canyon View Civic Center	
6 00	Dr. Wagner, Patient	
15	Management	
30		
45		

FIGURE 9-4

A daily schedule.

Establish a Daily Routine

Develop a routine in accordance with the guidelines established by the dental healthcare team. Certain tasks should be completed every day.

1. Pull patients' clinical records and review procedures that are going to be completed the following day.
2. Check patients' charts for any information that may not have been included on the schedule, such as need for premedication, payments due, or updated insurance and medical information.
3. Confirm the return of laboratory work.
4. Confirm or remind patients of their upcoming appointments.
5. Use the call list to fill any openings in the day's schedule.
6. Type the daily schedule (or print it from the computer).
7. Give patients' clinical records to the dental assisting staff to review before they see the patients.
8. Spend 5 to 10 minutes with the dental healthcare team and review the daily schedule. Review vital information about procedures and patients to help provide quality care and relieve stress factors before patients begin to arrive. If this cannot be done first thing in the morning because of staggered schedules, plan a time to meet the day before, when the entire dental healthcare team is together.
9. Update schedules throughout the day as changes occur.
10. Keep the dental healthcare team and patients informed of any changes that will affect their schedules.

KEY POINTS

- The development and implementation of an organized, functional schedule for a dental practice requires time, experience, and the cooperation of the entire dental healthcare team. There are two components to scheduling: the "mechanics of scheduling" and the "art of scheduling."
- The mechanics of scheduling involves selecting the appointment book or electronic scheduler that is best tailored to the daily schedule of the dental practice, and then matrixing it properly. The book

identifies who will perform which tasks, on what date, and at what time. The book outlines which treatment rooms are available and at what times. It identifies patients who will be seen and what treatment will be performed, including the amount of time required to complete the treatment. The appointment book is divided into days, and each day is divided into time segments. Time segments are referred to as *units*. Either four units per hour (15-minute intervals) or six units per hour (10-minute intervals) are used when scheduling patients.

- The art of scheduling includes establishing the rules for scheduling. The objective of this process is to determine when the dental healthcare team is the most productive, and how, through effective scheduling, the dental healthcare team can meet the financial goals of the dental practice.

- Effective scheduling takes into consideration the best time of day to perform procedures and how to meet the needs of patients while maintaining control of the appointment book.

 Web Watch

Dentist Info—Cyber Mall

http://www.dentistinfo.com/fdentcyb.htm

    Log on to Evolve to access additional web links!

 Critical Thinking Questions

1. Consider the following scenario: You have just started working for Canyon View Dental Associates. The dental practice employs two dentists, Dr. Edwards and Dr. Bradley, as well as two dental hygienists, Vivian and Diane. Dr. Edwards works 2 days per week and Dr. Bradley 3 days per week. Dr. Edwards works from 8 AM to 5 PM (2 days per week). Dr. Bradley works from 11 AM to 7 PM (2 days per week) and on Saturdays from 8 AM to 2 PM. The hygienists also work 2 days per week. Diane works 1 day with Dr. Edwards, and Vivian works 1 day with Dr. Bradley. Both dentists take 1 hour for lunch unless they are attending luncheon meetings.

- Identify what further information is needed to matrix an appointment book. With the information given in the scenario and the information you add, matrix a week in an appointment book for Canyon View Dental Associates. Use workbook, or instructor will provide appointment sheets.

- Schedule the following patients (listed on your worksheet) during 1 week in your matrixed appointment book. The number of patients listed will not fill the week. You may wish to add additional patients to the schedule and identify which dentist and hygienist each patient will see. For further practice, add emergency patients, study clubs, staff meetings, luncheon meetings, and other appointments that will need special consideration in the schedule.

Patient	Treatment	Units of Time	Tooth No.	Special Instructions	Telephone No.
Carol Aguilar	Recall	3		Hygienist	503-555-3376
Christopher Darling	Composite sealants	4	8 & 9 max and mand	After school	503-555-3256
Dawn Savage	AMAL	2	14		503-555-9987
Dorothy Starr	Comp	3	7, 8, & 9	Pre-medication	503-555-0087
Francisco Lopez	Cr Prep	3	18		503-555-0900
Frank Williams	Recall	3		Hygienist	503-555-3382
Jacob Henry	Cr prep	6	24	Pre-medication	503-555-3245
Jason Ward	Recall/Fl tx	2		Schedule with brother	503-555-7533
Jennifer Vail	NP	3		Early AM	503-555-6743
Jim Beckner	Extraction	4	14, 15, & 16	Schedule 15 min early	503-555-3356
Jim Butler	Recall	3		Hygienist	503-555-9923
Jon Ford	Recall	3		Hygienist	503-555-4428
Judy Carr	Recall	3		Hygienist	503-555-8833
Julie Singer	Check/po	$^1/_2$		Patient late	503-555-7774
Kathy Bader	Final Imp	4	FUD	PM	503-555-8763
Kathy Campbell	Recall	3		Hygienist	503-555-2245
Lloyd Barber	Try-in	2	FUD		503-555-6634
Louise Brooke	Final Imp	4	PUD	Before Noon	503-555-2953
Maria Gonzales	Prophy	3		Hygienist	503-555-7245
Maria Gonzales	Amalgam	4	2, 3	Following hygiene appt	503-555-7245
Mark Dyer	Check/adj	$^1/_2$		Late afternoon	503-555-1123
Martha Sterling	Bridge prep	8	12–14		503-555-6578
Michael Ward	Recall/Fl tx	2		Schedule with brother	503-555-7533
Pat Perez	Recall	3		Hygienist	503-555-4720
Mary Thomas	Amalgam composite	6	12, 14, 24, 25	Fearful of injections	503-555-5572
Carrie James	Prophy	3		Hygienist	503-555-8965

OUTLINE

KEY TERMS AND CONCEPTS

Combination Recall System

Computerized Recall System

Mail Recall System

Prescheduled Recall System

Recall Appointment

Recall System

Telephone Recall System

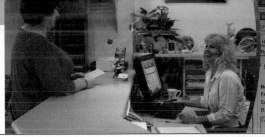

10

Recall Systems

LEARNING OBJECTIVES

The student will:

1. List the benefits to a patient of a recall appointment. List the benefits to the dental practice.
2. Discuss the elements that are necessary for an effective recall system.
3. List the different classifications of recalls.
4. Describe prescheduled, telephone, mail, and combination recall systems.
5. Describe the barriers to prescheduled, telephone, and mail recall systems.
6. Discuss solutions to the barriers of prescheduled, telephone, and mail recall systems.
7. List the sections of a tracking form, and describe their intended purpose.

INTRODUCTION

A **recall system** is an organized method of scheduling patients for examinations, prophylaxis, or other dental treatments. The success of a recall system is dependent on several factors: (1) Patients must be willing to return to the dental practice for follow-up care and examinations. (2) The dental practice must follow the procedure consistently to schedule patients at the prescribed time. (3) The dental practice must have an efficient method for tracking and contacting patients who fail to return at the scheduled time.

The function of a dental **recall appointment** system is to automate the scheduling of a patient for preventive dental treatment or for reevaluation of other dental conditions. A routine recall appointment, for the purpose of an examination and prophylaxis (cleaning), is scheduled for every 6 months. The prescribed length of time between appointments may vary from patient to patient. The dentist and dental hygienist determine the appropriate length of time between appointments on the basis of the dental needs of each patient.

Patients must understand the importance of the recall appointment before they are compelled to follow the advice of the dentist. Patients who seek dental treatment only when they are in pain are not likely to follow through with a recall appointment. The dental healthcare team has an obligation to all patients to educate them about the benefits of good oral health. Once patients understand and accept the benefits of good oral health, they are more likely to return for regular check-ups and prophylaxis.

The role of a dental healthcare team is to provide comprehensive, professional treatments through a system of dental examinations, preventive care measures, restorative treatments, and education. By educating patients about the benefits of home dental care and of establishing good dental health habits, the dental healthcare team forms a partnership with patients. When a team approach is used, the patient, as a team member, is more likely to accept his or her role in the prevention of dental disease, which includes regular examinations and prophylaxis.

Conditions that lead to a successful recall system do not just happen. Organization and commitment from the patient and the dental healthcare team are required if they are to come about.

Benefits of a recall system for the patient include the following:
- By maintaining good oral health, the patient will be free from dental disease, pain, and discomfort.
- Once optimal oral health has been achieved, the patient's cost of dental care is minimal.
- Insurance carriers encourage preventive dentistry. Most insurance polices provide 100% coverage for preventive procedures (radiographs, prophylaxis, and examinations).
- Some insurance carriers offer the incentive of providing higher percentages of coverage in increments for dental treatment to reward patients when they undergo examinations and prophylaxis on a regular basis (70% the first year, 80% the second year, and 100% after 4 years).
- The amount of time a patient must spend at the dental office is reduced when dental disease is detected and treated early, preventing the need for more extensive treatment.

The benefits of a recall system for the dental practice include the following:
- It forms a partnership between the patient and the dental healthcare team (the patient is a person and not just a "mouth").
- It increases referrals from patients because they feel comfortable and satisfied with the quality of the dental care (accomplished through patient education) they are receiving.
- It ensures a steady flow of patients through regularly scheduled appointments.
- It results in a partnership with other dental professionals because the total care of the patient is shared. Patients who are referred to a dental specialist for treatment are then referred back to the general dentist when that treatment is completed. When treatment continues longer than a few months, the patient is referred back to the general dentist for a regular recall appointment.

CLASSIFICATION OF RECALLS

The average recall appointment includes an examination, radiographs (at the prescribed intervals), and prophylaxis. For children, the appointment may also include a fluoride treatment.

During recall appointments, the dentist reexamines patients and evaluates their dental health. If dental disease is detected, it can be treated while it affects only a small area, which saves the patient time and money. Dental flossing and toothbrushing techniques should be discussed to optimize patients' home care.

In addition to the routine recall appointment, patients may be scheduled for follow-ups of previous dental treatments or for monitoring of a dental condition. Treatments that may require follow-up appointments include the following:

- Endodontic treatments
- Dental implants
- Crowns and bridges
- Partial and full dentures
- Surgical procedures
- Orthodontic evaluations

Additionally, patients who have been referred to specialists for treatment should subsequently be seen by the general dentist for regular check-ups.

METHODS FOR RECALLING PATIENTS

Once patients have been educated about and motivated to participate in preventive dentistry, the next step in the recall system is to formulate a process that ensures that each patient has the opportunity to return to the dental practice at the prescribed time. Several different types of systems can be used to identify when a patient should be seen, the type of appointment needed, and whether the patient followed through with the appointment. Manual and computerized systems have been developed for these purposes and vary widely from practice to practice.

 REMEMBER

The best system is the one that works.

General Information Needed for a Recall System

- Type of recall
- Month the patient is due for an appointment
- Who the appointment should be scheduled with, the dentist or the hygienist

- The amount of time needed for the appointment, and what treatment is going to be performed
- What method of recall each patient prefers: prescheduled appointment, reminder by mail, or reminder by telephone call

Prescheduled Recall System

One of the most effective recall methods is to have patients schedule their next appointment before they leave the office, after their current recall appointment is finished. This method (the **prescheduled recall system**) is highly successful because patients have personally participated in the scheduling of their own appointment. Although schedules change and some appointments must be rescheduled, they are very seldom broken.

 REMEMBER

Once patients have failed to make or to keep a recall appointment, they are sometimes too embarrassed to call and reschedule a new appointment.

Barriers to the Success of Prescheduled Appointments

Barrier: The hygiene schedule is booked 6 months in advance, and it is difficult to work in other patients.

Solution: Do not completely fill any one schedule. Designate appointment times that are not to be filled until 1 to 2 weeks before the date. *Rationale:* This leaves space to schedule patients who are new to the practice. Patients do not like to wait for appointments and may seek another dentist if they cannot get an appointment in a reasonable length of time (2 weeks is the average). Keep a call list. If you get an opening sooner, you can call the patient and fill the opening.

 REMEMBER

When talking to patients, never tell them you have a cancellation. This only raises the questions, "Why was the appointment cancelled? Was something wrong?" Tell patients you have an opening in the schedule, or that you have rearranged the schedule.

Steps in Prescheduling the Recall Appointment

1. Have the patient self-address a recall postcard.
2. Mutually schedule the next appointment before the patient leaves the office.
3. Enter the date and time on the recall postcard (Figure 10-1, *Top*). If a computer system is used, the appointment time is entered into the computer and the recall postcard will be generated at a later date.
4. Place the recall postcard into a monthly filing system. File the card according to the month the patient is due back for the appointment. (The month, date, and time of the appointment should also be recorded in the clinical chart.)

5. Mail cards to the patients 2 to 4 weeks before their appointment. Patients who must reschedule their appointment will call the office, and a new appointment can be scheduled.
6. Enter pertinent information on the tracking form.
7. Call patients 2 days before their appointment to confirm the date and time. This lessens the chance that a patient will miss an appointment.

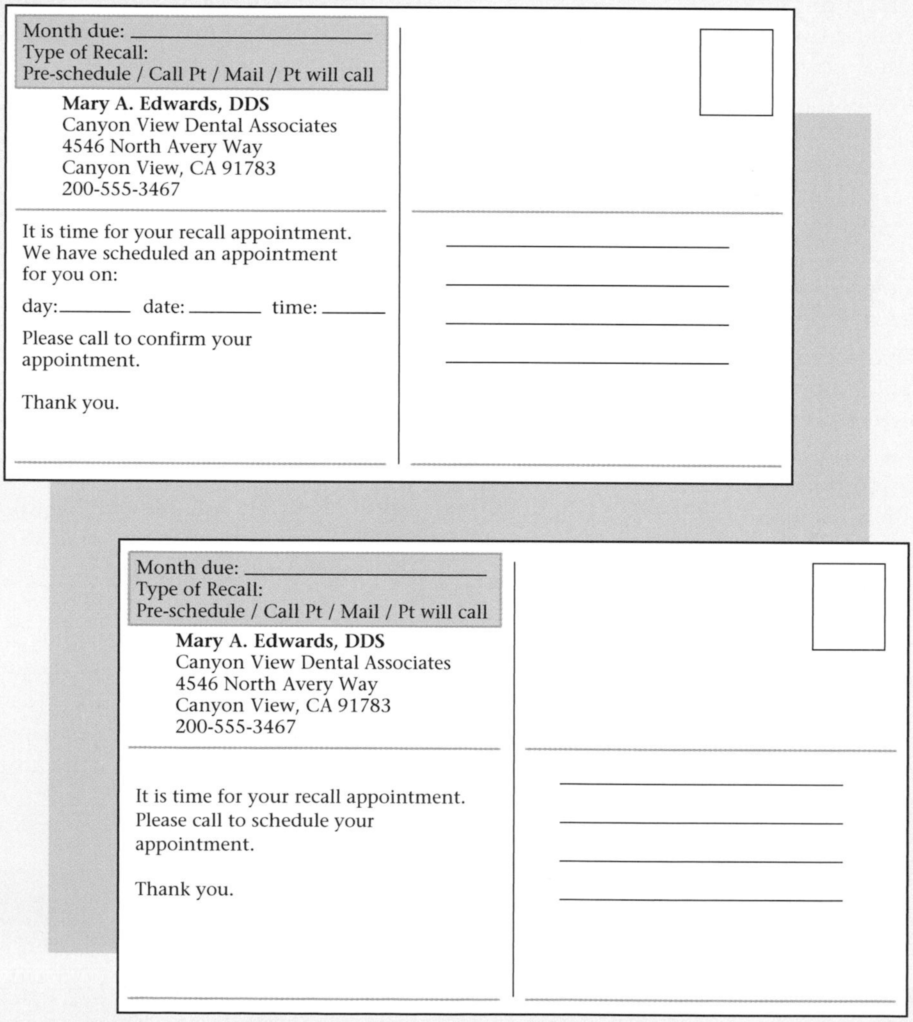

Month due: _____
Type of Recall:
Pre-schedule / Call Pt / Mail / Pt will call

Mary A. Edwards, DDS
Canyon View Dental Associates
4546 North Avery Way
Canyon View, CA 91783
200-555-3467

It is time for your recall appointment.
We have scheduled an appointment
for you on:

day: _____   date: _____   time: _____

Please call to confirm your
appointment.

Thank you.

Month due: _____
Type of Recall:
Pre-schedule / Call Pt / Mail / Pt will call

Mary A. Edwards, DDS
Canyon View Dental Associates
4546 North Avery Way
Canyon View, CA 91783
200-555-3467

It is time for your recall appointment.
Please call to schedule your
appointment.

Thank you.

Figure 10-1

Two types of messages are used on recall cards. Selection depends on whether a specific date and time has already been scheduled.

Steps in Using the Telephone Recall System

1. Select a time when you can make telephone calls with very few interruptions. (Remember to smile when you are talking to your patients. Smiles, as well as poor attitudes, travel over phone lines.)
2. Contact the patient and schedule an appointment.
3. Confirm the information you have, such as insurance coverage, and remind the patient to bring any necessary forms.
4. Follow up with a confirmation recall card.
5. Record the new information in the tracking system.

HIPAA

Privacy Rule: Confidential communications. Patient can request limitations to communications, including place and type of telephone calls and messages.

Telephone Recall System

The **telephone recall system** requires that an assistant call each patient before the month he or she is due for recall to schedule the appointment. This system provides immediate feedback about the needs of the patient.

Barriers to the Telephone System

Barrier: Patients are difficult to reach at home.

Solution: In today's society, it is difficult to reach patients at home. Often, both the husband and wife work. The best time to call is in the early evening, but then you may interrupt the dinner hour. With this type of recall system, it is best to know your patients' preferences. You may need to ask their permission to call them at work or in the early evening.

Barrier: The recall system is time consuming.

Solution: Select a time to make the phone calls when you have someone to answer the telephone and schedule patient appointments for you. Alternatively, schedule an evening when you can make the calls. Evenings are usually less hectic, and you can accomplish a great deal in a short time. You will find patients at home, and you will be free of interruptions.

Barrier: Only one person should make the calls.

Solution: Telephone scheduling is usually more successful if only one or two assistants are in charge of the calls. Although this may seem burdensome for one person, it does have an advantage. Patients are more comfortable when they are familiar with the assistant who is making the call. Over time, assistants get to know the needs and schedules of their patients, and this is comforting to patients. It eventually saves time in scheduling patients.

Barrier: Assistants can become frustrated after making several back-to-back calls. (They can begin to sound like a computerized message.)

Solution: Remember that this is not a telemarketing job. When you become frustrated, your patients easily detect it. It is best to pace yourself and not spend hours at a time on the telephone. If you develop a negative attitude while making the calls, go back to them when you feel more positive.

Mail Recall System

A **mail recall system** requires the mailing of recall cards to patients to remind them that they are due in the dental office for an appointment (see Figure 10-1, *Bottom*).

Barrier to the Mail Recall System

Barrier: Patients do not call.

Solution: This system relies on patients' taking the initiative to call the dental office to schedule an appointment. When patients are given sole responsibility, it is highly unlikely that they will call for the appointment. If you use this system, you will need to have a very good tracking system in place and to follow through often to ensure that patients are scheduling their appointments.

Steps in a Mail Recall System

1. Select recall cards that catch the eye of the receiver (Figure 10-2). Several companies print a wide selection of recall and other promotional cards.
2. Have patients self-address cards at the time of their appointment. If a computerized method is used, enter the date into the system and the computer will generate recall cards at the appropriate time.
3. Place the card in a card file according to the month the patient is due for recall.
4. Mail out the card before the month that the patient is due for recall.
5. Enter the information in a tracking system.

Tips for Maintaining a Successful Recall System

- Form a partnership with the patient. (Education = Motivation = Acceptance)
- Use the type of recall that works best for the individual patient.
- Follow through with a tracking system.
- Always remain flexible.
- Coordinate recalls with insurance coverage. If an insurance carrier will pay for a prophylaxis only very 6 months, do not schedule the patient for one in 5 months unless the dentist recommends that the patient be seen more often for dental health reasons, and only when the patient understands that the insurance company may not pay for the visit. *Always inform the patient.*
- Never lose contact with patients. They will not call you until they are in pain.
- Develop a system that can be used by all members of the dental healthcare team. Remember, the administrative dental assistant is the organizer of the system, but it takes a team effort to make it work smoothly.

Combination Recall System

Know your patients. What works well for one patient may not work for another patient. If one patient wishes to schedule an appointment 6 months in advance, schedule the appointment. Another patient may be unwilling to schedule an appointment in advance but does not mind if you call him or her at work to schedule the appointment closer to the actual appointment date. Another patient may be very good at scheduling an appointment as soon as he or she receives the card in the mail. By forming partnerships with your patients and respecting their preferences, you will have a very successful recall system. A **combination recall system** is shown in Figure 10-1.

Computerized Recall Systems

Many dental practices are beginning to use computers. Most software applications include a recall system. The **computerized recall system** can vary as widely as the manual systems.

Most software programs have a feature that recognizes procedures that require a recall. At the time the treatment is recorded, the program will automatically ask for the additional information needed to generate a recall card. For example, when you record that a patient has received a prophylaxis, the program will ask when the next appointment should

be. The program will automatically schedule the appointment according to the entered information, will print a recall card, and will place the patient's name on the recall list. If the patient does not return to the practice for the appointment, the program will automatically generate a reminder.

KEY POINTS

- A recall system is necessary to ensure that patients return to the dental practice at scheduled intervals for preventive treatment and examinations. The recall appointment benefits patients by helping them maintain good oral health, thus reducing their cost of dental treatment over the long term. It benefits the dental practice by promoting partnerships with patients, increasing referrals, and ensuring a steady flow of patients.

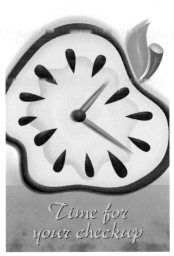
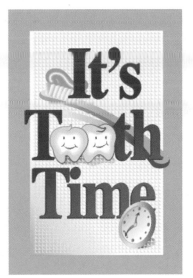
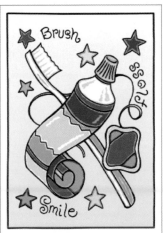

Figure 10-2
Recall cards are designed in a variety of styles and colors. (Courtesy Colwell, a Division of Patterson Dental Companies, Champaign, IL.)

- Types of recall systems include the following:
  - Prescheduled
  - Telephone
  - Mail
  - Combination
- Tips for maintaining a successful recall system include the following:
  - Customize the recall method for individual patients.
  - Follow through with a tracking system.
  - Remain flexible.
  - Coordinate recalls with insurance coverage.
  - Never lose contact with a patient.
- Computerized recall systems combine the elements of a manual system and are programmed to perform steps automatically.

STEPS FOR A COMBINATION RECALL SYSTEM

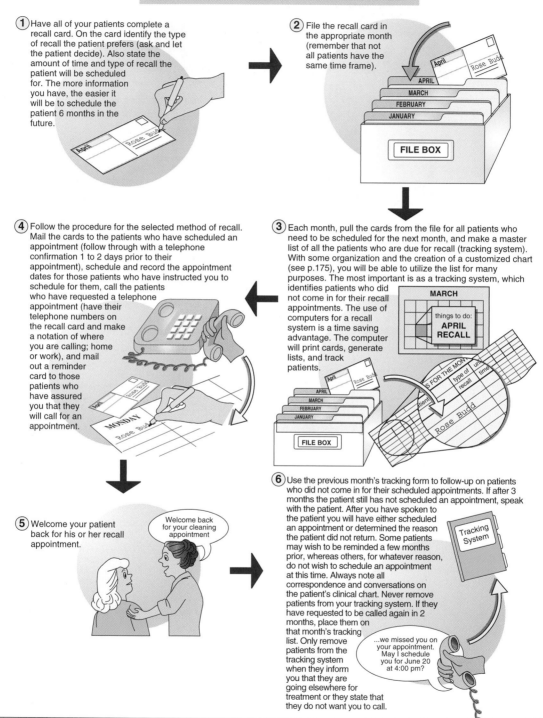

1 Have all of your patients complete a recall card. On the card identify the type of recall the patient prefers (ask and let the patient decide). Also state the amount of time and type of recall the patient will be scheduled for. The more information you have, the easier it will be to schedule the patient 6 months in the future.

2 File the recall card in the appropriate month (remember that not all patients have the same time frame).

3 Each month, pull the cards from the file for all patients who need to be scheduled for the next month, and make a master list of all the patients who are due for recall (tracking system). With some organization and the creation of a customized chart (see p.175), you will be able to utilize the list for many purposes. The most important is as a tracking system, which identifies patients who did not come in for their recall appointments. The use of computers for a recall system is a time saving advantage. The computer will print cards, generate lists, and track patients.

4 Follow the procedure for the selected method of recall. Mail the cards to the patients who have scheduled an appointment (follow through with a telephone confirmation 1 to 2 days prior to their appointment), schedule and record the appointment dates for those patients who have instructed you to schedule for them, call the patients who have requested a telephone appointment (have their telephone numbers on the recall card and make a notation of where you are calling; home or work), and mail out a reminder card to those patients who have assured you that they will call for an appointment.

5 Welcome your patient back for his or her recall appointment.

6 Use the previous month's tracking form to follow-up on patients who did not come in for their scheduled appointments. If after 3 months the patient still has not scheduled an appointment, speak with the patient. After you have spoken to the patient you will have either scheduled an appointment or determined the reason the patient did not return. Some patients may wish to be reminded a few months prior, whereas others, for whatever reason, do not wish to schedule an appointment at this time. Always note all correspondence and conversations on the patient's clinical chart. Never remove patients from your tracking system. If they have requested to be called again in 2 months, place them on that month's tracking list. Only remove patients from the tracking system when they inform you that they are going elsewhere for treatment or they state that they do not want you to call.

Figure 10-3

Steps used in a combination recall system.

ANATOMY OF A RECALL TRACKING SYSTEM

The ultimate purpose of the tracking system is to ensure that all patients who are in the recall system return for their recall appointment. It is easy for any member of the dental healthcare team to pick up the book and contact the overdue recall patients. Any member should be able to identify who has completed the recall and who has not. A system, manual or computerized, is set up that identifies the type of second notice, third notice, and so on until the patient is seen or removed from the system. When the system is used to its fullest extent, the status of the patient is always known and the patient is not lost.

				① Monthly Recall Tracking Form										
RECALLS FOR THE MONTH OF APRIL, 2000														
Patient	type of recall	unit time	x-rays	telephone #	prescheduled appointment	call patient	pt will call	recall completed	other work	appt Dr./Hyg.	1st notice	2nd notice	3rd notice
②	③	④	⑤	⑥	⑦	⑧	⑨	⑩	⑪	⑫	⑬	⑭	⑭
Rose Budd	prophy	3	no	555-1233(H)	4/4/99			4/4/99	bridge	hyg	####		
Bill Frank	endo	1	yes	555-4987(W)		x		4/22/99	crown	doctor	####		
Jose Gomez	prophy	3	bw/2	555-6794(VM)			x	4/18/99		hyg	####		
Sam Jones	prophy	3	FMX	555-0908(W)			x			hyg	####		

① **MONTH**
Identify the month and year the patient is due for recall.

② **PATIENTS' NAMES**
Patients' names are listed in alphabetical order. Adding an account number will help to locate the patient in the computer file, or the numerical number of the patient if the dental practice utilizes a numerical filing system.

③ **TYPE OF RECALL**
Identifies the category of recall needed.

④ **UNIT TIME**
States the amount of time that will be needed to complete the appointment.

⑤ **X-RAYS** (radiographs)
Indication of whether x-rays are needed and what type.

⑥ **TELEPHONE NUMBER**
The telephone number of the patient. Indicate if the telephone is home, work, voice mail, or message center.

⑦ **PRESCHEDULED**
Type of recall method. The appointment was made at the patient's last recall appointment. In a modified version of this system, the patient selects a general day of the week and time for the next appointment. When the recall cards are processed for a given month the assistant schedules the appointment. The patient is notified by mail and has the opportunity to keep the selected time or call the office to reschedule.

⑧ **CALL PATIENT**
Type of recall method. The patient has indicated that he or she wants to be called a few weeks prior to the recall to schedule an appointment.

⑨ **PATIENT WILL CALL**
Type of recall method. The patient has stated that he or she will call for an appointment after receiving a reminder in the mail.

⑩ **RECALL COMPLETED**
The date the patient is seen in the office for the recall. This is the most important element of the system. If this portion is not completed it will be impossible to determine if the patient has returned as scheduled. Time must then be taken to check the clinical record or the computer system.

⑪ **OTHER WORK**
Identify if there is any other treatment that needs to be scheduled at the time of the recall. It is also a good tracking tool for clinical treatment. Patients may delay treatment for a variety of reasons.

⑫ **APPOINTMENT WITH**
Identify which dental professional needs to see the patient.

⑬ **1ST NOTICE**
Record the date that the first recall card was sent or telephone call was made.

⑭ **2ND NOTICE, 3RD NOTICE**
The dates that follow-up contacts were made with the patient regarding the recall appointment. A system is designed by the dental practice to notify patients (via postcard, letter, or personal telephone call) that they need to schedule an appointment. For example, a 2nd notice is mailed if they have not returned to the dental practice within 3 months of their original recall month. At 6 months, a third attempt is made. This can be a combination of a reminder card or letter followed by a telephone call. At this point, patients on a 6-month recall have not had their teeth cleaned or examined for 1 year.

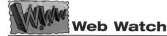 **Web Watch**

Dentist Info—Cyber Mall

http://www.dentistinfo.com/fdentcyb.htm

    Log on to Evolve to access additional
http://evolve.elsevier.com   web links!

 Critical Thinking Questions

1. A successful recall program depends on several factors. Describe the roles of the dental health-care team and the patient in developing a successful program.

2. List the steps in the combination recall system. Evaluate the system, state its barriers, and provide solutions.

Notes

OUTLINE

KEY TERMS AND CONCEPTS

Administrator
Allowable Charges
Assignment of Benefits
Attending Dentist's Statement
Audit
Balance Billing
Benefit Payment
Benefit Service
Birthday Rule
Capitation
Claim
Claims Payment Fraud
Claims Reporting Fraud
Closed Panel
Consolidated Omnibus Budget
  Reconciliation Act (COBRA)
Coordination of Benefits (COB)
Copayment
Corporate Dentistry
Covered Charges
Current Dental Terminology (CDT)
Current Procedural Terminology
Customary Fee
Deductible
Dental Insurance
Dental Service Corporation
Dependents

Direct Reimbursement
Downcoding
Electronically Submitted Forms
Encounter Forms
Exclusions
Expiration Date
Fee for Service
Fee Schedule
Fixed Fee Schedule
Franchise Dentistry
Gender Rule
Health Maintenance Organization
  (HMO)
Incentive Program
Indemnity Plan
Individual Practice Association
  (IPA)
Insured
Insurer
Least Expensive Alternative
  Treatment (LEAT)
Managed Care
Maximum Allowance
Maximum Benefit
Maximum Fee Schedule
Necessary Treatment
Nomenclature

Nonparticipating Dentist
Open Enrollment
Open Panel
Overbilling
Overcoding
Paper Claim Forms
Participating Dentist
Payer
Preauthorization
Precertification
Predetermination
Preexisting Condition
Preferred Provider Organization
  (PPO)
Prefiling of Fees
Reasonable Fee
Subscriber
Subscription Services
Superbills
Table of Allowances
Third Party
Union Trust Funds
Usual, Customary, and
  Reasonable (UCR) Plan
Usual Fee

11

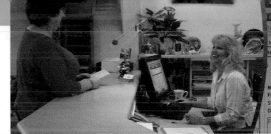

Dental Insurance Processing

LEARNING OBJECTIVES

The student will:

1. Classify and identify the various types of insurance coverage.
2. Discuss the purpose of insurance coding and differentiate between categories.
3. List the types of insurance information required to determine insurance coverage.
4. Identify the different methods of filing insurance claims and discuss the responsibility of the administrative dental assistant in filing dental claims.
5. Discuss part 5B of the ADA Code of Ethics, and identify how it applies to an administrative dental assistant.
6. Complete a dental claim form for manual submission.

INTRODUCTION

In the early days of dentistry, payment for dental treatment was arranged between the dentist and the patient. As dentistry progressed into a complex healthcare delivery system, with a wide range of treatment options, the need for financial assistance was recognized. In the middle of the 20th century, dental insurance was offered as a method of supplementing payment for dental treatment.

During the latter part of the 20th century, dentistry changed rapidly. The changes provided more comprehensive dental care, including preventive dentistry, advanced techniques for restorative dentistry, prosthodontics, orthodontics, dental implants, periodontics, and corrective surgical procedures. The dental insurance industry made changes to meet the new needs of policyholders. In addition to changes in dental treatment, the types of dental insurance changed. These changes expanded the scope of coverage and the delivery system. Today, employers and policyholders have a wide range of policy choices and can customize their coverage to meet their financial needs.

Whether only a few or many insurance claims are processed, the fundamental duties are the same. In a small dental practice, the administrative dental assistant may be in charge of the insurance process, along with several other assigned duties. In large dental practices, one or more insurance assistants may be responsible for processing insurance claims.

Before successfully processing a dental claim form, the assistant must to understand the types of dental insurance coverage available, insurance terminology (a glossary is provided later), and how to correctly code dental procedures. In addition, a clear-cut policy must be in place that outlines the requirements of the dental practice in relation to insurance billing, the patient's responsibilities, and the dental practice's responsibilities. It is extremely important, as it is in all phases of dental treatment, that patients have a clear and concise understanding of the treatment, what the insurance company will pay, and what their portion of the payment will be before any treatment is begun.

TYPES OF DENTAL INSURANCE

Dental benefits are determined by the type of dental insurance policy and the extent of the coverage.

Insurance coverage is calculated with specifications outlined in the insurance contract. Insurance contracts are between the carrier (insurance company), the purchaser of the insurance (group, in most cases employers), and the subscriber (individual or employee). Insurance policies are purchased for the subscriber, and additional coverage may be extended to the subscriber's dependents (spouse and children).

Insurance plans can be divided into several very broad categories. These categories are based on the types of coverage and the methods by which the dental office is paid.

Fee for Service

Fee for service is a method of payment that compensates the dentist according to individual services and procedures. Reimbursement is determined by established fee schedules.

Usual, Customary, and Reasonable Plans

Dental insurance companies establish fee schedules on the basis of a variety of information. The fee schedules in **usual, customary, and reasonable (UCR) plans** are based on the following criteria: **usual fee,** the fee the dentist uses most often for a given dental service; **customary fee,** the fee determined by the third party administrator from actual fees submitted for specific dental services; and **reasonable fee,** a determination by the third party administrator that a particular service for a given procedure has been modified to take into consideration unusual complications. This fee may vary from the dentist's usual fee and the administrator's customary fee. UCR fee schedules are calculated with distinct demographic information and criteria. Insurance companies survey dental practices within a geographic location and determine the average fee charged for each procedure code. Using this information, they establish a fee schedule. Each insurance company has its own criteria and method by which it determines the UCR fee.

Some insurance contracts require participating dentists to file a fee schedule. A review of the fee schedule determines whether the fees fall within the established UCR fee range. If the schedule is accepted, it will become the established fee schedule for that dental practice. If the fees do not fall within the established UCR, the schedule is not accepted and is returned to the dentist for revision. Once the

Dental Insurance Terminology

Administrator: A person or group of persons who represent dental benefits plans for the purpose of negotiating and managing contracts with dental service providers.

Allowable Charges: The maximum amount paid for each procedure.

Assignment of Benefits: Authorization given by the subscriber or patient to a dental benefit plan, directing the insurer to make payment for dental benefits directly to the providing dentist.

Attending Dentist's Statement: The form used by the dentist to request payment of services (dental claim form) from the dental benefit plan.

Audit: A method used by third parties to check the accuracy of dental claim forms by comparing patient clinical records with information submitted on the dental claim form.

Balance Billing: Billing the patient for the difference between the amount paid by the dental benefits plan and the fee charged by the dentist (according to the specification of the dental benefits plan contract).

Benefit Payment: The amount of the total bill paid by the dental benefits plan.

Benefit Service: A service that will be paid for by the dental benefits plan.

Birthday Rule: A method used to determine which parent is considered the primary provider of dental coverage. The rule simply states that the parent whose birth date comes first in the year is the primary provider. Gender rule states that the father is always the primary provider. These rulings are outlined in each individual insurance contract.

Capitation: A contract with a dental benefits plan that stipulates that payment will be made to the dentist per capita (per patient).

Claim: Also known as the Attending Dentist's Statement. Claims are a method used to request payment or authorization for treatment. Each claim provides necessary information about the patient, treating dentist, and treatment.

Claims Payment Fraud: Changing or manipulating information (by a dental benefits plan) on a dental claim form that results in a lower benefit being paid to the treating dentist (intentionally falsifying information and services).

Claims Reporting Fraud: Changing or manipulating information (by the dentist) on a dental claim form that results in a higher benefit being paid by the dental benefits plan (intentionally falsifying information and services).

Closed Panel: Panels are groups of dental providers who are under contract with third parties to provide dental services. Patients who receive benefits from the dental benefits plan must seek dental services only from members of the panel. Contracts also limit the number of panel members (dental providers) in a specified geographic area.

Code on Dental Procedures and Nomenclature (the Code): Code set adapted under the Administrative Simplification provisions of HIPAA used to identify dental procedures. The code is a listing of a five-digit code set and a description of the dental service. The Code is published by the American Dental Association.

Consolidated Omnibus Budget Reconciliation Act (COBRA): Legislation that mandates guaranteed medical and dental coverage for a period of 18 months after the loss of group benefits coverage. Individuals are given the option of purchasing their own coverage at a group rate under special COBRA contracts.

Coordination of Benefits (COB): A system that coordinates the benefits of two or more insurance policies. The total benefits paid should not be more than 100% of the original service fee.

Copayment: The portion of the service fee that remains after payment is made by the dental benefits plan.

Corporate Dentistry: Dental facilities that are owned and operated by companies for the purpose of providing dental care to their employees and dependents.

Covered Charges: Allowable services outlined in dental benefits plan contracts, fee schedules, or tables of allowance, provided by the dental provider and paid for, in whole or part, by the third party dental benefits plan.

Current Dental Terminology (CDT): A standardized list of terms and codes established by the American Dental Association (ADA) for the purpose of consistency in reporting dental services and procedures to dental benefits plans.

Current Procedural Terminology: A standardized list of codes and procedures developed by the American Medical Association (AMA) for the purpose of consistency in reporting medical treatment and services.

Dental Insurance Terminology—cont'd

Deductible: The service fee that the patient is responsible to pay before the third party will consider payment of additional services. The deductible may be payable annually, during a lifetime, or as a family.

Dental Benefit Plan: Provides dental service to an enrollee in exchange for a fixed, periodic payment made in advance of the dental service. Such plans often include the use of deductibles, coinsurance, and maximums to control the cost of the program to the purchaser.

Dental Benefit Program: Dental benefit plan being offered to the enrollees by the sponsor.

Dental Insurance: A method of financial assistance (provided by a dental benefits service) that helps pay for specified procedures and services concerning dental disease and accidental injury to the oral structure.

Dental Service Corporation: A legally formed, not-for-profit organization that contracts with dental providers for the sole purpose of providing dental care (e.g., Delta Dental Plans and Blue Cross/Blue Shield).

Dependents: Persons who are covered under another person's dental benefits policy, including, but not limited to, spouses and children. The terms of dependent coverage are stated in the dental benefits contract for each coverage group.

Direct Reimbursement: A plan that allows an organization to be self-funded for the purpose of providing dental benefits. The plan is administered by the individual provider or by an outside organization for the purpose of processing claims and distributing service benefit payments. These plans allow the patient to seek dental care and treatment at a facility of their choice, and in most states, this is not yet regulated by the insurance commission.

Downcoding: A method of changing a reported benefits code by third party payers to reflect a lower cost for the procedure.

Dual Choice Program: An insurance policy (benefit plan) that provides the eligible individual the choice of an alternative dental benefit program or a traditional dental benefit program.

Eligibility Date: The effective date of dental coverage:

Established Patient: Patient who has received dental care recently.

Exclusions: The option in a dental benefits program to exclude dental services and procedures (as outlined in the patient contract book).

Exclusive Provider Organization (EPO): A dental benefit plan or program that will cover dental services only if they are provided by an institutional or professional provider with whom the dental benefit plan has a contract.

Expiration Date: Date that the patient is no longer eligible for dental benefits based on expiration of the dental contract or termination of the patient's employment.

Family Deductible: A deductible that can be satisfied when combined deductibles of the family have been met. This deductible will be less than the total of the individual family members' deductibles.

Fee for Service: Dental benefits paid for each dental service or procedure performed by the dental practitioner, instead of payment that is salary based or capitation based.

Fee Schedule: A list of charges for dental services and procedures established by the dentist or a dental benefits provider and mutually agreed upon.

Franchise Dentistry: A method of providing dental care under a common name, with regional or national advertising, contract agreements with dental benefits providers, and financial and managerial support.

Health Insurance Portability and Accountability Act of 1996 (HIPAA): A federal law that requires all health plans, health care clearinghouses, and providers of health care who transmit PHI electronically to use a standard transaction code set. The official code set for dental services is the *Code for Dental Procedures and Nomenclature,* published by the American Dental Association.

Health Maintenance Organization (HMO): A healthcare delivery system with a network of providers who will accept payment for services on a per capita basis or a limited fee schedule. The purpose of the HMO is to contain costs through control of services provided. Patients who are enrolled in an HMO must seek dental treatment from the assigned provider. The period of time that a patient must stay with the provider varies according to the individual contract. Usually, patients cannot change providers without authorization from the HMO.

Dental Insurance Terminology—cont'd

Incentive Program: The copayment percentage changes when patients follow a preset standard of treatment. For example, a dental benefits plan may offer new enrollees a 70%-30% copayment arrangement for the first year of coverage (with the patient responsible for 30%). If the patient receives preventive care at set intervals during the first year, the dental benefits plan will increase the insurance company's copayment percentage to 80%-20% the following year (with the patient responsible for 20%). The increase will continue as long as the patient follows the preset standard of treatment. If the patient fails to follow the standard, the copayment percentage will revert backward (never to be lower than the original ratio).

Indemnity Plan: Dental benefits plan that uses a schedule of allowance, table of allowance, or reasonable and customary fee schedule as the basis of payment calculation.

Individual Practice Association (IPA): Legally formed organization that enters into contracts with dental benefits plans to provide services to the dental benefit plans' enrollees. The IPA is composed of individual dental practitioners.

Insured: A person who has enrolled with an insurer (third party) to provide payment for dental services and procedures.

Insurer: The third party (not the dentist or the patient) that assumes the responsibility for payment of dental services and procedures for enrollees in the program.

Least Expensive Alternative Treatment (LEAT): A provision in dental benefits plans that allows payment for dental services and procedures to be based on the least expensive treatment available. For example, a patient chooses to have a composite restorative material placed in a posterior tooth. The dental benefits plan will base payment on the least expensive restorative material, amalgam. The patient is responsible for the difference in payment.

Managed Care: A method employed by some benefits plans designed to contain the costs of healthcare, including limitations in access to care (enrollees are assigned healthcare providers), covered services and procedures, and reimbursement amounts.

Maximum Allowance: The total amount of specific dental benefits (dollars) that will be paid toward dental services and procedures. Maximums are determined by the provisions of individual group contracts.

Maximum Benefit: The total amount of dental benefits that will be paid for an individual or family for the purpose of dental services and procedures. This amount is determined by the individual group contract and may be a yearly maximum or a lifetime maximum.

Maximum Fee Schedule: The total acceptable fee for a dental service or procedure that can be charged by a dental provider under a specific dental benefits plan (e.g., preset fee schedules that have been accepted by the dental provider and the dental benefits plan).

Necessary Treatment: Dental services and procedures that have been established by the dental professional as necessary for the purpose of restoring or maintaining a patient's oral health. Treatment is based on established standards of the dental profession.

Nonduplication of Benefits: This applies if a subscriber is covered by more than one benefit plan. In the case of dual coverage, the subscriber will never receive payment for more than 100% of the covered benefit.

Nonparticipating Dentist: A dental professional who is not under contract with a dental benefits plan to provide dental services and procedures to enrollees.

Open Enrollment: A period during the year when a member of a dental benefits program has the option of selecting the type of coverage and the provider of dental services.

Open Panel: A type of dental benefits plan in which any licensed dentist can participate. The enrollee (insured) can seek treatment from any licensed dentist, with benefits being paid to the enrollee or to the dentist. The dentist may accept or refuse any enrollee.

Overbilling: Fraudulent practice of not disclosing the waiver of patient copayment to benefits plan organizations.

Overcoding: Billing dental benefits plans for higher-paying procedures than the service or procedure that was actually performed.

Participating Dentist: A dentist who has contracted with a dental benefits organization to provide dental care to specific enrollees.

Dental Insurance Terminology—cont'd

Payer: Insurance companies, dental benefits plans, or dental plan sponsors (direct reimbursement, unions) that make payments on behalf of patients.

Preauthorization: Confirmation by a dental benefits plan that a pretreatment plan has been authorized for payment according to the patient's group policy.

Precertification: Confirmation by a dental benefits plan that a patient is eligible to receive treatment according to the provision of the contract.

Predetermination: A process in which a dentist submits a pretreatment plan and documentation to a dental benefits plan organization for approval. The dental benefits plan organization will establish the patient's eligibility for payment of the procedure and will approve the fees to be charged according to the patient's contract. The document returned by the payer will state the benefit that will be paid, limitations if any, and the amounts of the copayment and deductible. Some contracts mandate that all treatments over a set dollar amount require predetermination.

Preexisting Condition: A clause in most dental benefits plans that limits coverage for conditions that existed before the patient enrolled in the benefits plan.

Preferred Provider Organization (PPO): A contract between a dental benefits plan organization and a provider of dental care that states that, in return for the referral of dental patients, the dentist will provide services and procedures at a reduced fee or according to a preestablished fee schedule. The purposes of this contract are to cut costs for the dental benefits plan organization and to provide a patient base for the dental professional.

Prefiling of Fees: A procedure in which a dental professional files a fee schedule with the dental benefits plan organization for the purpose of receiving preauthorization of fees. If the fee schedule is accepted by the dental benefits plan organization, the schedule will be the basis for coverage of enrolled patients. If an enrollee is charged a fee higher than that on file, the difference is not allowed and cannot be charged to the enrollee.

Subscriber: The holder of the dental benefits (insurance). Usually, this is the person whose name is on the policy, and additional coverage is extended to the spouse and children. Other terms used to describe the subscriber are *enrollee, insured,* and *certificate holder.*

Table of Allowances: A list of the services and procedures that will be paid by the dental benefits plan, with a dollar amount assigned to each procedure. Tables of allowance are also referred to as *schedules of allowance* and *indemnity schedules.*

Third Party: A group or organization that has the capacity to collect insurance premiums, accept financial risk, and pay dental claims (the patient is the first party, and the healthcare provider is the second party). Also known as the *administrative agent, carrier, insurer,* or *underwriter,* the third party also performs other administrative services.

Usual, Customary, and Reasonable (UCR) Plan: A dental plan that uses the following criteria to establish a fee schedule: **usual fee,** the fee the dentist uses most often for a given dental service; **customary fee,** the fee determined by the third party administrator from actual submitted fees for specific dental services; and **reasonable fee,** a determination by the third party administrator that a particular service for a given procedure has been modified to take into consideration unusual complications. This fee may vary from the dentist's usual fee and the administrator's customary fee.

---

fee schedule has been established, it becomes the basis for reimbursement from that insurance company.

Table of Allowances

Tables of allowances, schedules of allowances, and indemnity schedules are lists of procedures covered by an insurance company and their respective dollar amounts. These fees are the same for all dentists, regardless of location. The dental practice submits the dental practice fee for service, and reimbursement is calculated with the amount listed on the table of allowances. The difference between the fees is charged to the patient.

Fixed Fee Schedule

Government assistance programs and other programs establish a **fixed fee schedule.** These fee schedules include preestablished fees that are charged by all dentists, regardless of geographic area. If the usual fee charged by the dental practice is higher than the fixed fee, the difference between fees cannot be charged to the patient.

Capitation Programs

Capitation programs are programs in which the dental practice is paid a set amount for each patient who is enrolled in the program. Payment is made for each enrolled patient, regardless of whether he or she receives treatment. In addition to the monthly fee paid to the dentist under some contracts, the dentist can charge the patient a copayment. Copayments apply to each visit and may be applied to designated procedures.

Closed Panel Programs

Closed panel programs are programs that dictate to patients where they can receive their dental treatment. Under closed panel programs, dentists and dental entities enter into an agreement to provide services for a select group of patients. Contracts for closed panel programs are limited to a preset number in a geographic area. This limitation provides a larger patient pool for those dental practices or entities with contracts.

Another type of closed panel program is provided by large corporations that provide dental clinics for their employees and families. The dentist and the dental auxiliary are employees of the corporation.

Franchise Dentistry

Franchise dentistry is a method that allows a corporation (formed by a dentist or other entity) to own several dental practices (most states have very specific regulations and laws dealing with the ownership of medical and dental practices). The benefits of this type of dental practice are a common name and the means for a large advertising budget. Some franchise dental practices offer supplemental dental insurance to their patients to pay that portion of the fee that is not paid by their primary dental insurance. This type of insurance pays only when the patient is seen in one of the franchise dental prac-

tices. Dentists and staff members work for the corporation.

Direct Reimbursement

Direct reimbursement is a method of payment that bypasses an insurance company and pays fees directly from a fund established by an employer.

Preferred Provider Organization

The **preferred provider organization** (PPO) is a plan that establishes a list of dentists who have a contract with the insurance company. The contract states that the dentist will use only the fee schedule preapproved by the third party (insurance company). In exchange for the fixed fee schedule, the third party places the dentist's name on the preferred list, thus supplying a patient base for the dental office.

Patients who belong to PPOs have the option of receiving treatment from approved providers or from a dentist outside of the program. When treatment is performed by a nonmember dentist, the fee schedule is different and may result in a greater out-of-pocket expense for the patient.

Health Maintenance Organization

A **health maintenance organization** (HMO) accepts responsibility for payment of dental procedures and services for its members. Members enter into HMOs for the purpose of having all of their medical or dental fees covered. Members of HMOs can receive treatment only from assigned dentists. If they receive treatment outside of the HMO, the fees are not covered and become the responsibility of the patient. Patients are assigned contract HMO dentists and cannot make changes easily. Each month, the HMO sends the dental practice a roster of patients. The dental practice is paid a capitation for each patient on the roster.

Additional payment for treatment or a copayment is collected for covered expenses according to the individual contract. When an HMO patient is seen, the dental practice is required to submit an encounter claim form to the HMO. Supplemental payment to the dental practice is made according to services rendered. Patients may be required to pay a copayment at the time of the appointment. Copayments may be assessed according to a visit charge or for individual services. Each group has a different protocol for the collection of copayments and the filing of encounter forms.

Managed Care

Managed care is a program that is designed to contain the costs of dental procedures and services. This is accomplished by restricting the types and frequencies of procedures and services, preestablishing where a patient may seek dental care (contract dentist or dental entities), and controlling fee schedules.

Individual Practice Association

An **individual practice association** (IPA) is an organization that has been legally established by a group of dentists to enter into third party contracts. The objective of the association is to work collectively to secure third party contracts. The IPA usually consists of a small staff and an administrator.

Union Trust Funds

Union trust funds administer the distribution of their members' benefits. They are not insurance companies and are not mandated to follow the same rules as insurance companies. They establish their own fee schedules (table of allowances) that outline the amount of money paid for each procedure. Depending on the type of contract and on the program offered by the union, payment may be made from a fee for service, PPO, or capitation program.

INSURANCE CODING

Current Dental Terminology, CDT-2005, is published by the American Dental Association (ADA) and is recognized by the federal government as the standard for reporting dental services in compliance with the Health Portability and Accountability Act of 1996 (HIPAA). *CDT-2005* is the fourth in a series of publication by the ADA. The first list of procedures was produced in 1969, and revisions and additions to the code have been made on an ongoing basis. The code is maintained by the Code Revision Committee (CRC). This committee comprises members of the ADA and representatives from major health insurance plans and government programs.

Although the primary use of the *CDT-2005* is to identify and define the various transactions codes, it also contains information useful to the dental healthcare team in the compilation of dental claim forms. The *CDT-2005* is cross–referenced, so it is easy to locate a procedure numerically by procedure code or alphabetically by procedure nomenclature, in addition to the full description of the procedure code and nomenclature. Each time the Code is revised and updated, a section of the manual is used to identify and explain the new and revised codes. Another section of the manual answers common questions, to help clarify various codes and procedures. A detailed explanation of how to complete the dental claim form is included, along with applicable charts and tooth numbering systems. The final section of the manual is a glossary of common dental insurance terms. The first section of the manual contains the Code on Dental Procedures and Nomenclature (the Code). This section of the manual divides procedure codes into 12 categories (Table 11-1). Procedure codes are identified by a five-digit alphanumeric code, constituting the only approved coding system for the submission of dental claim forms that cannot be changed. The first digit of the code will be "D," which identifies the code as a dental service code. The second digit describes the category, and the remaining digits describe the nature of the procedure or service. For example, code D1110 is interpreted as follows. The first digit (letter), D, indicates a dental service. The second digit, 1, indicates a preventive procedure or service (see Table 11-1). The last three digits identify the procedure or service performed. Following each dental procedure

TABLE **11-1 CDT-2005 Categories**

I.	Diagnostic	D0100-D0999
II.	Preventive	D1000-D1999
III.	Restorative	D2000-D2999
IV.	Endodontics	D3000-D3999
V.	Periodontics	D4000-D4999
VI.	Prosthodontics, Removable	D5000-D58999
VII.	Maxillofacial Prosthetics	D59900-D5999
VIII.	Implant Services	D6000-D6199
IX.	Prosthodontics, Fixed	D6200-D6999
X.	Oral Surgery	D7000-D7999
XI.	Orthodontics	D8000-D8999
XII.	Adjunctive General Services	D9000-D9999

code is a brief literal definition. This definition is referred to as the **nomenclature.** When the procedure is defined on a dental claim form, the nomenclature can be abbreviated. When necessary, a written narrative of the dental procedure may follow the nomenclature.

The most current CDT Manual is used to code dental claims. When claims are processed manually, it is the responsibility of the insurance clerk to enter correct codes by referencing the CDT Manual. This procedure requires that the insurance clerk be familiar with the outline of the Manual. When claims are processed by computer, the code is entered into the computer database by the developer of the software or the insurance clerk. When a procedure is coded and entered during transaction posting, the software converts the transaction code into the proper CDT code. When a dental claim form is printed, the proper CDT code will appear. It is the responsibility of the administrative dental assistant to check the accuracy of the codes to ensure that the correct conversion has taken place. Table 11-2 lists some commonly used codes.

SNODENT, Systematized Nomenclature of Dentistry, is a combination of medical (SNOMED) conditions and dental conditions used to define dental diseases in an electronic environment. SNODENT is a comprehensive coding system used to identify diseases, diagnoses, anatomy, conditions, morphology, and social factors that may affect the outcomes of diagnosis and treatment. The use of these codes enables the dentist to describe conditions and other factors that relate to a given diagnosis. Currently, the use of the codes is optional. It is hoped that the codes will be used in the future in place of narrative reports to describe extenuating conditions when insurance claim forms are submitted.

ORGANIZING INSURANCE COVERAGE FOR EACH PATIENT

Because of the large number of dental claims processed by dental practices, it has become a full-time task in some practices to work with insurance claims. When a patient arrives for the first time, it is the task of the administrative dental assistant to determine insurance coverage. A process should be developed to help the assistant gather all needed information quickly and efficiently. A number of

methods have been established to organize this process. The administrative dental assistant can develop and keep a manual system, use a computer database, subscribe to a service, or use the information given by each insurance company.

Manual System

A manual system can be kept with a notebook and preprinted insurance information sheets. The notebook is organized according to insurance carrier and group number. When a patient comes to the office, his or her insurance information can be accessed, and coverage can be estimated according to the recorded information. This type of book is often referred to as a *blue book* and can be either manually or computer generated.

Computer Databases

Some practice management software programs may use a type of blue book by sorting and categorizing information as it is entered by the administrative dental assistant. In this type of software, the assistant enters information as it is received from Explanation of Benefits forms. When new patients come to the dental practice, the name of their insurance company and group number are entered, and further information is requested. The program may have the ability to supply basic information from other databases, including mailing address, contact person, percentage of coverage, and allowable fees. This information is based on information gathered by the assistant and may not be current.

Subscription Services

Subscription services provide information on a large number of insurance carriers and groups. The service compiles the same information for a wide range of third party carriers, employers, and other dental groups into one easy reference system. This information includes the maximum allowable, covered expenses, billing address, and recommended protocol in filing claims (Figure 11-1). The information is available on computer disks or online. The value of the service is that it is continually updated. In addition, the service has a staff that can research unlisted groups and provide technical assistance to the administrative dental assistant. Searches can be made by employer, group, or insurance carrier.

TABLE **11-2 Dental Terminology Coding**

Current Dental Terminology

Current Dental Terminology (CDT) is recognized by the federal government as the standard for reporting dental services in compliance with the Health Insurance Portability and Accountability Act of 1996 (HIPAA).

Although the primary use of the CDT is to identify and define the various transaction codes, it also contains information useful to the dental healthcare team in the compilation of dental claim forms. The procedure codes are divided into 12 categories and are identified by a five-digit alphanumeric code, constituting the only approved coding system for the submission of dental claim forms that cannot be altered.

The first digit of each code is the letter "D," identifying the code as a dental service code. This is followed by a second digit, which signifies the category of the code. The remaining digits of each code reflect the individual procedure or service.

Dental Claims

When processing dental claims manually, the insurance clerk is responsible for entering codes correctly by referencing the CDT Manual. When processing claims via computer, the insurance clerk or software developer enters the code into the computer database. For procedures coded and entered into the database during transaction posting, the insurance software converts the transaction code into the proper CDT code. This code will appear on the printed dental claim form. Below is more detailed information on the code categories.

I. Diagnostic   D0100-D0999

Diagnostic codes apply to procedures common to patient examination and diagnosis and those which form the basis for treatment planning. These procedures typically fall into one of four diagnostic areas:

1. Oral evaluations are conducted by the dental healthcare team to assess overall health status of new patients, check the evolution of existing patients, and diagnose and track progress of acute oral conditions.

2. Radiographs document intraoral and extraoral conditions using a variety of diagnostic imaging techniques and materials.

3. Biologic tests examine viral organisms and patients' vulnerability or predisposition to oral diseases.

4. Pathologic evaluations diagnose conditions of oral tissues.

TABLE **11-2 Dental Terminology Coding—cont'd**

II. Preventive	D1000 D1000

Codes in the preventive category refer to procedures conducted by the dental healthcare team designed to prevent the occurrence or recurrence of oral diseases:

- Prophylaxis treatment, through which plaque, calculus, stains, and other accumulated substances are removed from the clinical crowns of the teeth.

- Fluoridization of the teeth.

- Preventive counseling to encourage healthy dietary and hygienic habits and discourage the use of products that increase the risk of oral diseases.

- Installation and management of space-maintaining appliances designed to preserve the space created by the premature loss of a tooth

III. Restorative	D2000-D2999

Restorative codes apply to procedures concerned with the reconstruction of the hard tissues of a tooth or a group of teeth injured or destroyed by trauma or disease. These procedures are primarily classified by the restorative materials used in the reconstructive process. Common forms include the following:

- Amalgam

- Resin-based

- Gold

- Porcelain (for some crowns)

IV. Endodontics	D3000-D3999

Codes for endodontics involve the diagnosis, prevention, and treatment of diseases of the dental pulp. Typical procedures performed by the dental healthcare team include the following:

- Capping pulp with material that protects it from external influences.

- Surgical amputation of the pulp.

- Surgical removal of the apex of a root.

- Complete pulp removal from the pulp chamber and root canal.

Continued

TABLE **11-2 Dental Terminology Coding—cont'd**

V. Periodontics	D4000-D4999

Periodontal considerations concern the care of the supporting structures of the teeth. Coding for periodontics is usually assigned to procedures such as the following:

- Gingival surgery and treatment
- Crown extension
- Osseous replacement grafting
- Scaling and root planning

VI. Prosthodontics—Removable	D5000-D5899

Codes pertaining to the restoration and maintenance of oral function, comfort, appearance, and health through replacement of missing teeth fall under prosthodontics. Procedures used in conjunction with removable prosthodontics include the following:

- Creation and maintenance of complete, partial, and interim dentures
- Conditioning of dental ridge tissue
- Surgical prosthesis modification

VII. Maxillofacial Prosthetics	D5900-D5999

Maxillofacial prosthetics codes apply to procedures used in the prosthetic restoration of facial structures that have been affected by disease, injury, surgery, or congenital defect. Some of these extensive procedures include the following:

- Fabrication of prosthetic pieces that restore damaged or missing areas of the nose, eyes, ears, or jaw
- Surgical lifts of the jaw
- Surgical shielding or splinting

TABLE **11-2 Dental Terminology Coding—cont'd**

VIII. Implant Cervices	D6000 D6100

Oral implantation procedures performed by the dental healthcare team involve the surgical insertion of materials or devices into the patient's jaw. Codes in this category can apply to either occlusal rehabilitation or cosmetic dentistry, such as the following:

- Surgical installation of implants in the alveolar and/or basal bone

- Surgical installation of open-mesh frames designed to fit over the surface of the bone

- Surgical installation of implants threaded through the bone and into the oral cavity

IX. Prosthodontics—Fixed	D6200-D6999

Fixed prosthodontics codes concern procedures performed by the dental healthcare team that replace or restore teeth via artificial substitutes that are not readily removable. Typical procedures in this category include the following:

- Insertion of an artificial tooth on a fixed partial denture, replacing a missing natural tooth

- Reuniting the abutment tooth with the suspended portion of the bridge

- Anchoring of a removable overdenture prosthesis

- Installation of a stress-relieving connector

X. Oral And Maxillofacial Surgery	D7000-D7999

Surgical procedures pertaining to facial extractions or closures are coded under oral and maxillofacial surgery. Classifications include the following:

- Removal of teeth, tissue-retained remnants, or other tooth structures by means of elevators and/or forceps

Continued

TABLE **11-2 Dental Terminology Coding—cont'd**

- Surgical shaping and smoothing of the margins of the tooth socket in preparation for placement of prosthesis

- Surgical restoration of the alveolar ridge height through lowering of the jaw muscles

- Surgical removal of bone and/or lesions

- Fracture treatment

- Trauma repair

XI. Orthodontics	D8000-D8999

Any procedures performed by the dental healthcare team concerned with the guidance and correction of growing and/or mature dentofacial structures are coded under orthodontics, including the following treatments:

- Management of transitional dentition

- Prevention of dentofacial malformations

- Removable or fixed appliance therapy

- Appliance maintenance and replacement

XII. Adjunctive General Services	D9000-D9999

Any general procedures not classified in the previous categories or coded under adjunctive general services. Common procedures found in this category include the following:

- Administration of anesthesia

- Diagnostic consultation not involving treatment

- House calls

- Pharmaceutical administration

- Cosmetic bleaching

- Behavior management

Major insurance companies provide a reference book to all of their member dentists that contains information about each of their groups. The handbook (reference book) is categorized by group and lists the percentages of coverage for each type of service, maximum payable benefits, deductibles, and other valuable information.

Whatever method is used to collect insurance data, a simple form or sticker can be used to record the insurance information for future reference. The sticker or form is placed in each patient's clinical record for easy access by any member of the dental healthcare team. This information helps the dentist and the patient to reach a mutually agreed upon treatment plan.

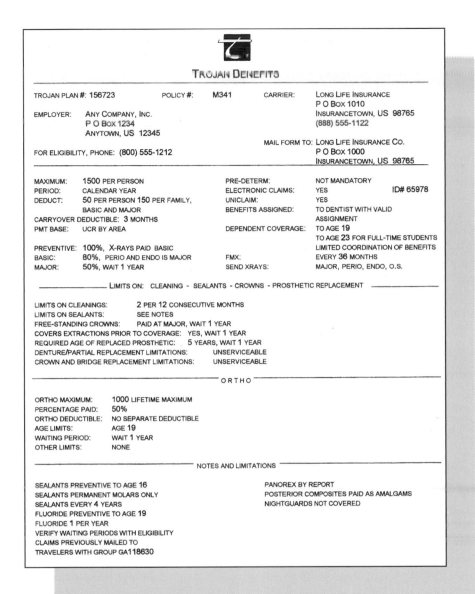

TROJAN BENEFITS

TROJAN PLAN #: 156723   POLICY #: M341   CARRIER: LONG LIFE INSURANCE
P O Box 1010
INSURANCETOWN, US 98765
EMPLOYER: ANY COMPANY, INC.   (888) 555-1122
P O Box 1234
ANYTOWN, US 12345
MAIL FORM TO: LONG LIFE INSURANCE CO.
P O Box 1000
FOR ELIGIBILITY, PHONE: (800) 555-1212   INSURANCETOWN, US 98765

MAXIMUM: 1500 PER PERSON   PRE-DETERM: NOT MANDATORY
PERIOD: CALENDAR YEAR   ELECTRONIC CLAIMS: YES   ID# 65978
DEDUCT: 50 PER PERSON 150 PER FAMILY,   UNICLAIM: YES
             BASIC AND MAJOR   BENEFITS ASSIGNED: TO DENTIST WITH VALID
CARRYOVER DEDUCTIBLE: 3 MONTHS   ASSIGNMENT
PMT BASE: UCR BY AREA   DEPENDENT COVERAGE: TO AGE 19
                                                         TO AGE 23 FOR FULL-TIME STUDENTS
PREVENTIVE: 100%, X-RAYS PAID BASIC   LIMITED COORDINATION OF BENEFITS
BASIC: 80%, PERIO AND ENDO IS MAJOR   FMX: EVERY 36 MONTHS
MAJOR: 50%, WAIT 1 YEAR   SEND XRAYS: MAJOR, PERIO, ENDO, O.S.

———————————— LIMITS ON: CLEANING - SEALANTS - CROWNS - PROSTHETIC REPLACEMENT ————————————

LIMITS ON CLEANINGS: 2 PER 12 CONSECUTIVE MONTHS
LIMITS ON SEALANTS: SEE NOTES
FREE-STANDING CROWNS: PAID AT MAJOR, WAIT 1 YEAR
COVERS EXTRACTIONS PRIOR TO COVERAGE: YES, WAIT 1 YEAR
REQUIRED AGE OF REPLACED PROSTHETIC: 5 YEARS, WAIT 1 YEAR
DENTURE/PARTIAL REPLACEMENT LIMITATIONS: UNSERVICEABLE
CROWN AND BRIDGE REPLACEMENT LIMITATIONS: UNSERVICEABLE

———————————————————————— O R T H O ————————————————————————

ORTHO MAXIMUM: 1000 LIFETIME MAXIMUM
PERCENTAGE PAID: 50%
ORTHO DEDUCTIBLE: NO SEPARATE DEDUCTIBLE
AGE LIMITS: AGE 19
WAITING PERIOD: WAIT 1 YEAR
OTHER LIMITS: NONE

———————————————————— NOTES AND LIMITATIONS ————————————————————

SEALANTS PREVENTIVE TO AGE 16   PANOREX BY REPORT
SEALANTS PERMANENT MOLARS ONLY   POSTERIOR COMPOSITES PAID AS AMALGAMS
SEALANTS EVERY 4 YEARS   NIGHTGUARDS NOT COVERED
FLUORIDE PREVENTIVE TO AGE 19
FLUORIDE 1 PER YEAR
VERIFY WAITING PERIODS WITH ELIGIBILITY
CLAIMS PREVIOUSLY MAILED TO
TRAVELERS WITH GROUP GA118630

FIGURE 11-1
Insurance benefit information sheet. (Courtesy Trojan Professional Services, Inc., Los Alamitos, CA.)

TYPES OF INSURANCE INFORMATION REQUIRED

Maximum Coverage

Maximum coverage is the total dollar amount that an insurance company will pay during a year. It is important to determine when the year begins and ends. Most companies use a calendar year, but some use a fiscal year, which can be any 12-month period.

Deductible

Most patients must pay a set dollar amount toward treatment each year (the deductible) before the third party will consider payment for additional services. This deductible may be payable annually, during a lifetime, or as a family.

Percentage of Payment

Not all services are covered by insurance at the same percentages. Preventive procedures and services are covered at higher percentages than restorative and prosthetic services. It is very important to determine how each percentage is calculated (different percentages may be used to calculate different categories of service). The percentage of coverage is determined by the provisions of each insurance group and varies from group to group and from company to company. Some insurance policies have provisions that pay services at a higher percentage if the patient has followed the established protocol for preventive care. For example, during the first year the patient is covered, the insurance company may pay 70% of expenses. If the patient is seen in the dental practice for routine preventive care during the year, the policy can increase to 80% coverage for the second year. This type of coverage is referred to as an **incentive program.** Each year that the patient receives the approved type and frequency of preventive care, the percentage is raised, until he or she is covered at 100%. If the patient does not follow the guidelines, the percentage is dropped (never below the original amount).

Limitation to Coverage

To keep the costs of dental insurance down, most companies establish limitations to coverage. They will pay for basic dental services, but any work that is considered more than basic is limited, or is not a covered benefit. For example, if a patient wants to have porcelain crowns placed on posterior teeth, an insurance company may determine that the teeth can be restored with metal crowns (the use of porcelain crowns on posterior teeth is considered cosmetic). Patients who choose porcelain over metal are responsible for the difference in fees. These types of limitations must be discussed with patients before dental treatment is begun.

Eligibility

Sometimes, the administrative dental assistant will have to determine eligibility by contacting the insurance carrier and asking for verification. Eligibility can refer to the employer, patient, or dependent. It is not uncommon for employers to change their dental coverage yearly. A family who had dental coverage last year may have a different carrier this year, as well as different benefits. It is prudent to check eligibility often.

Preauthorization/Pretreatment

When a treatment exceeds a specified dollar amount, or if there is any question about the amount of coverage, it is wise to submit a pretreatment form (a requirement of some third party carriers). Once pretreatment approval has been obtained, a financial plan can be established between the dentist and the patient.

It is important to remember that the estimated amount of coverage is just that, an estimate. Some companies give an estimate of coverage and do not check the eligibility of the patient. Before actual treatment is begun, check with the insurance company and reconfirm that the patient is eligible for the treatment. Insurance companies calculate eligibility on a monthly basis. Eligibility is determined by the payment of policy premiums, continued employment, and remaining benefits. If any of these conditions have changed between the time the original claim was submitted for authorization and the date of actual treatment, the third party carrier may no longer be liable for payment for treatment.

REMEMBER

There should be no surprises: all work and financial responsibility must be disclosed before treatment.

METHODS OF FILING INSURANCE CLAIMS

Paper Dental Claim Forms

Paper dental claim forms are generated by computer and printed in the office or are typewritten by the assistant and sent from the dental office to the correct carrier via mail. The forms used should be approved by the ADA, as well as by the third party carrier.

REMEMBER

When ordering computerized dental claim forms, make sure that they are compatible with the dental software package.

Superbills and Encounter Forms

Superbills and **encounter forms** are used to communicate the same type of information that is contained on a dental insurance claim form. Each superbill or encounter form contains patient information, subscriber information, billing dentist information, and signatures for assignment of benefits and release of information. The purpose of the superbill is to consolidate several different functions of the business office onto one form. It provides a means by which to communicate what treatment procedures were completed and a method to track treatment (with routing slips); it is helpful in controlling the posting of dental procedures and services. It is also a quick method of supplying the patient with needed insurance information because the patient can use the superbill to bill the insurance company directly for services. Superbills are designed to be used with computer software programs and in manual posting systems (e.g., pegboard).

Encounter forms are used by third party carriers for reporting of services rendered to policyholders. These forms are similar to superbills and are preprinted for manual or computerized billing. The configuration of the information varies from carrier to carrier. Superbills and encounter forms are typically forms that consist of multiple copies for the patient, the dentist, and the insurance carrier.

When superbills and encounter forms are ordered for the first time, all dentist billing information and the codes to be included on the preprinted forms must be supplied. Most companies will help the dental practice design superbills and encounter forms to best meet its requirements.

Electronically Submitted Forms

Electronically submitted forms contain the same information as a paper dental claim form, except that they are "mailed" via electronic transfer. When documentation of dental services is ready to be submitted to an insurance company for payment or preauthorization, the software program will prepare the electronic dental claim form. If supporting documents are required, such as digital radiographic images, scanned documents, photographs, letters, and intraoral images, these are electronically attached and included with the dental claim form. There are many different insurance companies, and protocols vary for the submission of electronic dental claim forms; thus, electronic formatting of the submitted claims is required. Electronic claims are first sent to a clearinghouse that translates the submitted electronic claim and supporting documents into the required protocol that is used by the insurance company's computers. Although this sounds like a very difficult and time-consuming job, the process is very rapid because it is done electronically. Claims can be sent electronically from the office to the clearinghouse and translated and forwarded to the insurance company within seconds.

When supporting documents are requested for electronically submitted claims and they cannot be attached electronically (e.g., radiographs, models), the documents are assigned an identification number and are mailed to the insurance company.

The turnaround time (amount of time it takes to pay a claim) is much longer for paper claims than for electronic claims. All paper claims must first be opened in the mail room. From the mail room, claims are scanned and are entered into a computer databank or placed on microfiche (for the purpose of storage). They are then transferred to the claim center, where they are processed by insurance clerks. The turnaround time for a paper claim is about 1 week. Electronically submitted claims can be turned around in 1 to 2 days. Additional turnaround time can be avoided if the dental practice participates in a direct deposit program. Direct deposits are made from the insurance company into the checking account of the dental practice. Documentation is then forwarded to the dental practice to complete the bookkeeping process.

INSURANCE PAYMENTS

When insurance vouchers arrive at the office, they are attached to an Explanation of Benefits (EOB) form. EOBs identify the name of the patient and the group number or other identification number. Depending on the type of insurance and stipulations outlined in an insurance contract, the form may contain an adjustment of any fee that was charged that was over the allowed amount. Normally, the EOB is self-explanatory regarding the breakdown of payment. The total fee is listed, including the amount the insurance company pays and the amount the patient must pay.

Some companies list several patients on a single voucher, and care must be taken to post each patient correctly. Once the payment has been received, checked, and posted, the final step in the tracking system is completed. If a manual system is used, an entry is made in the insurance log, or the claim is pulled from the file and stapled to the EOB.

INSURANCE TRACKING SYSTEMS

The objective of an insurance tracking system is to monitor the status of insurance claims. It is easy to overlook unpaid claims if they are forgotten. Patients usually will not pay their portion until the insurance company pays. It is important to remember that the amount of money that flows through the dental practice depends on the amount of money that is billed to insurance companies. Each day that a claim goes unpaid, the dental practice loses money. Develop a routine that is easy to follow, and take the time to work the system. This will improve cash flow.

Computerized systems that process claims produce electronic forms for submission. Tracking is done through the computer. Once a claim has been marked for submission, it is placed in a databank. Reports can be generated that identify the patient, amount of the claim, date filed, and date paid. Processing of reports in the same manner as for the manual system allows the assistant to track all claims.

Following are helpful hints for insurance processing:

- Know the details of each insurance group, such as coverage, deductibles, limitations, and special handling instructions.
- Know the details of contracts with insurance companies for PPOs and HMOs.
- Use the appropriate fee schedule for each company (make sure the patient is charged the

Steps in an Insurance Tracking System

1. Place a copy of the dental claim form in a file for the month that the claim was generated. Each claim filed during a given month is kept in a single file.
2. When payment is received, the copy of the claim is pulled from the file and stapled to the EOB. If the claim has a secondary carrier, the information can be entered on the claim and forwarded to the second insurance carrier for payment. A copy of the secondary claim is placed in the insurance file for the current month.
3. After 1 month, review any remaining claims for that month. If necessary, track the claim and determine why it has not been paid. After 2 months, further tracking is necessary. Claims should never remain in the file for longer than 2 months without the assistant's knowledge. Sometimes, payment has been delayed because some information is missing. When additional information is sent, a notation should be made directly on the original dental claim form and in the patient's clinical record.
4. Place all paid claims in a file for the month in which the claim is paid (chronological filing system). These files can be stored in an area with easy access, in case they are needed during the year. If EOBs must be checked, they can be easily located by the date of payment. After 1 year, these files can be placed in permanent storage. Check the established recommendations for the amount of time that this type of record must be kept.

same fee that is submitted to the insurance company).
- Check each claim for accuracy. Procedures not listed will not be paid. If information is missing or the claim is not sent to the correct address, payment will be delayed.
- Develop a tracking system. Computer software programs will include functions to track the insurance billing from the time the claim is generated to the time it is paid. Sophisticated programs will also generate reports to identify unpaid claims or treatments that have not been billed.

- Work the tracking system to follow up on unpaid claims.
- Use the tracking system to help identify work that has been authorized but not completed.
- Bill patients for their portions upon receiving the insurance payment (do not wait for the monthly billing cycle to generate the first bill).
- Do not keep copies of dental claim forms in the clinical record. Copies of claims and EOBs should be kept in a separate file.

OTHER TYPES OF INSURANCE COVERAGE

Secondary Coverage

Often, patients have more than one insurance plan to cover their dental expenses. This occurs when husband and wife both have insurance coverage and the spouse is included in the policy. The person who is the patient is the primary carrier, and the spouse is the secondary carrier. The primary carrier is always billed before the secondary. The patient does not have the option to determine who is going to be the primary carrier.

Secondary coverage for children is determined by the gender rule or the birthday rule. The **gender rule** determines the primary and secondary coverage of the child by assigning primary coverage to the father and secondary to the mother. The **birthday rule** designates primary coverage to the parent whose birthday comes first in the year. Coverage can become very confusing when step-parents and parents with custody have dental insurance. It is advisable to check with the third party carrier to help determine who is considered primary.

Once the primary carrier pays, the secondary company is billed. When billing the secondary insurance company, send the same information that is contained in the first claim. In addition to the information asked on the dental claim form, a copy of the EOB is attached. The secondary insurance company will not pay more than the balance that was not paid by the primary carrier. It is hoped that the secondary carrier will pay the full amount not paid by the primary carrier. Because of stipulations in some insurance policies, this is not always the case, and care should be taken not to imply to the patient that the full amount will be paid by the carrier. Patients

with dual coverage (primary and secondary coverage) should check with their carriers before treatment if they have any questions regarding the amounts that will be paid.

Government Assistance

Government assistance programs are administered by the US government and by state and local governments. Special filing procedures and dental claim forms are used. Check with each state to determine available programs and correct protocols. Insurance companies that process claims hold seminars on how to file.

Workers' Compensation

Workers' Compensation programs cover employees who sustain dental injuries while working; these require special handling and authorization. Patients who have a work-related claim also must provide billing information. It is wise to contact the insurance carrier and receive clear instructions before any work is begun.

Auto Accidents

Similar to Workers' Compensation cases, cases involving auto accidents and auto insurance must be handled according to specific procedures. These must be determined before any treatment is provided.

Other Accidents

Some claims can be processed through medical insurance instead of dental insurance. Be sure that you understand all procedures involved before treatment is begun.

COMPLETING A DENTAL CLAIM FORM

There are two basic ways to file a dental claim form: the first is to mail the form (paper copy) directly to the insurance company, and the second is to send the claim electronically (see page 213). When a paper dental claim form is submitted, the form will be generated electronically or manually. The electronically prepared form will be generated by a software program, printed, and prepared for submission. The administrative assistant will check the dental claim form for completeness, obtain the necessary signatures, and attach documentation, if required. When it is necessary for the administrative assistant to complete the dental claim form (handwritten or typed), he or she must enter the information onto an approved claim form. It is the responsibility of the administrative dental assistant to know how to correctly complete the dental claim form. This requires an understanding of what information goes into each of the 58 specific data items on the form.

The ADA Dental Claim Form (Figure 11-2) is the form accepted by all insurance carriers in submitting dental treatment for preauthorization and payment. The form is organized into ten related sections, with a total of 58 data items (see Anatomy of a Dental Claim Form for detailed information of each of the data items).

Sections of the ADA Dental Claim Form

Header Information (1, 2)

The header contains information about the type of transaction; statement of actual treatment; predetermination/preauthorization; Early and Periodic Screening, Diagnosis and Treatment program (EPSDT); and the predetermination/preauthorization number.

Primary Payer Information (3)

Contains information about the insurance company, or the third party payer. If the patient is covered by more than one insurance company, the primary insurance company information is entered in this section.

Other Coverage (4–11)

Describes additional insurance coverage information. This may include additional dental or medical insurance coverage. The purpose of this section is to help the insurance company determine whether there is additional insurance and the need for coordination of benefits.

Primary Insured Information (12–17)

Contains information about the insured person (subscriber), who may or may not be the dental patient.

Patient Information (18–23)

Contains information about the patient.

Record of Services Provided (24–35)

This section records information about each of the services being submitted for payment or predetermination/preauthorization (do not enter dates for predetermination/preauthorization).

Authorization (36, 37)

This section requests the signature of the patient or guardian stating consent to the treatment plan, acceptance of financial responsibility, and permission to release protected health information (PHI) to the insurance company or third party payer. In addition, the subscriber signs to authorize the insurance company to send payment for treatment directly to the dentist or dental business entity.

Ancillary Claim/Treatment Information (38–47)

This section contains additional information needed by the insurance company or third party payer to determine patient coverage.

Billing Dentist or Dental Entity (48–52)

This section provides information about the individual dentist or dental entity that is submitting the claim for payment. The information may or may not pertain to the treating dentist. This section will not be completed if the patient is submitting the claim directly to the insurance company for payment.

Treating Dentist and Treatment Location Information (53–58)

The information in this section pertains to the dentist who has provided the treatment.

Before you begin the process of completing the dental claim form, you will need to gather specific information. This information will be found in the patient's record (see mock patient file folder in Chapter 7).

Text continued on p. 224

ADA. Dental Claim Form

HEADER INFORMATION

1. Type of Transaction (Check all applicable boxes)

☐ Statement of Actual Services   ☐ Request for Predetermination/Preauthorization

☐ EPSDT/Title XIX

2. Predetermination/Preauthorization Number

PRIMARY PAYER INFORMATION

3. Name, Address, City, State, Zip Code

OTHER COVERAGE

4. Other Dental or Medical Coverage?   ☐ No (Skip 5-11)   ☐ Yes (Complete 5-11)

5. Other Insured's Name (Last, First, Middle Initial, Suffix)

6. Date of Birth (MM/DD/CCYY)   7. Gender ☐M ☐F   8. Subscriber Identifier (SSN or ID#)

9. Plan/Group Number   10. Patient's Relationship to Other Insured (Check applicable box)   ☐ Self ☐ Spouse ☐ Dependent ☐ Other

11. Other Carrier Name, Address, City, State, Zip Code

PRIMARY INSURED INFORMATION

12. Name (Last, First, Middle Initial, Suffix), Address, City, State, Zip Code

13. Date of Birth (MM/DD/CCYY)   14. Gender ☐M ☐F   15. Subscriber Identifier (SSN or ID#)

16. Plan/Group Number   17. Employer Name

PATIENT INFORMATION

18. Relationship to Primary Insured (Check applicable box)   ☐ Self ☐ Spouse ☐ Dependent Child ☐ Other

19. Student Status   ☐ FTS   ☐ PTS

20. Name (Last, First, Middle Initial, Suffix), Address, City, State, Zip Code

21. Date of Birth (MM/DD/CCYY)   22. Gender ☐M ☐F   23. Patient ID/Account # (Assigned by Dentist)

RECORD OF SERVICES PROVIDED

	24. Procedure Date (MM/DD/CCYY)	25. Area of Oral Cavity	26. Tooth System	27. Tooth Number(s) or Letter(s)	28. Tooth Surface	29. Procedure Code	30. Description	31. Fee
1								
2								
3								
4								
5								
6								
7								
8								
9								
10								

MISSING TEETH INFORMATION

34. (Place an 'X' on each missing tooth)

Permanent: 1 2 3 4 5 6 7 8 9 10 11 12 13 14 15 16 / 32 31 30 29 28 27 26 25 24 23 22 21 20 19 18 17

Primary: A B C D E F G H I J / T S R Q P O N M L K

32. Other Fee(s)

33. Total Fee

35. Remarks

AUTHORIZATIONS

36. I have been informed of the treatment plan and associated fees. I agree to be responsible for all charges for dental services and materials not paid by my dental benefit plan, unless prohibited by law, or the treating dentist or dental practice has a contractual agreement with my plan prohibiting all or a portion of such charges. To the extent permitted by law, I consent to your use and disclosure of my protected health information to carry out payment activities in connection with this claim.

X_____

Patient/Guardian signature   Date

37. I hereby authorize and direct payment of the dental benefits otherwise payable to me, directly to the below named dentist or dental entity.

X_____

Subscriber signature   Date

ANCILLARY CLAIM/TREATMENT INFORMATION

38. Place of Treatment (Check applicable box)   ☐ Provider's Office ☐ Hospital ☐ ECF ☐ Other

39. Number of Enclosures (00 to 99)   Radiograph(s)   Oral Image(s)   Model(s)

40. Is Treatment for Orthodontics?   ☐ No (Skip 41-42)   ☐ Yes (Complete 41-42)

41. Date Appliance Placed (MM/DD/CCYY)

42. Months of Treatment Remaining   43. Replacement of Prosthesis? ☐ No ☐ Yes (Complete 44)   44. Date Prior Placement (MM/DD/CCYY)

45. Treatment Resulting from (Check applicable box)   ☐ Occupational illness/injury   ☐ Auto accident   ☐ Other accident

46. Date of Accident (MM/DD/CCYY)   47. Auto Accident State

BILLING DENTIST OR DENTAL ENTITY (Leave blank if dentist or dental entity is not submitting claim on behalf of the patient or insured/subscriber)

48. Name, Address, City, State, Zip Code

49. Provider ID   50. License Number   51. SSN or TIN

52. Phone Number (   )

TREATING DENTIST AND TREATMENT LOCATION INFORMATION

53. I hereby certify that the procedures as indicated by date are in progress (for procedures that require multiple visits) or have been completed and that the fees submitted are the actual fees I have charged and intend to collect for those procedures.

X_____

Signed (Treating Dentist)   Date

54. Provider ID   55. License Number

56. Address, City, State, Zip Code

57. Phone Number (   )   58. Treating Provider Specialty

©2002, 2004 American Dental Association
J515 (Same as ADA Dental Claim Form – J516, J517, J518, J519)

Cat. #590154 Rev. 2-05

FIGURE 11-2

Dental claim form. (Courtesy The American Dental Association, Chicago, IL.)

ANATOMY OF A DENTAL CLAIM FORM

ADA Dental Claim Form

HEADER INFORMATION

1. Type of Transaction (Check all applicable boxes)

☐ Statement of Actual Services   ☐ Request for Predetermination/Preauthorization

☐ EPSDT/Title XIX   **(1)**

2. Predetermination/Preauthorization Number   **(2)**

HEADER INFORMATION

(1) **Type of Transaction (Check all applicable boxes):**
Statement of Actual Services: This box is checked when the services listed have been completed.
Request for Predetermination/Preauthorization: This box is used to request an estimate of dental benefits before treatment begins. Some insurance carriers ask that all treatment for a specified procedure or dollar amount be submitted. It is best to have complete information about the insurance coverage before treatment is started in order to make financial arrangements with the patient. **REMEMBER:** *There should be no surprises — insurance coverage and patient financial responsibility must be disclosed and agreed upon before treatment begins.*

CAUTION: Pre-estimate figures are not a guarantee of payment by the insurance carrier. The final payment may change due to previous unpaid claims and current enrollment status of the patient.
EPSDT/Title XIX: This box is checked if the patient is part of a *special* program through the Early and Periodic Screening, Diagnosis, and Treatment Program.

(2) **Predetermination/Preauthorization Number:** This box is used when a claim has been previously preauthorized and you are now submitting it for payment. The preauthorization number will be provided by the insurance company.

PRIMARY PAYER INFORMATION

3. Name, Address, City, State, Zip Code

Cigna   **(3)**
P.O. Box 467
Denver CO 76452

PRIMARY PAYER INFORMATION

(3) **Name, Address, City, State, Zip Code:** This item must always be completed. The information is provided by the patient and will be used to mail the insurance claim form to the insurance company. If the patient is covered by more than one insurance plan, this information will be for the primary carrier. **REMEMBER:** *Each insurance company may have several different offices that process claims. Check the patient's insurance identification card for the correct billing address.*

OTHER COVERAGE

4. Other Dental or Medical Coverage?   ☐ No (Skip 5-11)   ☒ Yes (Complete 5-11)   **(4)**

5. Other Insured's Name (Last, First, Middle Initial, Suffix)

(5)   Rogers, Doris

6. Date of Birth (MM/DD/CCYY)   **(6)** 12/02/1950

7. Gender   **(7)**   ☐ M ☒ F

8. Subscriber Identifier (SSN or ID#)   632-24-7654   **(8)**

9. Plan/Group Number   **(9)** 63467

10. Patient's Relationship to Other Insured (Check applicable box)   ☐ Self   ☐ Spouse   ☒ Dependent   ☐ Other   **(10)**

11. Other Carrier Name, Address, City, State, Zip Code

Delta Dental   **(11)**
P.O. Box 3333
San Francisco CA 90234

OTHER COVERAGE

④ Other Dental or Medical Coverage:
No (Skip 5-11): If there is not any additional coverage you can skip the completion of data items 5-11.
Yes (Complete 5-11): If this box is checked you will need to complete data items 5-11. This information is used to determine primary coverage liability when multiple coverage is indicated.

⑤ Other Insured's Name (Last, First, Middle Initial, Suffix):
In this box you will identify the person who has additional dental or medical insurance. The additional coverage could be through a spouse, domestic partner or, if a child, through both parents. In some cases the secondary coverage could be through a second policy of the patient.

⑥ Date of Birth (MM/DD/CCYY): The birth date entered pertains to the person identified in Item 5. Enter the full date (eight digits): two for the month, two for the day of the month, and four for the year.

⑦ Gender: Enter the gender for the person identified in Item 5.

⑧ Subscriber Identifier (SSN or ID#): Enter the number that has been assigned to the subscriber (Item 5) by the insurance carrier. **REMEMBER:** You must use the number issued by the insurance company. The use of the SSN may not be permitted as an identifier in some states.

⑨ Plan/Group Number: Enter the group plan or policy number of the person in Item 5. This number will be on the patient's insurance card.

⑩ Patient's Relationship to Other Insured (Check applicable box): Enter the relationship between the person identified in Item 5 and the patient.

⑪ Other Carrier Name, Address, City, State, Zip Code:
Enter the information for the insurance carrier of the person identified in Item 5.

PRIMARY INSURED INFORMATION

12. Name (Last, First, Middle Initial, Suffix), Address, City, State, Zip Code

Rogers, Donald S
8176 Hillside Dirve
Riverville CA 90070   ⑫

13. Date of Birth (MM/DD/CCYY) ⑬ 02/08/1947	14. Gender ⑭ ☒ M ☐ F	15. Subscriber Identifier (SSN or ID#) ⑮ 012-34-5678
16. Plan/Group Number 43216 ⑯	17. Employer Name Riverville Police Department ⑰	

PRIMARY INSURED INFORMATION

⑫ Name (Last, First, Middle Initial, Suffix), Address, City, State, Zip Code: Enter the full name and address of the primary insured (employee).

⑬ Date of Birth (MM/DD/CCYY): This is the birth date of the insured, identified in item #12 (this may or may not be the patient). Enter the full date (eight digits): two for the month, two for the day of the month, and four for the year.

⑭ Gender: This information applies to the insured, identified in item #12 (who may or may not be the patient).

⑮ Subscriber Identifier (SSN or ID#): Enter the assigned identifier issued by the insurance company. This information will be located on the patient's insurance identification card.

⑯ Plan/Group Number: Enter the plan or group number of the primary insurance company. This information will be located on the patient's insurance identification card.

⑰ Employer Name: If applicable, enter the name of the insured's employer.

PATIENT INFORMATION

18. Relationship to Primary Insured (Check applicable box) (18)   **19. Student Status** (19)

[ ] Sell   [ ] Spouse   [X] Dependent Child   [ ] Other   [X] FTS   [ ] PTS

20. Name (Last, First, Middle Initial, Suffix), Address, City, State, Zip Code

Roges, Jason
8176 Hillside Drive
Riverville CA 90070   (20)

21. Date of Birth (MM/DD/CCYY)	22. Gender (22)	23. Patient ID/Account # (Assigned by Dentist)
(21) 03/12/1980	[X] M [ ] F	(23) R349877

PATIENT INFORMATION

(18) Relationship to Primary Insured (Check applicable box):
Check the box that identifies the relationship of the primary insured to the patient. If the patient is also the insured, check the "Self" box and skip to item #23.

(19) Student Status:
Check the box that identifies the dependent student as an FTS (full-time student) or PTS (part-time student). With most insurance policies this box does not pertain to dependents less than 18 years of age. If neither applies you can skip to item #20.

(20) Name (Last, First, Middle Initial, Suffix), Address, City, State, Zip Code: Enter the complete name of the patient.

(21) Date of Birth (MM/DD/CCYY):
This is the birth date of the patient identified in item 20. Enter the full date (total of eight digits): two for the month, two for the day of the month, and four for the year.

(22) Gender:
This information applies to the patient.

(23) Patient ID/Account # (Assigned by Dentist):
Enter the patient ID# that has been assigned by the dental practice (this is not required to process the claim).

RECORD OF SERVICES PROVIDED

	24. Procedure Date (MM/DD/CCYY)	25. Area of Oral Cavity	26. Tooth System	27. Tooth Number(s) or Letter(s)	28. Tooth Surface	29. Procedure Code	30. Description	31. Fee
1	12/10/2006	10				D0220	Periapical First Film	$40:00
2	12/10/2006	20				D0230	Additional Film	$28:00
3	12/10/2006	00				D1110	Prophylaxis	$93:00
4	12/18/2006		JP	2	MO	D2150	Amalgam	$92:00
5	12/18/2006		JP	7		D2720	Crown-Resin /High Noble	$435:00
6								
7								
8								
9								
10								

MISSING TEETH INFORMATIOIN

Permanent / Primary

34. (Place an 'X' on each missing tooth) (34)

Permanent: X 2 3 4 5 6 7 8 9 10 11 12 13 14 15 X
32 31 30 29 28 27 26 25 24 23 22 21 20 19 18 X

Primary: A B C D E F G H I J
T S R Q P O N M L K

32. Other Fee(s) (32)	
33. Total Fee (33)	$688:00

35. Remarks (35)

RECORD OF SERVICES PROVIDED

NOTE: Items 24-31 apply to each dental service and will be repeated if multiple services are being billed. There is space for 10 services on each dental claim form; if additional space is needed it will be necessary to complete additional claim forms. Each additional claim form will need to be fully completed (all information will be repeated on the second claim form).

(24) Procedure Date (MM/DD/CCYY):
Enter the date for each completed procedure. Enter the full date (eight digits): two for the month, two for the day of the month, and four for the year. If the claim is for preauthorization the date is left blank.
Remember: *You cannot combine "actual services" and a request for "predetermination/preauthorization" on the same dental claim form.*

(25) Area of Oral Cavity: The use of this data item will depend on the type of service or procedure being reported. You will not need to complete this item if:
• The procedure requires the identification of a tooth number, or a range of teeth.
• The procedure identifies a specific area. For example, complete denture—mandibular
• The procedure does not relate to any portion of the oral cavity. For example, sedation/general anesthesia.

Two-digit Codes Used to Identify Specific Areas of the Oral Cavity	
Code	**Area of Oral Cavity**
00	Entire oral cavity
01	Maxillary arch
02	Mandibular arch
10	Upper right quadrant
20	Upper left quadrant
30	Lower left quadrant
40	Lower right quadrant

26 **Tooth System:** Enter "JP" when the tooth designation system being used is the ADA's Universal/National Tooth Designation System (1-32 for permanent dentition and A-T for primary dentition). Enter "JO" when using the International Standards Organization System (see Chapter 2 for full details of the various tooth designation systems).

27 **Tooth Number(s) or Letter(s):** Enter the number or range of numbers that applies to the procedure. If the procedure does not involve a specific tooth or range of teeth leave item #27 blank.
REMEMBER: *If the same procedure has been completed more than one time, each repeated procedure will have to be entered on a separate line.* When entering a range of teeth numbers (and it is appropriate to enter them on the same line) the teeth numbers can be separated with a comma, for example: 2,3,5, or for a continual range of numbers 3-6.

28 **Tooth Surface:** When a procedure requires that the tooth surface be identified, the following is a list of the single abbreviations (see Chapter 2 for a complete list of tooth surfaces)

Surface	Code
Buccal	B
Distal	D
Facial (or Labial)	F
Incisal	I
Lingual	L
Mesial	M
Occlusal	O

29 **Procedure Code:** Enter the appropriate procedure code found in the latest version of the *Code on Dental Procedures and Nomenclature.*

30 **Description:** Briefly describe the service. You can abbreviate the description. CAUTION: Use standard abbreviations that are common with dental terminology.

HIPAA

Code on Dental Procedures and Nomenclature lists the code sets that are recognized by HIPAA for the electronic submission of dental claims.

REMEMBER

Incorrect coding causing an overpayment of services is an act of fraud.

31 **Fee:** Enter the full fee charges by the dentist.

32 **Other Fee(s):** Enter other charges that may be applicable to the dental service. Charges may include state tax and other charges imposed by regulatory bodies.

33 **Total Fee:** The sum of all fees from lines in item #31, plus any fee(s) entered in item #32.

34 **Missing Teeth Information:** Chart missing teeth when reporting periodontal, prosthodontic (fixed and removable), or implant procedures.

35 **Remarks:** Enter additional information for procedure codes that require a report, or when you believe additional information will help in the processing of the claim (for example, the amount the primary carrier paid on the claim).

AUTHORIZATIONS

36. I have been informed of the treatment plan and associated fees. I agree to be responsible for all charges for dental services and materials not paid by my dental benefit plan. unless prohibited by law, or the treating dentist or dental practice has a contractual agreement with my plan prohibiting all or a portion of such charges. To the extent permitted by law, I consent to your use and disclosure of my protected health information to carry out payment activities in connection with this claim.

X _Jason Rogers_   **36**   _12-18-06_
Patient/Guardian signature   Date

37. I hereby authorize and direct payment of the dental benefits otherwise payable to me, directly to the below named dentist or dental entity.

X _Donald Rogers_   **37**   _12-18-06_
Subscriber signature   Date

AUTHORIZATIONS

36 **Patient Consent:** The patient, or patient's parent, caretaker, guardian, or other individual as appropriate under state law, must sign the form stating that they have been informed of the treatment, accept financial responsibility, and have established a professional relationship with the dentist for the delivery of dental health care.

37 **Insured's Signature:**
The signature and date, or signature on file, is required when the insured wishes to have benefits paid directly to the dentist.

HIPAA

Privacy Rule

The patient authorizes release of PHI to the insurance company for the purpose of processing the insurance claim.

ANCILLARY CLAIM/TREATMENT INFORMATION

38. Place of Treatment (Check applicable box) **38**	39. Number of Enclosures (00 to 99) **39**

38. Place of Treatment (Check applicable box) **38**
[X] Provider's Office [ ] Hospital [ ] ECF [ ] Other

39. Number of Enclosures (00 to 99) **39**
Radiograph(s) [02] Oral Image(s) [01] Model(s) [00]

40. Is Treatment for orthodontics? **40**
[ ] No (Skip 41-42) [ ] Yes (Complete 41-42)

41. Date Appliance Placed (MM/DD/CCYY) **41**

42. Months of Treament Remaining **42**

43. Replacement of Prosthesis **43**
[ ] No [X] Yes (Complete 44)

44. Date Prior Placement (MM/DD/CCYY) **44**
02/14/2000

45. Treatment Resulting from (Check applicable box) **45**
[ ] Occupational illness/injury [ ] Auto accident [ ] Other accident

46. Date of Accident (MM/DD/CCYY) **46**

47. Auto Accident State **47**

ANCILLARY CLAIM/TREATMENT INFORMATION

38 **Place of Treatment (Check applicable box):**
Check the box that identifies the location of the dental treatment.

39 **Number of Enclosures (00 to 99):**
This item is completed whether or not radiographs, oral images, or study models are submitted with the claim. The rationale for entering the information in the box is to alert the insurance company that information was (or was not) included with the claim. Two digits will be entered in the box; if less than 10 is entered, 0 is used in the first position (02). **Radiograph(s).** When procedures require that radiographs be sent, attach to the claim and enter the number in the box (if none are sent, enter 00) **Oral Image(s).** Include digital radiographic images and photographs. Enter the number of images submitted with the claim (if none, enter 00). **Model(s).** When models are included with the claim, enter the number in the box (if none are sent, enter 00). **REMEMBER:** *If claims are electronically submitted, follow the guidelines established by the insurance carrier for the submission of supplemental material.*

40 **Is Treatment for Orthodontics:**
No (Skip 41 and 42): If the treatment is not for orthodontics check the box and skip to item #43.
Yes (Complete 41 and 42): If this box is checked you will need to complete data items 41 and 42.

41 **Date Appliance Placed (MM/DD/CCYY):**
Indicate the date an orthodontic appliance was placed. This information should also be reported in this section for later orthodontic visits.

42 **Months of Treatment Remaining:**
Enter the estimated number of months required to complete the orthodontic treatment.

43 **Replacement of Prosthesis?:**
This item applies to crowns and all fixed or removable prostheses (bridges and dentures). There are three statements to guide in the completion of the item.
   1. If the claim **does not involve a prosthetic restoration**, *mark the box NO* and proceed to item #45.
   2. If the claim is the **initial placement** of a crown or a fixed or removable prosthesis, *mark the box NO* and proceed to item #45.
   3. If the patient **previously had these teeth replaced** by a crown or a fixed or removable prosthesis, *mark the box YES* and complete item #44.

44 **Date of Prior Placement (MM/DD/CCYY):**
Enter the date of the prior placement of the crown or the fixed or removable prosthesis.

45 **Treatment Resulting From (Check applicable box):**
If the dental treatment is the result of an accident or injury, check the applicable box and complete items #46 and #47. If the dental treatment is not the result of an accident or injury, this item does not apply; proceed to item #48.

46 **Date of Accident (MM/DD/CCYY):**
Enter the date of the accident or injury.

47 **Auto Accident State:**
If the accident was an auto accident (item #45), enter the state in which the auto accident occurred. If not an auto accident, leave item #47 blank.

BILLING DENTIST OR DENTAL ENTITY (leave blank if dentist or dental entity is not submitting claim on behalf of the patient or insured/subscriber)

48. Name, Address, City, State, Zip Code **48**
Canyon View Dental
4546 North Avery Way
Canyon View CA 91783

49. Provider ID **49**
DDS34569

50. License Number **50**
CA123567

51. SSN or TIN **51**
95-7689321

52. Phone Number (000) 555-8976 **52**

© 2002, 20004 American Dental Association
J515 (Same as ADA Dental Claim Form = J516, J517, J518, J519)

BILLING DENTIST OR DENTAL ENTITY
If the patient is submitting the dental claim form directly and has not signed item #37, do not complete items 48-52.

48 **Name, Address, City, State, and Zip Code:**
Enter the information of the billing dentist or dental entity.

49 **Provider ID:**
Enter the provider identifier assigned to the billing dentist or dental entity. This number **is not** an SSN or TIN number. The identifier is assigned by the Insurance company or third party payer. This item can be left blank if an identifier has not been assigned.

IIIPAA

National Provider Identifier (NPI)

Beginning as early as May 23, 2005 providers will be eligible to apply for their NPI. All HIPAA-covered entities must use NPIs by the compliance dates: May 23, 2007 for most groups and May 23, 2008 for small health plans. The personal NPI will be the only allowable identifier (accepted by all insurance companies and third party payers) and must be included on all claims submissions.

50 **License Number:**
Enter the license number of the billing dentist. If a dental entity is entered in item #48, leave this item blank.

51 **SSN or TIN:**
   1. If the billing dentist is an individual (unincorporated) enter the SSN or TIN.
   2. Enter the TIN if the individual dentist is incorporated or billing for an incorporated dental entity.
   3. Enter the TIN if the billing dentist or dental entity is a group practice or dental clinic.

52 **Phone Number:**
Enter the business phone number of the billing dentist or dental entity.

TREATING DENTIST AND TREATMENT LOCATION INFORMATION

53. I hereby certify that the procedures as indicated by date are in progress (for procedures that require multiple visits) or have been completed and that the fees submitted are the actual fees I have charged and intend to collect for those procedures.   **53**

X _____ *Mary Edwards* _____   *12-22-06*
Sighed (Treating Dentist)   Date

| 54. Provider ID **54** DDS89765 | 55. License Number **55** CA7834983 |

56. Address, City, State, Zip Code

4546 North Avery Way
Canyon View CA 91783   **56**

| 57. Phone Number (**000**) **57** 555-8976 | 58. Treatling Provider Specialty **58** 122300000X |

TREATING DENTIST AND TREATMENT LOCATION INFORMATION

53 **Certification:**
Have the treating dentist (can be different from the billing dentist) sign the certification statement. By signing the certification the treating dentist is verifying the following:
   1. The procedures and services listed on the claim have been completed or are in progress.
   2. The fee submitted is the actual fee charged and will be the fee collected for the procedures.

54 **Provider ID:** Enter the provider identifier assigned to the treating dentist. This number is not an SSN or TIN number. The identifier is assigned by the insurance company or third party payer. This item can be left blank if an identifier has not been assigned.

55 **License Number:**
Enter the license number of the treating dentist.

56 **Address, City, State, and Zip Code:**
Enter the mailing address of the treating dentist.

57 **Phone Number:**
Enter the business telephone number of the treating dentist.

58 **Treating Provider Specialty:**
Enter the number that identifies the treating dentist. The following list is a code set that has been assigned to members of the dental healthcare team. The code comes from the ***Dental Service Providers'*** section of the ***Healthcare Providers Taxonomy Code*** list used in all HIPAA transactions.

The Provider Taxonomy is a unique alphanumeric code, ten characters in length. The code list is structured into three distinct "Levels" including Provider Type, Classification, and Area of Specialization. (See page 224.)

Dental Provider Toxonomy

Dental Providers
- Dental Assistant - **126800000X**
- Dental Hygienist - **124Q00000X**
- Dental Laboratory Technician - **126900000X**
- Dentist - **122300000X**
  - Dental Public Health - **1223D0001X**
  - Endodontics - **1223E0200X**
  - General Practice - **1223G0001X**
  - Oral and Maxillofacial Pathology - **1223 P0106X**
- Oral and Maxillofacial Radiology - **1223 X0008X**
- Oral and Maxillofacial Surgery - **1223 S0112X**
- Orthodontics and Dentofacial Orthopedics - **1223X0400X**
  - Pediatric Dentistry - **1223P0221X**
  - Periodontics - **1223P0300X**
  - Prosthodontics - **1223P0700X**
- Denturist - **122400000X**

Steps in Processing a Dental Claim Form

1. *Obtain information from the patient.* Have the patient complete the *registration* form, and check for completeness. Also, photocopy and check the patient's insurance card. The card provides information such as an ID number, group number, and billing addresses for claims.
2. *Verify coverage* by contacting the insurance carrier, consulting an insurance information service, or using the office blue book (computerized or manual).
3. *Discuss the coverage with the patient, and determine the patient's portion.* Stress that the patient is responsible for the full amount if the insurance company does not pay. File the treatment plan for preauthorization if required by the patient or the insurance company.
4. *Complete the dental claim form.* If submitting a paper claim, complete the dental claim form for completed dental procedures (use the patients chart to identify completed treatment). Check the form for accuracy, and make sure that the correct codes have been used and that all treatments have been listed. When submitting electronic claims, confirm the dental procedures and check the dental claim form for completeness, making sure all data items have been completed.
5. *Include documentation* such as radiographs, oral images, models, or pocket measurements as requested by the insurance company. If you are not sure what needs to be included, check the insurance handbook, call the insurance company, or check with the insurance information service. When you submit electronically, follow the protocol of the insurance company for needed documentation.
6. *Record in the patient's clinical record* the date the claim was submitted and the treatment included.
7. *Record the information into a tracking system.* A tracking system helps to organize insurance information and provides a means for the administrative dental assistant to check on the status of claims.
8. *Post insurance payments, and bill the patient for the balance.* If an adjustment must be made, it is done at this time. For example, a claim filed with Delta Dental is over the preset fee schedule for a prophylaxis. According to the contract, you cannot charge the patient the difference; therefore, adjust the disallowed amount from the patient's balance.

REMEMBER

You cannot write off the patient balance.

9. *Record the payment in your tracking system.* When a claim has been paid, it should be removed from the tracking system. Develop a method to flag claims that have both primary and secondary insurance carriers. It is necessary to enter the amount paid by the primary carrier before billing the secondary insurance.
10. *Follow up on any unpaid claims within 30 days of submission.* The purpose of the tracking system is to ensure that claims are not forgotten when they are not paid. The longer you wait to follow up, the longer it will take the dentist to receive a payment.

REMEMBER

The dentist has a legal and ethical obligation in the submission of dental claims. Review The ADA Principles of Ethics and Code of Professional Conduct (page 201).

FRAUDULENT INSURANCE BILLING

No matter what the intention, when false information is given on a dental claim form, it becomes a concern to the dentist, the insurance carrier, and the patient. The ADA addresses this issue in section 5B of its Principles of Ethics and Code of Professional Conduct with official advisory opinions revised to January 2005.

5.B. Representation of Fees

Dentist shall not represent the fees being charged for providing care in a false or misleading manner.

Advisory Opinions

5.B.1 Waiver of Copayment

A dentist who accepts a third party* payment under a copayment plan as payment in full without disclosing to the third party that the patient's payment portion will not be collected is engaged in overbilling. The essence of this ethical impropriety is deception and misrepresentation; an overbilling dentist makes it appear to the third party that the charge to the patient for services rendered is higher than it actually is. (A third party is any party to a dental prepayment contract that may collect premiums, assume financial risks, pay claims, and/or provide administrative services.)

5.B.2 Overbilling

It is unethical for a dentist to increase a fee to a patient solely because the patient is covered under a dental benefits plan.

5.B.3 Fee Differential

Payments accepted by a dentist under a governmentally funded program, a component or constituent dental society sponsored access program, or a participating agreement entered into under a program of a third party shall not be considered as evidence of overbilling in determining whether a charge to a patient, or to another third party in behalf of a patient not covered under any of the aforcited programs, constitutes overbilling under this section of the Code.

5.B.4 Treatment Dates

A dentist who submits to a third party while reporting incorrect treatment dates for the purpose of assisting a patient in obtaining benefits under a dental plan, which benefits would otherwise be disallowed, is engaged in making an unethical, false, or misleading representation to such third party.

5.B.5 Dental Procedures

A dentist who incorrectly describes to a third party a dental procedure in order to receive a greater payment or reimbursement or incorrectly makes a noncovered procedure appear to be a covered procedure on such a claim form is engaged in making an unethical, false, or misleading representation to such third party.

5.B.6 Unnecessary Services

A dentist who recommends and performs unnecessary dental services or procedures is engaged in unethical conduct.

KEY POINTS

- Dental insurance processing requires an understanding of different types of insurance coverage (insurance plans), insurance terminology, and effective insurance coding.
- Insurance coding is accomplished by reference to the current *CDT Users Manual*. This Manual provides standardized claim forms, procedure codes, and nomenclature. The codes are divided into 12 categories, and each category is subdivided into specific procedures.
- To determine each patient's insurance coverage, you must identify the insurance carrier and the details of the coverage, including:
  - Maximum coverage
  - Type of deductible
  - Percentage of payment
  - Limitation to coverage

- Eligibility
- Preauthorization/pretreatment specifications
- Forms for filing insurance claims include paper claims (manually and computer generated), superbills, encounter forms, and electronically submitted forms. Manual and electronic tracking systems monitor the status of each claim. This helps the administrative dental assistant to locate and follow up on unpaid claims.
- A correctly completed dental claim form will contain all information requested in each data item. This information is taken from the patient's clinical chart (review the clinical chart in Chapter 7).

Web Watch

Discussion of Dental Benefits for Consumers

http://www.toothinfo.com/ibsplit.htm

Consumer Guide to Dental Insurance

http://www.cda.org/public/dentalcare/consumer.htm

 Log on to Evolve to access additional web links!

http://evolve.elsevier.com

Critical Thinking Questions

Based on the information given in the boxes for Jason Rogers, complete the following exercises:

1. List the information you would place on an the attending dentist's claim form for the following boxes: 8, 12, 18, 19, 20, 21, 22, 28, 31, 32, 33, 34, 37, and total fee. The policy uses the birthday rule.
2. Correctly code the treatments listed for Jason.

Personal Information

Birth date	3-12-80
Soc. Sec. #	321-68-2173
Name	Jason Rogers
Sex	Male
Address	8176 Hillside Drive, Riverville, CA
Employer	Full Time Student, UCLA

Responsible Party

Name	Donald Rogers
Relationship to Patient	Father
Birth Date	2/8/47
Address	8176 Hillside Drive, Riverville, CA
Employer	Riverville Police Department
Occupation	Captain
Work Phone	261-324-9111
Home Phone	261-483-6217

Dental Insurance Information

Name of Insured	Donald Rogers
Relationship to Patient	Father
Insurer's Birth Date	12/8/47
Soc. Sec. #	012-34-5678
Employer	Riverville Police Department
Date Employed	Jan. 1970
Occupation	Police Captain
Insurance Company	Northwest
Group #	43216
Employee Certificate #	7321456790
Ins. Co. Address	P.O. Box 467, Denver, CO
Max. Annual Benefit	$2000.00

Additional Dental Insurance Information

Name of Insured	Doris Rogers
Relationship to Patient	Mother
Insurer's Birth Date	12/2/50
Soc. Sec. #	632-24-7654
Employer	Riverville School District
Date Employed	Sept. 1981
Occupation	Teacher
Insurance Company	Delta Dental
Group #	634567
Employee Certificate #	632-24-7654
Ins. Co. Address	P.O. Box 3333, San Francisco, CA
Max. Annual Benefit	$1500.00

Treatment

Date	Tooth and Surface	Treatment	Fee
2/10/06		3 Periapical X-rays	40.00
2/10/06	2 MO	Amalgam	92.00
2/10/06	3 O	Amalgam	81.00
2/10/06	4 MOD	Amalgam	108.00
2/24/06	8 MI	Composite	140.00
2/24/06	9 M	Composite	110.00
3/8/06	17	Extraction Full Bony Impaction	195.00
3/8/06	18	Extraction Partially Bony	110.00

OUTLINE

KEY TERMS AND CONCEPTS

Back Order
Consumable Supplies and Products
Disposable
Expendable Products

Hazardous Communication Program
Lead Time
Major Equipment
Material Safety Data Sheet

Nonconsumable Products
Products
Rate of Use
Supplies

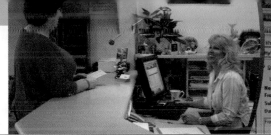

12

Inventory Management

LEARNING OBJECTIVES

The student will:

1. List the information needed to order supplies and products, and discuss how this information will be used. Define rate of use and lead time.
2. Describe the role of an inventory manager.
3. Analyze the elements of a good inventory management system, and describe how elements relate to the organization and overall effectiveness of a dental practice.
4. Compare the advantages and disadvantages of catalog ordering and supply house

services. Discuss when it is appropriate to use the two services.
5. List the information that should be considered before an order is placed for supplies and products.
6. Describe the various sections of a Material Safety Data Sheet, and discuss what information is important to an inventory manager.

INTRODUCTION

Ordering and managing supplies in a dental practice requires organization, communication, and the cooperation of the entire dental healthcare team. Inventory control is not limited to supplies in the clinical area. Those in the laboratory and business office must be managed as well. Tempers flare and frustration levels climb when needed supplies are not readily available. To ease tensions between team members, a systematic and well-organized inventory management system must be implemented and practiced.

INVENTORY MANAGEMENT SYSTEMS

Like any system, the one that works the best is the one that everyone will use. When a well-organized and well-defined system is in place, it is easy to know when products and supplies have to be ordered, who will order, and how long it will take to receive the order. Several different types of inventory management systems are available—both computerized and manual.

Computerized Inventory Management Systems

Computers and online services now allow dental practices to be linked directly to a supply house. Because it is directly linked to the database of a large supply house, a small dental practice has access to a much larger system for the management of inventory. If bar codes are used, the staff can scan supplies as they are used and the system will keep track of stock on hand. At the predetermined reorder point, the system will automatically produce a report that identifies the supplies needed. It is then possible, with the simple click of a mouse, to reorder the supplies.

The use of an in-house computer system also allows for the tracking and control of inventory. Practice management systems are designed with a database that the assistant can use to record supplies and products used and to track their consumption. This software will predetermine reorder points and generate order lists for sales representatives. When supplies are received, the information is entered into the system to complete the manage-

ment procedure. A computer system can be used only for the tasks that it is programmed to perform with the data that have been entered. If you are working with a very limited program that has not been designed to perform all tasks required to track and record inventory, it will be of little use to the dental practice without some other method such as a manual system.

Manual Inventory Management Systems

Without the use of a computer or in conjunction with a limited computer program, manual systems can be used. A manual system is effective but in most cases is far more time consuming than a good computer program.

A simple card index system can be used to track the use of supplies and products (Figure 12-1). An index card is formatted to include all the vital information needed to track and reorder the correct supplies and products.

Information Needed for Ordering
• Name of product (generic)
• Brand name
• Supplier (vendor)
• Telephone number, fax number
• Minimum or maximum number to be ordered
• Amount and date of order
• Unit price

Determining Reorder Points

One of the most important tasks in inventory management is the determination of when a supply or product has to be ordered. If inventory is not properly maintained, you may often find that you have run low or are out of a needed product. To prevent this, a critical part of inventory management is to tag, track, or otherwise identify when it is time to reorder.

Manual systems use a form of identification to flag a supply or product when it is time to reorder. This can be a small card, a tag, or colored tape. When the supply or product that has been flagged is removed from the inventory, the team member who has removed it has the responsibility to notify the inventory management coordinator. Systems

ORDER (ITEM NAME) PATIENT TOWELS **ON ORDER**

ORDER QUANTITY 1000 REORDER POINT 300

ORDER	QTY	REC'D	COST	PREPAID	ON ACCT	ORDER	QTY	REC'D	COST	PREPAID	ON ACCT

INVENTORY COUNT

	JAN	FEB	MAR	APR	MAY	JUNE	JULY	AUG	SEPT	OCT	NOV	DEC
19 ___												
19 ___												

ORDER SOURCE UNIT PRICE

Acme Dental Supply

1-800-942-8000

FORM 2450 COLWELL CO., CHAMPAIGN, ILLINOIS

FIGURE 12-1

One type of inventory control card. (Courtesy of Colwell Systems, Champaign, IL.)

Steps in Determining When to Reorder

1. Determine how much of the product is used and how quickly it is used **(rate of use).** Some supplies arrive in quantities that will last at least 1 week, and other supplies will last much longer, depending on how frequently they are used. The dental healthcare team can help determine how rapidly supplies and products are used.
2. Determine how long it will take for supplies to arrive to the office once the order has been placed **(lead time).** Depending on the product and the supplies, this time will vary. It is a good management skill to establish a list of your vendors and record their average delivery times. Remember to add in a few extra days for a margin of safety.

will fall apart at this point if the proper protocol is not followed. Once the information has been given to the inventory manager, the manager will continue with the established ordering process (Figure 12-2).

Master List of Supplies and Products

Another type of manual system is the master list. A master list can be customized for each dental practice. The master list should be separated into broad categories (infection control, disposable supplies, restorative materials, and so forth). Depending on the needs of the dental practice, the categories can be as simple as the clinical area and the business office. An alphabetical list can also be used.

In addition to the name of the supply or product, the list may include such information as a code or name of the vendor, the manufacturer, and the quantity to be ordered. The list should be posted in a place that is convenient for all members of the dental healthcare team to access. When it is time to reorder a supply or product, a mark can be made on the order form. When sales representatives and ordering assistants preview the list, they can quickly identify which items are needed. This list can be permanently posted on a white board or other type of material that can be marked with a marker and erased when the item has been ordered. Another method is to cover a typed list with heavy plastic laminate. To identify what needs

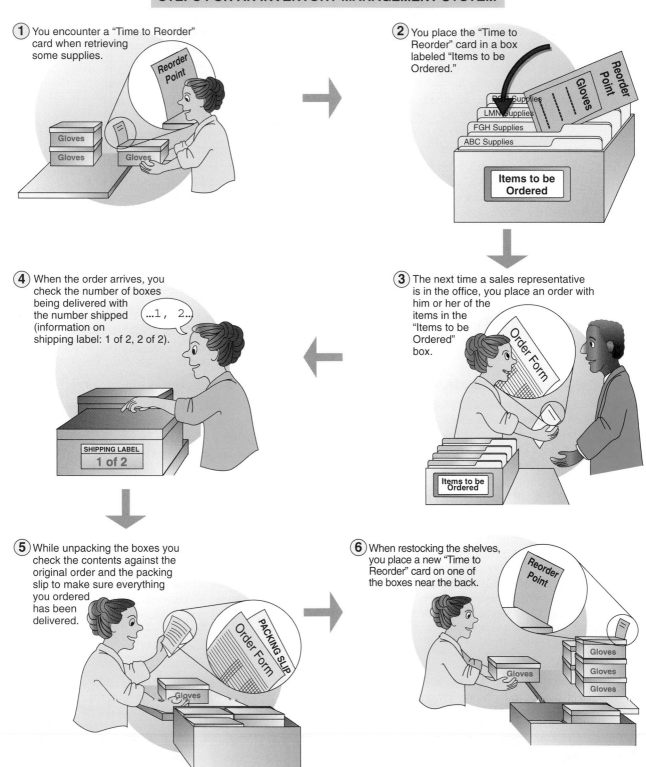

FIGURE 12-2
Steps to be followed in an inventory management system.

to be ordered, the item is identified with an erasable marker. Once the order has been placed, the mark is erased.

A record of items that have been ordered must be kept for verification when the order is received. A copy of the order can be placed in a file until the shipment is received, at which time it is used to verify that the correct items have been shipped. At times, it will be necessary for the vendor to place items on **back order.** This means that the items ordered were not available for shipping and will be sent at a later date. When items are placed on back order, the inventory manager must make a notation in a tracking system. If items are not received within a reasonable length of time, the inventory manager will have to call the vendor and check on the status of the supply or product. It may be necessary to place the order with another vendor if the product cannot be shipped before it is needed. To prevent inventory from being completely depleted of a needed supply or product, this tracking system must be carefully monitored.

A few vendors will supply the information needed for reordering. For example, a vendor who supplies preprinted office supplies will include with each order a "reorder form" that includes the information needed for printing and the quantity that is normally ordered. An envelope and the reorder form can be tucked between sheets of stationery or in another location that is easily found at the point that a new order should be placed. If the reorder is not received in a specified length of time, the vendor will send a reminder to the office that it is time to reorder. This method can be easily implemented by any office. A reminder card or an order form with the needed information can be placed at the appropriate reorder point. This method not only serves as a reminder that it is time to reorder, it also provides all of the information needed to place the order.

Selecting an Inventory Manager

It is easy to turn over all of the responsibility to one member of the dental healthcare team and simply say "handle it," but this method is not always a good dental business strategy. There is much more to a well-organized and efficient system. It is acceptable to have one person in charge, but he or she must be given direction, guidance, and cooperation from other members of the dental healthcare team. Each

---

Personal Characteristics of an Inventory Manager

- Is organized
- Has time to carry out duties
- Is able to communicate with others
- Is a team player
- Is a good shopper

Duties of an Inventory Manager

- Develops and maintains an accurate inventory system
- Seeks input from other members of the dental healthcare team
- Monitors inventory
- Processes orders
- Receives orders and verifies invoices
- Organizes and maintains storage areas
- Tracks back orders

Elements of a Good Inventory Management System

- A qualified inventory manager is in charge.
- Supplies and products that are used in the dental practice can be identified quickly via a computer system, organized list, or card index.
- Products are stored according to the manufacturer's and OSHA's requirements (cool dry place, refrigerated, away from heat).
- Supplies are located for easy access by all members of the dental healthcare team (a master list identifies the location of each product or clearly labeled cabinets and shelves).
- Reorder points are clearly identified with labeled tags, cards, or tape.
- A protocol has been clearly defined for notifying the inventory manager when a product or supply should be ordered.
- A process is in place for identifying which products need to be ordered, have been ordered, or are on back order (tracking system).

---

member of the team has the duty and responsibility to help maintain the inventory management system. This includes selecting products and following the established protocol for the management of inventory.

Inventory Management System Protocol

Several points must be considered when an inventory management system protocol is developed. It may be the primary duty of one person to maintain the system, but cooperation from the entire dental healthcare team is required to develop the protocol.

Steps in Developing an Inventory Management System Protocol

1. Identify products and supplies that are needed.
2. Select the vendor or vendors to be contacted.
3. Develop ordering guidelines.
4. Establish a receiving protocol.
5. Organize the storage area.
6. Check for compliance with OSHA regulations.

TYPES OF SUPPLIES, PRODUCTS, AND EQUIPMENT

Consumable Supplies and Products

Consumable supplies and products are those items that are used and must be replenished. In the clinical area, such items as x-ray film, anesthetics, dental materials, and infection control products are used or consumed (not eaten). When the product is gone, it has to be replaced with fresh material. In addition, **disposable** supplies are used only once. These products include needles, saliva ejectors, and suction tips. Usually, for health and safety reasons, these supplies are not reused. The only time that a supply that comes in direct contact with a patient can be reused is if it can be sterilized (complete destruction of all living organisms; not to be confused with disinfecting, which is only partial destruction of organisms).

Supplies for the business office include paper, envelopes, insurance forms, business cards, patient billing statements, business checks, clinical records forms, and charts. Impression material, gypsum products, and wax are among the supplies needed in the dental laboratory.

Nonconsumable Products

Nonconsumable (expendable) products are supplies and products that can be reused for a specific length of time before they must be replaced. Instruments, handpieces, and small equipment fall into this category. These items can be used for a year or two before they must be replaced because of wear and tear.

Major Equipment

Major equipment includes equipment that can be used for longer than 1 to 2 years. This equipment, such as dental chairs, radiology units, computers, office equipment, and laboratory equipment, can be depreciated on the business's tax returns.

SELECTING AND ORDERING SUPPLIES, PRODUCTS, AND EQUIPMENT

Selecting Supplies and Products

Supplies and *products* are terms that are sometimes interchangeable. For the purpose of this discussion, **supplies** are defined as consumable goods that are used in support of dental treatment. Examples include infection control supplies, paper towels, 2 × 2 gauze, disposable suction tips, mixing sticks, and business office supplies. **Products** are defined as materials used in direct patient care. They include dental materials and dental therapeutics.

The first step in the ordering process is to decide which supplies and products will be used. Some supplies are very generic and do not require research before their purchase. Other products, such as restorative materials, require that the dental healthcare team research them before a decision is made as to which ones to use.

By attending trade shows and dental conventions, the dental healthcare team is able to speak with several different vendors. Each manufacturer has representatives available to answer questions and to demonstrate the correct application and use of products.

Networking is one of the most valuable sources of information. Information can be exchanged through study clubs, membership in professional organizations, and continuing education programs. These organizations help members of the dental health-care team reach their own conclusions by providing a wide range of opinions and shared experiences.

Manufacturers and vendors of dental products send representatives (detail persons) into the field (individual dental practices) for the purpose of introducing new products. During their visit to the dental practice, they explain the intended usage, instruct the dental healthcare team, and answer questions about the products they represent.

Common Terms Associated With Ordering of Supplies and Products

Manufacturer: Company that produces goods.

Vendor: Company that sells goods.

Consumer: Company or person who uses goods.

ADA approved: Products that have been tested and meet the standards of the American Dental Association (ADA Seal).

Dental supply house: Company that sells several different manufacturers' goods (supplies, products, and equipment).

Brand name: Manufactured supplies and products that are identified by a specific given name (registered trademark).

Generic name: Name of a product that is based on its composition—not the brand name. For example, *aspirin* is the generic name of a drug—not the brand name.

Dental salesperson: A representative for a dental supply house who visits dental practices for the purpose of selling supplies and products (also known as a "sales rep").

Purchasing Major Equipment

The purchasing of major equipment is time consuming and involves large sums of money. The cost of a dental chair ranges from $3,000 to $10,000. When new equipment is needed, several factors must be considered:

- What is the budget (how much can be spent)?
- What features must be present (what is the minimal function)?
- What features would be advantageous (would like to have but are not necessary)?
- What features should not be included (would not consider even if they were free)?

The dentist and other team members should attend trade shows or dental conventions, where they can meet with several different manufacturers with samples of their equipment. Once a decision on the manufacturer is decided, it may be necessary to shop for the best price and service. Manufacturers usually do not sell directly to individual dental practices. Instead, equipment must be purchased through a supply house. This is similar to purchasing a new automobile. After you decide on the make and model of the automobile, you must purchase it through an authorized dealer. The price of the automobile will be competitive, and you must decide which dealer is going to give you the best price and service.

Once major equipment has been purchased and installed, a file must be set up that contains all vital information about the equipment. This information includes equipment name and manufacturer, owner's manuals, maintenance schedules, serial and model numbers, date and price of purchase, and telephone numbers for technical assistance.

Information about equipment can be organized for quick reference with an index card file, Rolodex, or computerized database. This information is needed when someone calls for service and technical assistance and should be easy to access by any member of the dental healthcare team.

Selecting the Vendor

Several different dental supply houses are generally available. Small local supply houses are tailored to the individual needs of their clients and are personally involved in local community projects (somewhat like an extended family). Other types of supply houses include regional, national, and international organizations. Each type has its advantages and disadvantages. The choice may be determined by the individual needs of each dental practice. It is not necessary to purchase all of your supplies and products from the same dental supplier. Individual suppliers may not provide all of the products you use or may not offer the best price.

Supplies can be ordered through a sales representative from the supply house or by placing orders through a catalog service. The method of ordering will be determined by the dental practice, and both systems have advantages and disadvantages. Most often, it is best to use more than one type of supply house.

Catalog Ordering

Advantages	Disadvantages
• Lower prices	• Very little personal
• Large selection	service
• Easy to compare	• Limited technical
several products	support
while browsing	• Takes time to complete
through the catalog	order forms
• Direct online	• Returns require
computer service	packaging and
	reshipping

Supply House Services

Advantages	Disadvantages
• Personal service	• Higher prices (although
• Technical support	some are very
• Share knowledge	competitive)
about specific	• Shipping can be slower
products and	• Selection of products
feedback about	is limited
what other	• No comparison
offices are	shopping with catalogs
using (networking)	
• Know your	
ordering pattern	
• Know your	
preferences in	
supplies and	
products	
• Advise on	
quantities to be	
ordered	

Dental supply houses that use sales representatives typically schedule their representatives to visit dental practices weekly or biweekly. The use of sales representatives can be advantageous, depending on the nature of the product. When representatives visit the office, they provide more than an opportunity to place an order. They also provide valuable information concerning new products and specials they are running, and they can help determine the quantity of items you need to purchase. The type of

service that is required by the dental practice varies from office to office.

Similar to retail services, dental services may be provided in varying degrees. Depending on the type of service, the products needed, and the budget constraints, each service has its advantages and disadvantages. Therefore, it is up to each individual dental practice to decide on the type of service needed, to consider the costs of products, and to determine the amount of time they are willing or able to spend on ordering supplies and products.

Information to Consider Before Placing an Order

Before placing an order for supplies and products, you must consider several factors. Following is a list of questions that should be answered before orders are placed:

1. *What is the shelf life of the product?*

The shelf life is the length of time that a product will continue to meet the manufacturer's specifications for use. After a certain amount of time, x-ray film will become foggy and will not produce diagnostically clear radiographs, anesthetic will not be as effective, and chemical compositions will change. Products that have a shelf life will have an expiration date printed on the box or container. The length of time before a product expires varies from product to product. When ordering, you should know the expected shelf life and not order more than can be used in the prescribed time. Caution should be taken when ordering specials on products that are known to have a shelf life. Companies will place products on sale because they want to sell them before the expiration date. This type of sale is an advantage to the dental practice only if all of the product can be used before the expiration date is reached.

2. *What are the storage requirements?*

The amount of available storage space is also a factor to consider when one is determining the quantity of a product to be ordered. If space is limited, it is not advisable to order large quantities. Health and safety codes may dictate where supplies can be safely stored. It is not safe to store combustible materials close to a heat source or in an area that can become very warm. Additionally, some products have very specific storage requirements, such as in cool dry places, refrigerators, or dark areas.

3. *Will technology change before the product is used?*

Because of rapid changes in research and technology, it is best not to order large quantities of products that are constantly being changed and updated.

4. *Has the product been tried and tested in the office?*

Many products remain on the shelf because the dentist and staff did not research the product sufficiently. It is sometimes difficult to use new products because they require training in their proper manipulation and application. In most cases, it is awkward to change from one product to another. If a change is going to be successful, the dental healthcare team must be patient and expect that it will take time to learn to use the new product efficiently.

5. *Will information provided in printed material change before a new order can be used up?*

When ordering stationery and other printed forms, make sure that no changes in the information printed will occur before a new order is placed.

6. *What is the return policy?*

When trying new products, check with the dental representative to clarify your options if the product fails to live up to its claims, or if the dentist decides it is not in the patients' best interests to use the product. Some companies provide sample kits that contain a few applications of a product so the dentist can try the material before purchasing a larger amount. Other companies will trade the product for a different product if it does not meet the needs and expectations of the dentist.

7. *Is it economically advisable to invest in a large quantity order?*

Before expending money for a year's supply of something, check other options. Is a sufficient amount of money going to be saved that will not be better spent elsewhere?

REMEMBER

All products used in direct patient care should meet the standards established by the American Dental Association.

Receiving Supplies and Products

After you have received supplies and products, the next step is to verify your order. Included with all orders are packing slips. These slips are used by the vendor to verify that the goods you ordered have been packaged. It is not uncommon to receive more than one box or package. If you have placed a large order, the goods will arrive in several boxes. Usually, the labels on the boxes indicate the total number of boxes shipped and the individual number of the box. For example, you have placed a large order and the shipping company delivers four boxes. When you check the labels, you notice that they indicate that a total of five boxes were shipped. To help determine which box you are missing, check each of the labels for the box number. Upon additional checking, you can account for box 1 of 5, box 3 of 5, box 4 of 5, and box 5 of 5. You can then assume that box 2 is missing.

Steps in Accepting Shipments

1. Sign for the shipment.
2. Check for the correct number of boxes or items shipped.
3. Inventory the contents of each box, and verify them with the shipping invoice.
4. Check the invoice against your original order.
5. File the shipping invoice, which will be used to verify the billing statement.
6. Record any back ordered supplies.
7. File any new Material Safety Data Sheets that are needed.
8. Enter the quantities of the new supplies into the inventory control system.
9. Place supplies in the appropriate storage areas.

Most shipping companies have very sophisticated methods of tracking their shipments. They can tell you what time the box left the warehouse, was loaded on a plane or truck, and was delivered. Because of their tracking system, they will be able to locate your missing box and give you an estimated time of arrival.

Storage Areas

Areas where supplies and products are to be stored are determined by several factors. The chemical compositions of certain products will determine what type of storage environment they require. Accessibility is also important: How often is the product used? Is it stored near the area where it will be used? Can it be safely removed from the area (considering its weight and height)? These are all factors that must be considered before supplies and products are stored.

Another consideration is how easily a supply or product can be located. If supplies are not stored in a common area, a method of locating the supply must be established. To assist in the location of supplies, a master list is established. The list can be organized alphabetically or divided into broad categories. Once the desired supply is located on the list, directions to where it is stored can be followed. With this type of organization, all storage areas can be easily accessed by any member of the dental health-care team.

When a large storage room is used, shelves should be marked and supplies arranged in a way that can be easily understood by all members of the dental healthcare team. If the room is large and the design does not allow for categorizing supplies, a master list should be posted that states what supplies are located in the storage area and where they are located.

REMEMBER

Make sure that the storage areas comply with OSHA regulations.

OCCUPATIONAL SAFETY AND HEALTH ADMINISTRATION (OSHA)

It is the responsibility of the employer to instruct each and every employee about all areas of safety. The Occupational Safety and Health Administration

(OSHA) mandates that a protocol be established that alerts employees to health hazards and instructs them about the proper ways to safely perform their assigned duties. A written hazard communication program must be maintained by the employer, and annual training sessions should be held. Each employee must know:

- Which chemicals are hazardous
- What risk is involved when one is working with specific chemicals
- How to use the chemicals safely to minimize exposure
- How to handle the chemicals safely after an accident
- Where to find information about hazards (Material Safety Data Sheets)

For employees to gain this knowledge, they must be given product information. This information is communicated in the form of a **Material Safety Data Sheet** (MSDS). The MSDS is made available to the employer by the manufacturer of the product and is usually sent with the product when it is delivered. MSDSs should be maintained in a notebook that can be easily accessed by all employees. In addition, all product containers should be labeled with the proper warnings and information. It is the responsibility of the inventory manager to forward MSDSs to the proper location when products are received. The complete **hazardous communication program** for each dental practice will outline the established protocol, which must be followed by each employee.

ANATOMY OF A MATERIAL SAFETY DATA SHEET

SECTION I—IDENTIFICATION OF THE SUBSTANCE/ PREPARATION AND OF THE COMPANY/UNDERTAKING
Contains product and manufacture information, the product name, and emergency contact information.

SECTION II—COMPOSITION/ INFORMATION ON INGREDIENTS
Lists the hazardous ingredients of the material.

SECTION III—HAZARDS IDENTIFICATION
Identifies the adverse human hazards, effects, and symptoms.

SECTION IV—FIRST AID MEASURES
Describes what actions need to be taken if exposure occurs.

SECTION V—FIRE-FIGHTING MEASURES
List the fire-fighting criteria.

SECTION VI—ACCIDENTAL RELEASE MEASURES
Describes what is affected, personally and environmentally, if an exposure incident were to occur and the clean-up protocol.

SECTION VII—HANDLING AND STORAGE
Describes how to safely handle the material and the correct storage.

SECTION VIII—EXPOSURE CONTROLS/PERSONAL PROTECTION
Lists what safety precautions should be taken to protect yourself in case of an exposure.

SECTION IX—PHYSICAL AND CHEMICAL PROPERTIES
List the physical and chemical properties of the material.

SECTION X—STABILITY AND REACTIVITY
Describes how the chemical will react with other chemicals.

SECTION XI—TOXICOLOGICAL INFORMATION
States what will happen to the body if it is exposed to the chemical.

SECTION XII—ECOLOGICAL INFORMATION
States the effect of the material on the environment.

ULTRADENT PRODUCTS, INC.
MATERIAL SAFETY DATA SHEET
Controlled Product Yes ☐ No ☑

SECTION I IDENTIFICATION OF THE SUBSTANCE/PREPARATION AND OF THE COMPANY/UNDERTAKING

Material Name Ultra-Blend⁺ *plus*™	Manufactured by Ultradent Products, Inc. 505 West 10200 South South Jordan, Utah 84095 USA
Material Use Calcium hydroxide dentin liner and protective base.	Emergency Contact 1-800-552-5512 or 1-801-572-4200 (Outside USA)
Date June 4, 1997	EC Representative
Prepared by: Steve Jensen, Chemist	

SECTION II - COMPOSITION/INFORMATION ON INGREDIENTS

Active Ingredients	Approximate Concentration %	LD_{50}/LC_{50} Specify Species and Route	C.A.S. N.A. or U.N. Numbers
Urethane dimethacrylate	58%	N/A	109-16-0
Calcium hydroxide	10%	LD_{50} 7340 mg/kg Oral – Rat	1305-62-0

SECTION III - HAZARDS IDENTIFICATION

Adverse Human Effects and Symptoms Not defined.

SECTION IV - FIRST AID MEASURES

Inhalation N/A	Eye Contact Flush with lots of water.
Skin Contact Wash thoroughly with soap and water.	Ingestion In large volumes, induce vomiting.

SECTION V - FIRE-FIGHTING MEASURES

Flammability Yes ☐ No ☑ If Yes, Under Which Conditions:

Means of Extinction Water spray, foam, CO_2	Protective Equipment for Firefighters Not defined.

SECTION VI - ACCIDENTAL RELEASE MEASURES | **SECTION VII - HANDLING AND STORAGE**

Personal & Environmental Precautions Not defined.	Handling Precautions Not defined.
Methods for Cleaning Wipe up as much as possible with dry cloth, clean remaining material with alcohol.	Storage Requirements Refrigerate when not in use.

SECTION VIII - EXPOSURE CONTROLS/PERSONAL PROTECTION

Respiratory Protection N/A	Eye Protection Protective eyewear.
Hand Protection Latex gloves.	Skin Protection Lab coat.

SECTION IX - PHYSICAL & CHEMICAL PROPERTIES

Appearance Tinted paste.	Solubility in Water Not defined.	Melting Point/Range N/A
Odor Slight acrylic odor.	pH Basic.	Other Data None.

SECTION X - STABILITY AND REACTIVITY

Chemical Stability Yes ☑ No ☐ Conditions and Materials to Avoid Light exposure initiates polymerization.	Hazardous Decomposition Products N/A

SECTION XI - TOXICOLOGICAL INFORMATION

Route of Entry Skin Contact ☑ Skin Absorption ☑ Eye Contact ☐ Inhalation Acute ☐ Inhalation Chronic ☐ Ingestion

Effects and Symptoms of Short-Term Exposure Eye contact: irritation. Skin contact: slight irritation.

Chronic Effects and Symptoms of Long-Term Exposure Eye contact: irritation. Skin contact: slight irritation.

Sensitization Not defined.	Irritancy of Product Slight.

SECTION XII - ECOLOGICAL INFORMATION | **SECTION XIII - DISPOSAL CONSIDERATIONS**

Biodegradability Yes.	Method of Waste Disposal Dispose of according to local and government regulations.
Further Details None.	

SECTION XIV - TRANSPORT INFORMATION | **SECTION XV - REGULATORY INFORMATION**

Not regulated.	N/A

SECTION XVI - OTHER INFORMATION

FOR DENTAL USE ONLY. Use as directed.
The information and recommendations are taken from sources (raw material MSDS(s) and manufacturer's knowledge) believed to be accurate; however, Ultradent Products, Inc., makes no warranty with respect to the accuracy of the information or the suitability of the recommendation and assumes no liability to any user thereof. Each user should review these recommendations in the specific context of the intended use and determine whether they are appropriate.

(Courtesy Ultradent Products, Inc., South Jordan, Utah)

SECTION XIII—DISPOSAL CONSIDERATIONS
States how the material should be disposed.

SECTION XIV—TRANSPORT INFORMATION
Lists regulations and limitations in the transportation of the material.

SECTION XV—REGULATORY INFORMATION
List specific regulation if any.

SECTION XVI—OTHER INFORMATION
Special instructions and the intended use of the material.

KEY POINTS

- Ordering and managing supplies for the laboratory, business, and clinical areas in a dental practice requires organization, communication, and the cooperation of the entire dental healthcare team.
- Inventory management systems can be computerized or manual. Inventory systems use a variety of methods to identify when a product or supply needs to be ordered, who will place the order, and which vendor will fill the order.
- Elements of a good inventory management system include the following:
  - A qualified inventory manager
  - Identification of what supplies and products are used in the dental practice
  - Proper storage
  - A master list of all supplies and products that provides their locations
  - Easy access to storage areas with clearly marked shelves
  - A clearly defined protocol for ordering
  - Inventory includes supplies, products, and equipment. These items are purchased from vendors. The types of vendors and delivery methods used will vary depending on the needs of the dental practice.

 Web Watch

OSHA (Occupational Safety and Health Administration)

http://www.osha.gov

Material Safety Data Sheet Searches

http://msds.ehs.cornell.edu/msdssrch.asp

Where to Find MSDS on the Internet

http://www.ilpi.com/msds/index.html

    Log on to Evolve to access additional web links!
http://evolve.elsevier.com

 Critical Thinking Questions

1. As the inventory manager, you have been given the task of developing a system for your office that identifies when a product needs to be ordered. Describe your system, and identify the different elements that helped you design it.
2. Where can you find information to help you store supplies safely?
3. A sales representative informs you that his or her company is running a special on x-ray film. The film will be discounted 25% when you order 10 or more boxes. The current price of the film is $32.00 per box. You check your order card and find that you currently have 5 boxes of film in stock. After reviewing your order history, you find that the office uses 2.5 boxes of film per month. You question the reason for the discount, and the sales representative informs you that the expiration date on the film is 1 year from now.
   - What would be the price for 10 boxes of film?
   - How long will it take to use the film you have in stock?
   - How many boxes of film are used in 1 year?
   - Should you take advantage of the sale?
   - If yes, how many boxes of film should you order?
   - What will be the cost of your order?

Notes

OUTLINE

KEY TERMS AND CONCEPTS

Account Aging Reports
Credit Reports
Divided Payment Plans
Extended Payment Plans

In-House Payment Plans (Budget
  Plans)
Insurance Billing Plans
Outside Payment Plans

Payment in Full Plans
Skip Tracing

13

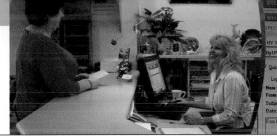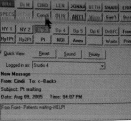

Financial Arrangement and Collection Procedures

LEARNING OBJECTIVES

The student will:

1. List the elements of a financial policy and discuss the qualifying factors for each of the elements.
2. Describe the different types of financial plans and explain how they can be applied in a dental practice.
3. State the purpose of managing accounts receivable. Describe the role of the administrative dental assistant in managing accounts receivable.
4. Classify the different levels of the collection process.
5. Place a telephone collection call.
6. Process a collection letter.
7. Interpret aging reports and implement proper collection procedures.

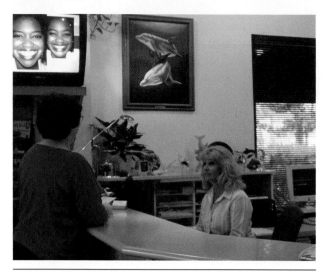

FIGURE 13-1
Administrative dental assistant asking a patient for payment.
(Courtesy of William C. Domb, DMD, Upland, CA.)

INTRODUCTION

The responsibility for collecting fees is shared by all members of the dental healthcare team. The team will establish the policies and then follow them. The administrative dental assistant has the most visible task (Figure 13-1). After a treatment plan has been drawn up, the administrative dental assistant will write the financial plan, present the plan to the patient, and then monitor compliance with the plan. If the plan is not followed, it is usually the administrative dental assistant who initiates collection procedures.

DESIGNING A FINANCIAL POLICY

Elements of a Financial Policy

- Community standards
- Practice philosophy
- Business principles

Community Standards

The community or area where the dental practice is located and the people served by the practice are factors in the financial policy. The policy in an affluent area will be different from that in an economi-

cally disadvantaged one. The types of dental insurance accepted are among the other factors that enter into financial policy making. It is conceivable that practices that accept a variety of insurance plans and that treat people from different socioeconomic levels will have more than one payment plan option. These options are designed to meet the needs of the practice's patients while providing for the economic welfare of the employees and the dentist.

Practice Philosophy

The philosophy of the dental practice is described in its mission statement. The goals and objectives of the dental practice summarize the attitudes of the dentist and staff toward patient care and financial policy. This information is a component of the policy and procedure manual and is communicated to the patient in the dental practice's brochure.

Business Principles

A dental practice is a business, and it must be run according to sound business principles. Those who work in the healthcare industry provide help to patients by being caring and understanding. Asking for money naturally makes us uncomfortable, and healthcare workers are reluctant collectors. An accountant or business manager can provide valuable financial information and can set guidelines that must be followed.

FINANCIAL POLICIES

The dental practice of the 21st century is faced with many challenges. Dentists must constantly strive to improve the quality of dental care, provide for their employees, and meet the expectations of their patients. Several surveys have indicated that patients will accept a dentist according to the types of financial plans that are offered. For dentists to meet these challenges, they must be flexible in the types of financial plans they provide to their patients. They may need to customize financial plans to meet the needs of each patient while practicing prudent business strategies.

Payment in Full

The payment in full policy requires that the patient pay in full after each visit. Payment may be given in the form of cash, check, or credit card. **Payment**

in full plans are beneficial to the dental practice because they provide a constant cash flow. For this type of financial policy to be successful, you must follow several steps:

- Inform patients of the expected amount to pay in advance of treatment. Patients should always know the estimated fee for each dental visit. This information can be given when they call for their appointment, or it can be outlined in the treatment plan.
- Be direct in asking for payment: "Ms. King, The fee for today's visit is $234.00."
- Know your patients: If they have insurance, and according to their policy, the insurance company should be billed first, ask for the patient's portion: "Ms. King, The fee for today is $234.00. I will bill your insurance company. According to our records, your company will pay 80% of the fee, leaving a balance of $46.80, which is due from you today."
- When patients are unprepared to pay, give them a walk-out statement (itemization of charges) and a return envelope, and instruct them to send the payment as soon as possible.
- Offer cash discounts to patients who pay for a treatment plan in advance of the treatment. This policy is attractive to those who view the discount (5% or less) as a savings.

Insurance Billing

Insurance billing plans are considered types of payment plans that have established polices that must be followed. Some dental practices will bill the insurance company first and then bill the patient for the balance. Again, it is very important that patients understand the process and that they are made aware of the approximate balance they will be paying. When the balance is going to be large, a financial payment plan can be drawn up, and patients can start paying their portion before the work is completed.

Copayment represents that portion of the dental treatment for which the patient is responsible for payment. For example, some insurance policies state that the patient will pay a $10.00 copayment for each visit. These fees should be considered due and payable at the time service is provided. Other insurance policies clearly outline the patient portion

for each procedure. These charges should be discussed with the patient before treatment is begun and financial arrangements are made.

Extended Payment Plans

When it is necessary to allow payments for treatment over time, several different methods can be used to set up **extended payment plans. In-house payment plans (budget plans)** are established by the dental practice. A contract is drawn up, and the proper forms are completed (Figure 13-2). A payment coupon book may be given to the patient, or a computerized statement system can generate monthly bills for the agreed upon amount.

A variation of the payment plan is the **divided payment plan.** In this plan, payments are divided according to the length of treatment. For example, one third of the balance is due at the beginning of treatment, one third at the midpoint of treatment, and the balance at the completion of treatment.

Outside payment plans are arranged by the dental office and are administered by an outside agency. The dental practice may offer these types of plans to patients who need to extend payments over a longer period. Typically, the financial application is completed in the dental office and is sent to the agency for approval. The agency will approve the application for a preset amount. Some agencies issue a credit card that can be used only in the dental practice. Each time the patient receives treatment, the credit card is activated and the charges recorded. The agency will charge the dental practice a percentage of the total charge (the same is true for other credit card agencies such as Visa, MasterCard, American Express, and Discover Card). The agency deposits the discounted amount into the practice account. The advantage of this service is that the dental practice does not have to manage the account, and the agency assumes the risk for collecting the charges.

Credit Cards

Credit card payments are considered cash payments. Each time the patient receives treatment, the charge is posted to the credit card via an electronic modem (as in, for example, a department store). The discounted payment is deposited directly into the practice's account.

|3|2|6|5|7|0|
PATIENT NUMBER

© *1991 Wisconsin Dental Association*
(800) 243-4675

PATIENT'S NAME   *Budd*   *Rose*   *L*
                       Last   First   Initial

I   *Rose*   have had my treatment plan and options explained to me and hereby
authorize this treatment to be performed by Dr.   *Mary Edwards*

Patient's Signature   *Rose Budd*   Date   *7/23/2006*
(Parent or Guardian MUST sign if patient is a minor)

I also understand that the cost of this treatment is as follows and that the method of paying for the same
will be:

Total (Partial) estimate of treatment	$	*2708.⁰⁰*
Less:		
Initial Payment	−	*1000,⁰⁰*
Insurance Estimate if Applicable	−	*1000.⁰⁰*
Other _____	−	*θ*
Balance of Estimate Due	$	*708,⁰⁰*

Terms: Monthly Payment $ *236,⁰⁰* over a *3* month period.

PLEASE CONTACT THE BUSINESS OFFICE IF YOU ARE UNABLE TO MEET YOUR FINANCIAL OBLIGATION

The truth in lending Law enacted in 1969 serves to inform the borrowers and installment purchasers of the true Annual Interest charged on the amounts financed. This law applies to this office whenever the office extends the courtesy of Installment Payments to our patients, even when no finance charge is made.

The signature below indicate a mutual understanding of the ESTIMATE for treatment and the acceptable schedule of payment as noted.

Today's Date *7/23/2006*   *Rose Budd*
                              Signature of Responsible Party

                    Sharon Williams
                    Financial Advisor   Phone Number

Note: THIS IS AN ESTIMATE ONLY, if treatment plan should change please request an amended estimate should it not be offered by our staff. This estimate is valid for 90 days from the date above IF treatment has not begun within that period. A patient's voluntary termination of treatment makes this agreement invalid.

Form 260FA   **FINANCIAL ARRANGEMENTS**

FIGURE 13-2

Financial arrangement form and truth in lending statement. See clinical record on page 123. (Courtesy of The Dental Record, Wisconsin Dental Association, Milwaukee, WI.)

FINANCIAL POLICY COMMUNICATIONS

Once financial policies are created, they must be communicated to the patient. Patient communication begins the first time a patient calls the office to ask for information or to make an appointment. Office policy can be tactfully delivered to the patient without discomfort to the dental assistant. Verbal information should be followed by a written statement. This can be accomplished by sending the patient a copy of the practice brochure.

When a treatment plan is completed, it is the responsibility of the administrative dental assistant to complete a financial plan. This plan can be written on a simple form that illustrates the work to be performed, the fee for each service, and the desired method of payment (Figure 13-3).

MANAGING ACCOUNTS RECEIVABLE

Accounts receivable represents the amount of money patients owe the dental practice for services rendered. The dentist, accountant, or business manager will set a limit on the amount of money that can be outstanding. When the dollar amount exceeds the limit, a careful analysis of the system should be conducted. This analysis will reveal areas that need to be strengthened to keep the accounts within budget. Several steps must be followed in managing and controlling the accounts receivable.

Gather Financial Data

Financial information is obtained when the patient completes the Patient Registration Form (Figure 13-4). As discussed in Chapter 7, this document lists who is financially responsible for the account and pertinent insurance and employment information. It may be necessary to determine who is financially responsible for a child whose parents are divorced. This can be a complicated process and the situation should be thoroughly researched before a determination is made. When another parent or guardian is responsible, that person must be contacted to complete the financial portion of the registration form. The responsible party will need to be informed of the treatment and must authorize any payment plan before treatment is begun.

Credit reports are another tool used to gather credit information. These reports list the names of all creditors, all amounts owed, and payment history. Accounts that have been turned over for collection or a legal judgment are identified. Credit reports are available through a credit-reporting agency and can be used by the dental practice to determine payment patterns.

REMEMBER

Patients must give permission before reports are requested from the credit reporting agency.

Prepare a Treatment Plan

A treatment plan is an outline of the treatment that the dentist has recommended and the patient has agreed to (see Figure 13-3). The administrative dental assistant is responsible for preparing the written treatment plan. The assistant will present the written plan to the patient and discuss financial arrangements.

Payment Plans

Payment plans are confidential and should be discussed in a quiet area away from distractions. Once the plan has been presented, the administrative dental assistant will discuss the payment options with the patient or responsible party. After the patient and the administrative dental assistant agree on the payment plan, the appropriate paperwork can be prepared, such as Truth in Lending Statements (see Figure 13-2), Budget Plan Payment Coupons, and contracts.

Billing Statements

Billing statements are monthly accounts of business transactions. They contain important information and must be easy for the patient to understand. These statements should include the following:
- Date of each transaction (payments, charges, and adjustments)
- Name of the patient associated with each transaction

		3	2	6	5	7	0		

PATIENT NUMBER

© *2001 Wisconsin Dental Association*
(800) 243-4675

PATIENT'S NAME _____ *Budd* _____ *Rose* _____ *L* ____ 7-1-2006
Last   First   Initial   Date

DATE	TREATMENT PLAN	FEE	ALTERNATE TREATMENT	FEE	PROB # ASGN
7-1-2006	#3 Extraction	83⁻			2
7-1-2006	#2-4 3 unit Fix Br	2160	PUD	745⁻	3
7-1-2006	UR quad perio scaling	100⁻			4
7-1-2006	UL quad perio scaling	100⁻			4
7-1-2006	LL quad perio scaling	100⁻			4
7-1-2006	LR quad perio scaling	100⁻			4
7-1-2006	Prophy + polish	65⁻			5
7-1-2006	Patient selected Fix Br				
	Total	2708⁰⁰			

RELEASE:

I accept the above treatment plan. I understand that because of unexpected circumstances, the treatment, the fees for treatment and/or the materials required as explained to me at this time, may require some changes after actual care has begun.

PATIENT'S/GUARDIAN'S SIGNATURE _____ *Rose Budd* _____ DATE ____ 7-1-2006

ANEST.
yes

MED. ALERT
penicillin coleine

Form No. T201TP

TREATMENT PLAN

FIGURE 13-3

Treatment plan clearly stating treatment and fees. See clinical record on page 123. (Courtesy of The Dental Record, Wisconsin Dental Association, Milwaukee, WI.)

- Description of each transaction in terms that the patient will understand
- List of fees for each transaction
- Current balance for the account
- Statement of patient's balance; for example:

Budget plan balance due: $220.00
Patient portion after insurance paid: $14.00
Patient portion after insurance adjustment: $23.00
The statement should look professional yet attractive and should include a return envelope.

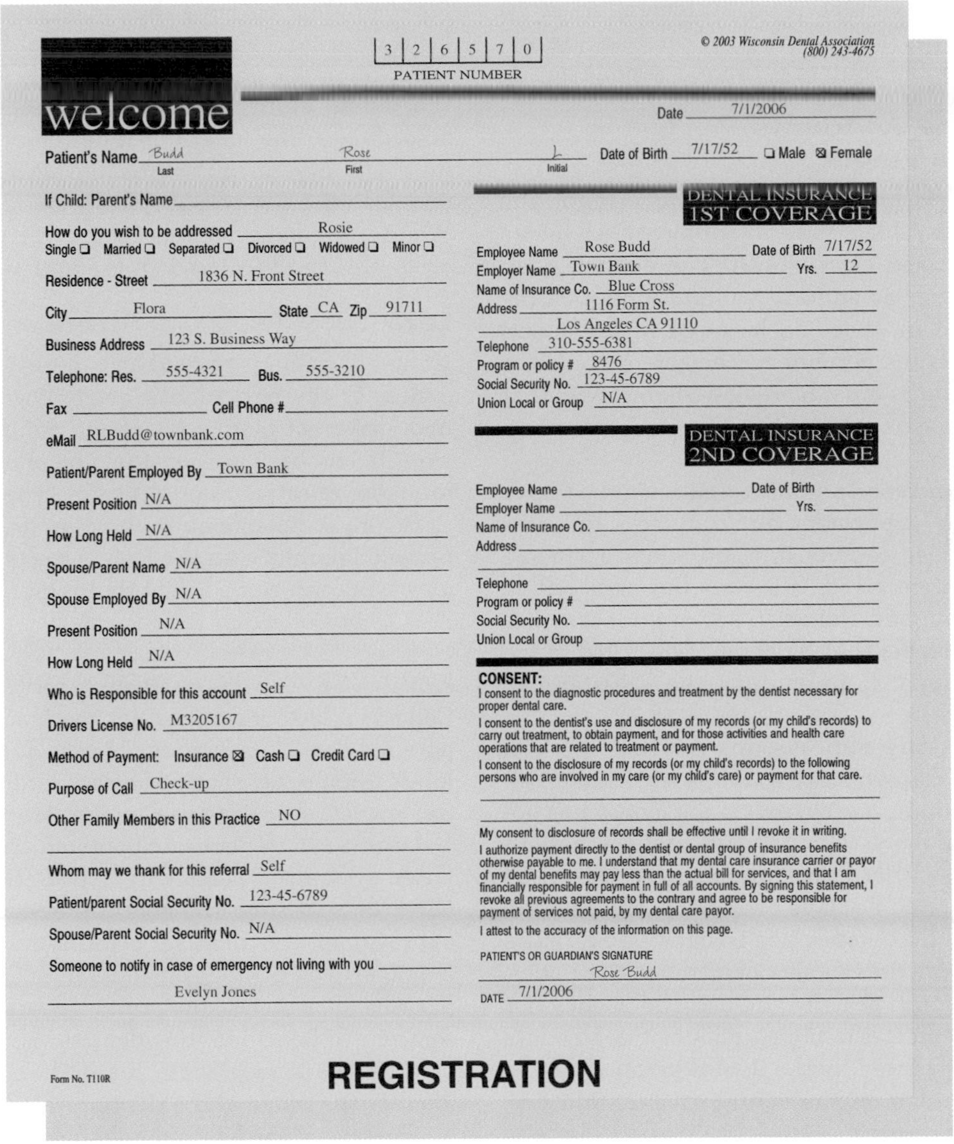

© 2003 Wisconsin Dental Association (800) 243-4675

welcome

3 2 6 5 7 0
PATIENT NUMBER

Date 7/1/2006

Patient's Name Budd (Last) Rose (First) L (Initial) Date of Birth 7/17/52 ☐ Male ☒ Female

If Child: Parent's Name

How do you wish to be addressed Rosie

Single ☐ Married ☐ Separated ☐ Divorced ☐ Widowed ☐ Minor ☐

Residence - Street 1836 N. Front Street

City Flora State CA Zip 91711

Business Address 123 S. Business Way

Telephone: Res. 555-4321 Bus. 555-3210

Fax Cell Phone #

eMail RLBudd@townbank.com

Patient/Parent Employed By Town Bank

Present Position N/A

How Long Held N/A

Spouse/Parent Name N/A

Spouse Employed By N/A

Present Position N/A

How Long Held N/A

Who is Responsible for this account Self

Drivers License No. M3205167

Method of Payment: Insurance ☒ Cash ☐ Credit Card ☐

Purpose of Call Check-up

Other Family Members in this Practice NO

Whom may we thank for this referral Self

Patient/parent Social Security No. 123-45-6789

Spouse/Parent Social Security No. N/A

Someone to notify in case of emergency not living with you
Evelyn Jones

DENTAL INSURANCE 1ST COVERAGE

Employee Name Rose Budd Date of Birth 7/17/52
Employer Name Town Bank Yrs. 12
Name of Insurance Co. Blue Cross
Address 1116 Form St.
Los Angeles CA 91110
Telephone 310-555-6381
Program or policy # 8476
Social Security No. 123-45-6789
Union Local or Group N/A

DENTAL INSURANCE 2ND COVERAGE

Employee Name Date of Birth
Employer Name Yrs.
Name of Insurance Co.
Address
Telephone
Program or policy #
Social Security No.
Union Local or Group

CONSENT:
I consent to the diagnostic procedures and treatment by the dentist necessary for proper dental care.
I consent to the dentist's use and disclosure of my records (or my child's records) to carry out treatment, to obtain payment, and for those activities and health care operations that are related to treatment or payment.
I consent to the disclosure of my records (or my child's records) to the following persons who are involved in my care (or my child's care) or payment for that care.

My consent to disclosure of records shall be effective until I revoke it in writing.
I authorize payment directly to the dentist or dental group of insurance benefits otherwise payable to me. I understand that my dental care insurance carrier or payor of my dental benefits may pay less than the actual bill for services, and that I am financially responsible for payment in full of all accounts. By signing this statement, I revoke all previous agreements to the contrary and agree to be responsible for payment of services not paid, by my dental care payor.
I attest to the accuracy of the information on this page.

PATIENT'S OR GUARDIAN'S SIGNATURE Rose Budd

DATE 7/1/2006

Form No. T110R

REGISTRATION

FIGURE 13-4
Registration form used to gather financial information. (Courtesy of The Dental Record, Wisconsin Dental Association, Milwaukee, WI.)

Information provided in the statement should be consistent with previous financial information given to the patient. The budget plan payment due must match the agreed upon amount. Insurance transactions must match the information sent to the patient from the insurance company (in Explanation of Benefits forms). Transactions and amounts should also be the same as those recorded on the walk-out statement given to the patient at the end of the appointment.

Billing cycles are used to process monthly statements in batches. For example, practice statements are divided into four batches, and one batch is generated and mailed during each week of the month. Statements will have information printed on the back summarizing the payment policy. If interest is charged, the correct legal statement must be included to notify the patient of the interest rate and whom they should contact if there is a problem.

Monitor the Accounts Receivable Report

It is a prudent business practice to monitor the accounts receivable. Several different elements should be checked each month. The dentist, business manager, or accountant will put a limit on the amount of money that can be owed to the dental practice. When the accounts receivable exceeds the limit, the accounts must be reviewed and areas that need attention must be identified (reports can reveal these areas).

Budget plan reports indicate patients who have failed to make a payment (or to make a full payment). Insurance reports indicate when payments have not been received, allowing the assistant to follow up on unpaid claims. Insurance reports also identify treatments that have not been billed to the insurance company, prompting the assistant to submit a claim.

Account aging reports analyze the length of time that has elapsed since a charge was made. Traditionally, accounts are current if the money has not been owed for more than 30 days and the patient has not received the first statement. Periods of 30 days, 60 days, and 90 days are used to indicate the length of time that money has been owed. Statistics show that money loses value over time. The inability of the dental practice to use the money for salaries or to meet the obligations of the accounts payable (money owed by the dental practice) places a financial burden on the dental practice and prevents financial growth.

Collection Process

When it becomes necessary to remind a patient that a payment is due, different methods and tools may be used. The collection process is a series of reminders that payment is past due. At each step, a different strategy is used with a different level of intensity. The objective of the process is to collect the payment from the patient.

Level One: "Friendly Reminders"

The first level of the collection process is the "friendly reminder." Several methods are available for reminding patients that their payment has not been received. If a computerized billing method is used, reminder notices can be printed directly onto the billing statement. These reminders will vary according to the length of time the account is past due. The system automatically ages the accounts and includes the correct phrase on the statement. When a manual system is used, a variety of stickers or stamps can be placed on the statement.

Level Two: "Telephone Reminders"

If the bill remains unpaid for a period of two billing cycles, or the patient has not followed the agreed upon payment plan, a telephone reminder is necessary. It has been proven that telephone reminders are more effective than letters or repeated bills.

Before a telephone call is made, review and become familiar with the legal aspects of contacting a patient concerning a debt that is owed. Consult the Fair Debt Collection Practices Act.

Level Three: "The Collection Letter"

Collection letters are another method of reminding patients that their account is past due. A collection letter should be short, concise, and to the point (review letter writing in Chapter 4).

Letters can be generated automatically by a computer system or personally typed. Letters should never be sent from the dental practice without the approval of the dentist, accountant, or business manager. The dentist, business manager, or administrative dental assistant can sign the letter. When someone other than the dentist signs the letter, identify the signer, state his or her position, and identify the name of the dental practice.

The tone of the letter should increase in intensity as time goes on. Letters should be sent in stages: Begin the first letter in a pleasing tone and increase the intensity in later letters (Figure 13-5).

Level Four: "The Ultimatum"

The final attempt by the dental practice to collect on an overdue account will also include a letter of increased intensity (see Figure 13-5). The letter will give the patient one more chance to pay the balance before the account is turned over to a collection agency, or a claim is filed in Small Claims Court. The letter should clearly outline what will happen if the account is not paid within 10 days. The letter should

Canyon View Dental Associates
4546 North Avery Way
Canyon View, California 91787

April 11, 2006

Ms. Jennifer Lyons
1256 Roanoke Avenue
Canyon View, CA 91787

Dear Ms. Lyons:

Two months ago you agreed to pay your account by the 15th of April. Our contract was based on two things: (1) your word that you would pay as agreed and (2) your ability to pay the total bill of $456.00.

You'll have to agree that we have kept our part of the agreement. Now, please keep your part by sending a check for the full amount of $456.00 within the next week.

We have enclosed a self-addressed, postage-paid envelope for your convenience.

Yours truly,

Diana Blangsted
Business Manager, Canyon View Dental Associates

DLG: sw
Enclosure

A

Canyon View Dental Associates
4546 North Avery Way
Canyon View, California 91783

April 11, 2006

Mr. James Spencer
1198 Berry Drive
Canyon View, CA 91787

Dear Mr. Spencer:

We recently reviewed your financial status and were surprised by your lack of response to our numerous attempts to collect final payment for treatment you received November 11, 1998.

According to our records, your remaining balance of $221.00 has now accumulated interest of $25.00. Please check your records and contact us immediately if they do not match ours, so we can correct any discrepancy.

If your records agree with ours, we regard this as a very serious situation. We certainly do not wish to be forced to seek other recourse to collect the money owed. We want to communicate with you. But if we do not hear from you within 10 days, we will turn your account over to a collection agency.

Sincerely yours,

Diana Blangsted
Business Manager, Canyon View Dental Associates

DLG: sw

B

FIGURE 13-5

A, Collection letter, moderate intensity. **B,** Collection letter used as an ultimatum. (Modified from Dietz E: SmartPractice: The Complete Dental Letter Handbook: Your Fingertip Resource for Practice Communications, Semantodontics, Phoenix, AZ, 1989)

Level One Collection Reminders

- Don't delay further; your payment of $75.00 was due last month.
- Now is the time to take care of this balance of $34.00.
- Prompt payments for your regular dental check-ups are appreciated.
- Don't delay. Please pay $123.00 today for last month's recall cleaning and exam.
- Have you overlooked this balance due? You agreed to send a check for $90.00 following your recall appointment.
- Remember that you agreed to pay for your dental exam and cleaning 30 days following your appointment.
- We took your word in good faith; you promised to pay the remaining $100.00 for your crown within 60 days.
- We are counting on you to pay the remaining balance of $120.00 due for dental services rendered on January 10th.
- If there is any reason for not paying this balance of $89.00, please contact us. Thank you.

From Dietz E: SmartPractice: The Complete Dental Letter Handbook: Your Fingertip Resource for Practice Communication. Semantodontics, Phoenix, AZ, 1989.

be sent registered mail with a return receipt. This will document that the patient received or refused the letter.

There will be times when patients will move and will not inform the dental practice of their new address. Steps can be taken to locate them. This procedure is referred to as **skip tracing.**

- Use envelopes with the words "address correction requested" below the return address. This will prompt the postal service to send a notice with the patient's new address.
- Call the patient's old telephone number; a forwarding number may be available.
- Contact the patient's friend or relative (from information on the patient's registration form).
- Contact the patient at work. The employer may be able to answer questions or relay messages.
- Send a registered letter and request a return receipt. Use a plain envelope without a return address (patients who are trying to avoid you will not know who sent the letter).

Level Five: "Turning the Account Over to Collections"

After you have tried all other methods of collecting the amount due and have not succeeded, your last resort is to turn the account over for collection. Collection agencies take over the process and collect a fee from the dental practice. The fee is a portion of the account, normally 30% to 50% of the balance due.

Accounts turned over to collection agencies should still be collectable. If a collection agency is used, it should be a reputable agency with a record of receiving payment. You can check on an agency's reputation by calling the Chamber of Commerce or the Better Business Bureau. Check with the local dental society and talk with other professionals. Professional organizations that monitor collection agencies include the National Retail Credit Association and the Associated Credit Bureau of America. Select a collection agency that follows the same ethical standards that the dental practice does.

Once the account is turned over to the agency, the agency controls the collection process. Payments are made directly to the agency, and then a percentage is forwarded to the dental practice. The agency will provide monthly statements and will keep the dental practice up to date with any progress. The agency should consult with the dental practice before turning the account over for legal action.

The use of a collection agency may cause additional problems for the dental practice. Patients may become irritated and alienate themselves and their family from the dental practice. Some patients will use this as an excuse to bring alleged charges of malpractice against the dental practice. Before turning accounts over to collection agencies or taking additional legal action, such as filing a lawsuit, make every effort to resolve the problem.

Use tact and diplomacy when discussing delinquent accounts with patients. Try to make arrangements with them by setting up a realistic financial plan.

Try to find outside financing that will help the patient spread payments out over a longer period.

Use final letters and notices to warn the patient that further action, such as a small claims suit or a collection agency, will be used if the account is not settled. Give the patient time to respond, generally

Fair Debt Collection Guidelines

When and how can you contact a debtor?

Calls cannot be made before 8 A.M. or after 9 P.M., unless directed by the debtor. Calls can be made to the responsible party at home or at work (unless the employer disapproves). Contact can be made in person, or by mail, telephone, telegram, or fax.

What type of debit collection practice is prohibited?

- *Harassment:* You may not harass, oppress, or abuse anyone.
  For example, you may not:
  - Use threats of violence or harm against the person, property, or reputation
  - Publish a list of consumers who refuse to pay their debts (except to a credit bureau)
  - Use obscene or profane language
  - Repeatedly use the telephone to annoy someone
  - Telephone people without identifying yourself
  - Advertise debts
- *False statements:* You may not use any false statements when collecting a debt.
  For example, debt collectors may not:
  - Use a false name
  - Falsely imply that they are attorneys or government representatives
  - Falsely imply that the debtor has committed a crime
  - Falsely represent that they operate or work for a credit bureau
  - Misrepresent the amount of the debt
  - Misrepresent the involvement of an attorney in collecting the debt
  - Indicate that papers being sent are legal forms when they are not
  - Indicate that papers being sent are not legal forms when they are
  - Send anything that looks like an official document from a court or government agency when it is not
  - Give false credit information to anyone
- *Threats.* You may not threaten to do something unless it is legal and you really intend to do it.
  For example, you may not state that:
  - They will be arrested if they do not pay
  - You will seize, garnish, attach, or sell their property or wages, unless the collection agency or creditor intends to do so, and it is legal to do so
  - Actions, such as a lawsuit, will be taken, which legally may not be taken, or which you do not intend to take
- *Unfair practices:* Collectors may not engage in unfair practices when they try to collect a debt.
  For example, collectors may not:
  - Collect any amount greater than the debt, unless allowed by law
  - Deposit a postdated check prematurely
  - Make the debtor accept collect calls or pay for telegrams
  - Take or threaten to take the debtor's property, unless this can be done legally
  - Contact the debtor by postcard

Who can be contacted?

The only person who can be contacted is the person or persons legally responsible for the account. If you are trying to locate patients, you can call a third party, but you cannot reveal that you are trying to reach them because of a debt they owe. You can usually contact them only one time.

---

10 days. Be prepared to follow through with the action if your demands are not met.

After the account is turned over, cooperate with the agency and notify someone if the patient contacts you to make payment arrangements (once the account is turned over, the payment must go to the agency).

Roadblocks to Effective Collections

There may be several reasons for poor or ineffective payments. It is important to identify the reason and to take action to correct the problem.

Patient attitudes and excuses can sometimes prevent effective collections. Common excuses for not paying a dental bill are:

- "I can wait to make this payment; dentists don't report late payments to credit agencies."
- "The doctor makes plenty of money. I will send only $20.00 a month."
- "It won't matter that I have not paid, the dentist has to see me to complete the work."
- The patient becomes defensive and angry when asked for payment.

Steps in Placing Collection Calls

1. *Plan the call.* Obtain the patient's clinical record, insurance information, and billing statement. If collection calls (or letters) have been made in the past, review your notes. Follow the correct protocol.
2. *Plan your questions.* Phrase questions in a way that will get you the answers you want. Open-ended questions are the best form to use because they require a person to provide specific information: "When can we expect to receive your payment? Is there a reason for the delay of your payment?" Closed-ended questions require only a yes or no answer: "Will you send a payment?" When the patient responds "yes," you still do not know how much will be sent and when.
3. *Place the call.* Select a time of day when you can place the call without interruptions. Know the name of the responsible party. When the call is answered, identify yourself and the name of the dental practice. Use a confident, professional voice. With your best professional voice, state the reason you are calling, pause, and give the patient a chance to respond before you continue. Remember, you will get better results with a voice that is professional, friendly, and sincere. Never sound timid, angry, embarrassed, annoyed, or rushed: "Hello, Mr. Jones, this is Diane from Canyon View Dental.

I am calling about the balance due for Susie's dental treatment."
4. *Be prepared to resolve the problem.* This may take some creative planning, but remember that the end result is to collect the money. You may find that the patient is having some financial difficulties and cannot send you the full amount; set up a payment plan. When the current payment plan is not working, renegotiate it. When patients owe the dentist money, they are not likely to continue with their scheduled treatment. Sometimes, they are embarrassed and will seek treatment elsewhere. During collection calls, it is not unusual for patients to become angry (this is a defensive reaction). It is important that you remain calm and professional.
5. *Review what is expected.* At the conclusion of the call, summarize what has been said and clearly state the expected outcome: "Thank you for taking the time to work out a new payment plan. I will expect your payment of $75.00 by Monday and then $75.00 by the 15th of each month until the balance is paid."
6. *Record what is expected.* Enter the results of your call in the patient's clinical record. Summarize the results of the telephone call in a letter and mail it to the patient.

Time Table for Collection Levels

- 0–30 days: Send statements, process insurance claims, monitor budget plans.
- 30–60 days: Level One: Use a friendly reminder on statements.
- 60–90 days: Level Two: Follow up with a telephone call. Identify the problem and provide a solution. Notify the patient in writing, summarizing the results of the telephone call.
- 90–120 days: Level Three: Send a collection letter and follow with a telephone call.
- Beyond 120 days: Level Four: Send a letter, giving the patient an ultimatum.
- No response to letter: Level Five: Turn the account over for collection, or file a suit in Small Claims Court.

Time intervals may vary, depending on the policies of the dental practice.

- The patient does not follow through with payment promises.

Excuses that should not be accepted are these:

- "I will pay the bill in full when all of the work is completed," or "I will pay the bill when I get my tax return." Tactfully explain the office payment policy. If the patient does not accept the financial policy, do not schedule a next appointment.
- "Let me talk to the dentist, he is an old friend." Explain that the dentist has given you the responsibility of making the financial arrangements. When patients demand to speak with the dentist, ask them to wait while you see if the dentist is available to speak with them. Tell the dentist the situation and have the dentist tell the patient that you are in charge. This formally returns control to you.

Sometimes, even the attitudes of the dental healthcare team can hamper effective collections. Some examples of this are:

- "I don't think they can pay the bill, so I won't ask and embarrass them."
- "I hate to ask for money. I hope they pay the bill after the insurance company pays."
- "I am the dentist. I will let someone else worry about collecting the money."
- "I don't have time to write letters and make telephone calls; there are other things that need to be done first."
- "I know they have lots of money. They will pay their account. I will just send them a statement."
- "I don't have time to write an aging report; it will just have to wait."

Even though these are natural feelings, you should make sure that they do not prevent you from performing this aspect of the job. Keep in mind that if collections are done with a professional attitude, you do not have to be mean or insulting.

KEY POINTS

- When designing financial policies, consider the community's standards, the practice's philosophy, and sound business principles.
- Types of financial policies include payment in full at time of service, insurance billing, and extended payment plans.
- Managing accounts receivable includes gathering financial data, preparing treatment plans, making financial arrangements, and monitoring accounts receivable reports.
- Collection procedures are a series of reminders that payment is past due. The objective of the process is to collect payment from the patient. There are five levels:
  - Level One: Friendly reminder
  - Level Two: Telephone reminders

- Level Three: Collection letter
- Level Four: The ultimatum
- Level Five: Turning the account over for collection

 Web Watch

Writing a Financial Policy

http://www.pcc.com/mc/seminars/policy.html

How to Improve your Chances of Receiving Payment From a Risky Customer

http://www.bernsteinlaw.com/publications/htimprov.html

Business Owner's Toolkit: Improving Your Collection Cycle

http://www.toolkit.cch.com/text/P062700.asp

Collection Techniques

http://www.onlinewbc.org/docs/finance/collect.html

 Log on to Evolve to access additional web links!

http://evolve.elsevier.com

 Critical Thinking Questions

1. List the elements of a financial policy, and describe how each element is applied to the policy.
2. State the purpose of managing accounts receivable. Describe the role of the administrative dental assistant in managing accounts receivable.
3. List the various levels of the collection process. Describe the steps that the administrative dental assistant must take to complete the collection process at each level.

OUTLINE

KEY TERMS AND CONCEPTS

Accounting
Accounts Payable
Accounts Receivable
Accounts Receivable Reports
Aging
Bookkeeping

Charge Slip
Daily Journal
Financial Reports
Financially Responsible
Insurance Information
Pegboard System

Posting Transactions
Production Reports
Profit and Loss Statements
Proof of Posting
Receipts
Routing Slips

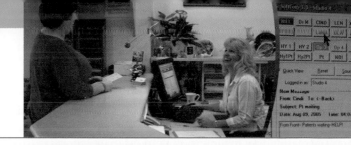

14

Bookkeeping Procedures: Accounts Receivable

LEARNING OBJECTIVES

The student will:

1. Discuss the role of the administrative dental assistant in the management of patient financial transactions.
2. Describe the different components of a pegboard system: daily journal, ledger card, and receipt and charge slips.
3. Describe the steps in posting transactions: charges, payments and adjustments, and proof of posting.
4. Discuss the importance of an audit report.
5. Describe a process for implementing an audit trail. Compare the audit trails used in a computerized bookkeeping system with those used in a manual bookkeeping system.

INTRODUCTION

Dentistry, like any business, is mandated by federal and state regulations to maintain a system that documents the collection of monies. Smart business practice also requires that a financial system be maintained, with both accounts receivable and accounts payable. **Accounts receivable** is the system that records all financial transactions between a patient and the dental practice. This system calculates the amount of money owed to the dental practice by accounting for charges and payments. **Accounts payable** is the system that records all monies the dental practice owes others. It is the responsibility of the administrative dental assistant to maintain accurate records in the management of accounts receivable and accounts payable.

Two separate procedures are required in the maintenance of financial records and reports. The administrative dental assistant is responsible for bookkeeping. **Bookkeeping** is the method of recording all financial transactions. The second procedure is accounting. **Accounting** is the method used to verify and classify all transactions (accounts payable and accounts receivable) and is usually the duty of an accountant. An accountant may be employed by large dental practices. Smaller dental practices usually seek the outside services of an accountant who will audit bookkeeping procedures, calculate taxes, and write financial reports.

COMPONENTS OF FINANCIAL RECORDS ORGANIZATION

Patient information
- Identifies person responsible for payment of the account
- Identifies insurance coverage

Method of recording transactions
- Computerized
- Manual bookkeeping, "pegboard" or "one write" system

Billing
- Patient
- Insurance company

Patient Information

The first step is to determine who is **financially responsible** for the account. Information can be obtained from the financial information section of a patient registration form (Figure 14-1). **Insurance information,** both primary (first coverage) and secondary (second coverage), is listed on the same form.

Methods of Recording Transactions

Computerized Bookkeeping Systems

Computerized bookkeeping uses a program to organize, track, and calculate the accounts receivable (Figure 14-2, *A*). This program is usually a main component in a full management system of the type used in most dental practices (discussed in Chapter 17). The advantage of using a comprehensive practice management system is that the information that has been recorded in an electronic clinical record is shared with other components of the system. Data that have been entered once into the system can be used for a variety of different financial tasks, including tracking treatment, billing insurance, billing patients, preparing deposit slips, formulating accounting reports, and forecasting the financial health of the dental practice. The system will also perform many of the daily tasks performed by the administrative assistant in managing patient transactions quickly and efficiently.

Manual Bookkeeping Systems

The most common manual bookkeeping system used in a dental practice is the **pegboard system.** This system uses a variety of forms designed to be placed one on top of another for the purpose of entering the information one time (also referred to as a "one write system"). As with the computer system, the same information is used to perform several different functions. Once the information is entered, it is the responsibility of the administrative assistant to calculate totals and balance the spreadsheets (Figure 14-2, *B*).

Use of a pegboard requires that the administrative assistant be familiar with each step and know how to properly make entries, use receipts and superbills, produce monthly statements, and use a 10-key adding machine or calculator (preferably with a tape for verification of entries).

3 2 6 5 1 0

© 2002 Wisconsin Dental Association
(800) 243-4675

welcome

Date 7/1/2006

Patient's Name Budd (Last) Rose (First) L (Initial) Date of Birth 7/17/52 Male Female

If Child: Parent's Name ____

How do you wish to be addressed Rosie

Single ☒ Married ☐ Separated ☐ Divorced ☐ Widowed ☐ Minor ☐

Residence - Street 1836 N Front Street

City Flora State CA Zip 91711

Business Address 123 S Business Way

Telephone: Res. 555-4321 Bus. 555-3210

Fax ____ Cell Phone # ____

eMail R.L.Budd@townbank.com

Patient/Parent Employed By Town Bank

Present Position N/A

How Long Held N/A

Spouse/Parent Name N/A

Spouse Employed By N/A

Present Position N/A

How Long Held N/A

Who is Responsible for this account Self

Drivers License No. M3205167

Method of Payment: Insurance ☒ Cash ☐ Credit Card ☐

Purpose of Call Check-up

Other Family Members in this Practice No

Whom may we thank for this referral Self

Patient/parent Social Security No. 123-45-6789

Spouse/Parent Social Security No. N/A

Someone to notify in case of emergency not living with you

Evelyn Jones

DENTAL INSURANCE 1ST COVERAGE

Employee Name Rose Budd Date of Birth 7/17/52

Employer Name Town Bank Yrs. 12

Name of Insurance Co. Blue Cross

Address 1116 Form St.
Los Angeles, CA 91110

Telephone 310-555-6381

Program or policy # 8476

Social Security No. 123-45-6789

Union Local or Group N/A

DENTAL INSURANCE 2ND COVERAGE

Employee Name ____ Date of Birth ____

Employer Name ____ Yrs. ____

Name of Insurance Co. ____

Address ____

Telephone ____

Program or policy # ____

Social Security No. ____

Union Local or Group ____

CONSENT:

I consent to the diagnostic procedures and treatment by the dentist necessary for proper dental care.

I consent to the dentist's use and disclosure of my records (or my child's records) to carry out treatment, to obtain payment, and for those activities and health care operations that are related to treatment or payment.

I consent to the disclosure of my records (or my child's records) to the following persons who are involved in my care (or my child's care) or payment for that care.

My consent to disclosure of records shall be effective until I revoke it in writing.

I authorize payment directly to the dentist or dental group of insurance benefits otherwise payable to me. I understand that my dental care insurance carrier or payor of my dental benefits may pay less than the actual bill for services, and that I am financially responsible for payment in full of all accounts. By signing this statement, I revoke all previous agreements to the contrary and agree to be responsible for payment of services not paid, by my dental care payor.

I attest to the accuracy of the information on this page.

PATIENT'S OR GUARDIAN'S SIGNATURE Rose Budd

DATE 7/1/2006

Form No. T110R

REGISTRATION

FIGURE 14-1

Completed patient registration form, including financial and insurance information. (Courtesy The Dental Record, Wisconsin Dental Association, Milwaukee, WI.)

ACCOUNTS RECEIVABLE REPORT

01/31/06

ACCOUNT	PATIENT	DESCRIPTION	CHARGE	PAYMENT	ADJ.	BALANCE	DOCTOR
326570	Budd, Rose	Insurance payment		98.00			
	Budd, Rose	Insurance adjustment			12.00	80.00	
436825	Williams, Frank	Nonsufficient funds	68.00				
		Service charge	12.00			80.00	
563261	Coulson, Jodi	Patient payment		62.00		+22.00	
421831	Johnson, Dawn	Restorative	230.00			240.00	Edw
234681	Gonzales, Maria	Prophylaxis	62.00				
		Cash payment		62.00		0	Viv
246392	Brown, Angela	Full mouth x-ray	80.00				Edw
		Patient payment		62.00		80.00	
136218	Vail, Mark	Composite restoration	246.00				Edw
		Prof. courtesy			24.60	221.40	
023815	Tract, Lois	Insurance payment		630.00			
		Insurance adjustment			20.00	171.00	
		Daily total	698.00	914.00			
					56.60		
		Month-to-date	3938.00	3077.00			
					35.50		
		Accounts receivable month-to-date	825.50				

A

FIGURE 14-2

A, Computer-generated daysheet.

BILLING

Billing is the procedure that notifies a responsible party (individual or insurance carrier) regarding the current status of an account. Insurance carriers are sent the attending dentist's statements (claim forms) and patients are sent statements. A statement indicates the date of service, identifies the patient, and lists all transactions (treatment and payment). The purposes of the statement are to inform the patient and to request payment for the balance due. It is important that statements are easy for patients to read and understand (Figure 14-3).

Patient billing is an organized procedure that should be performed at the same time each month. Several different methods may be used to produce and mail patient statements. A key to successful billing is to be consistent each month. Patients usually pay bills around their paydays. The most common pay periods are the 1st and 15th of each month. Therefore, if you want the bills to be paid

DAILY LOG OF CHARGES AND RECEIPTS

DATE 1/31/06 SHEET NUMBER _____ A B1 B2 C D

	DATE	FAMILY MEMBER	PROFESSIONAL SERVICES	CHARGE	CREDITS PYMTS.	CREDITS ADJ.	NEW BALANCE	PREVIOUS BALANCE	NAME
1	1/31	Rose	ins. pmt./adj.		98 00	12 00	80 00	190 00	Rose Budd
2	1/31	Frank	NSF	80 00	—	—	80 00	Ø	Frank Williams
3	1/31	Jodi	payment	—	62 00	—	‹22 00›	40 00	Jodi Coulson
4	1/31	Dawn	Restorative	230 00	Ø	—	240 00	10 00	Dawn Johnson
5	1/31	Maria	prophy/c.pmt.	62 00	62 00	—	Ø	Ø	Marie Gonzales
6	1/31	Angela	FMX		62 00	—	80 00	62 00	Angela Brown
7	1/31	Mark	Composite	246 00	—	24 00	221 40	Ø	Mark Vail
8	1/31	Lois	ins. pmt.	—	630 00	20 00	171 00	821 00	Lois Tract

TOTALS		Col. "A"	Col. "B-1"	Col. "B-2"	Col. "C"	Col. "D"
THIS PAGE		698 00	914 00	56 60	850 40	1123 00
PREVIOUS PAGE		3240 00	2163 00	‹21 10›	5419 10	4321 00
MONTH-TO-DATE		3938 00	3077 00	35 50	6269 50	5444 00

PROOF OF POSTING	
COL. D TOTAL	$ 1123.00
PLUS COL. A TOTAL	$ 698.00
SUB TOTAL	$ 1821.00
LESS COLS. B-1 & B-2	$ 970.60
MUST EQUAL COL. C	$ 850.40

ACCOUNTS RECEIVABLE CONTROL	
PREVIOUS DAY'S TOTAL	$ 1098.10
PLUS COL. A	$ 698.00
SUB TOTAL	$ 1796.10
LESS COLS. B-1 & B-2	$ 970.60
TOTAL ACCTS. REC.	$ 825.50

ACCOUNTS RECEIVABLE PROOF	
ACCTS. REC. 1ST OF MONTH	$ Ø
PLUS COL. A.-MO. TO DATE	$ 3938.00
SUB TOTAL	$ 3938.00
LESS B-1 & B-2 MO. TO DATE	$ 3112.50
TOTAL ACCTS. REC.	$ 825.50

FIGURE 14-2, cont'd

B, Pegboard daysheet.

STATEMENT

Mary A. Edwards, DDS
4516 North Avery Way
Canyon View, CA 91783

CLOSING DATE
September 10, 2006

RESPONSIBLE PARTY
Ms. Rose Budd
1836 N. Front Street
Flora, CA 91711

ACCOUNT NUMBER
120-345678-900

AMOUNT ENCLOSED

A

DATE	DESCRIPTION	CHARGES	CREDITS	BALANCE DUE
7-1-06	Initial examination	20.00		
	Full mouth x-rays	90.00		110.00
7-17-06	Gingival treatment	65.00		
	Patient payment, check		50.00	125.00
7-23-06	Gingival treatment	65.00		190.00
8-12-06	Insurance payment, Blue Cross		98.00	
	Insurance adjustment, per BC		12.00	80.00
8-22-06	Insurance payment, Blue Cross		54.00	26.00
9-10-06	Patient payment, check		26.00	0
				PAY LAST AMOUNT

FIGURE 14-3
A, Computer-generated statement.

around those dates, schedule your billing period so that patients receive their statements around the 10th or 23rd of each month. Not all statements need to be sent on the same day. If you are working in a very large office, statements can be divided and sent weekly or bimonthly.

Insurance companies are billed with the attending dentist's statements or encounter forms, as discussed in Chapter 11. In addition to billing of the insurance company directly, superbills can be given to patients, and it becomes the responsibility of the patient to bill the insurance company. Superbills can

be computer generated or may be completed with use of a pegboard system.

Pegboard System

Components of the pegboard system include NCR (no carbon required) paper with carbon strips placed on the backs of receipts. This system allows the administrative assistant to write the information one time. When all of the forms are aligned correctly, the information is transferred to the corresponding column on the receipt, ledger card, and **daily journal.** In addition, an NCR-treated deposit slip

STATEMENT

Mary A. Edwards, DDS
4516 North Avery Way
Canyon View, CA 91783

Ms. Rose Budd
1836 N. Front Street
Flora, CA 91711

DATE	FAMILY MEMBER	PROFESSIONAL SERVICE	CHARGE	CREDITS		BALANCE
				PAYMENTS	ADJ.	
				BALANCE FORWARD ⟶		Ø
7/1/06	Rose	EX, FMX	110.00	Ø		110.00
7/17/06	Rose	GT, CK	65.00	50 00		125.00
7/23/06	Rose	GT	65.00			190.00
8/12/06	Rose	CI–		98 00	12 00	80.00
8/22/06	Rose	CI–		54 00		26.00
9/10/06	Rose	CK		26 00		Ø
				PAY LAST AMOUNT IN THIS COLUMN ⟶		

B

B = Bording	CK = Check	NC = No Charge
BA = Broken Appointment	E = Extraction	OS = Oral Surgery
CB = Crown and bridge	EX = Examination	P = Prophylaxis
C = Composite restoration	FMX = Full Mouth X-rays	PER = Periodontal
CA = Cash	FT = Fluoride Treatment	R = Root Canal
CI = Check – Insurance	GT = Gingival Treatment	RC = Restoration Amalgam

FIGURE 14-3, cont'd
B, Pegboard statement (copy of ledger card).

ANATOMY OF A PEGBOARD ACCOUNTS RECEIVABLE SYSTEM

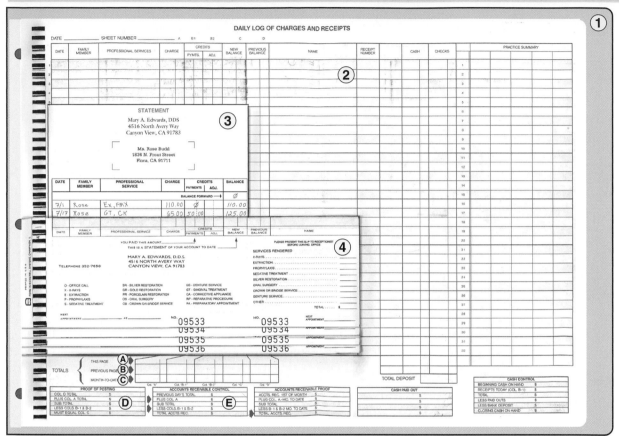

(Forms courtesy of Colwell Systems, Champaign, IL.)

① PEGBOARD
The pegboard is a flat board with a series of pegs on the left-hand side of the board. The pegs align and hold the forms in place. The alignment facilitates the "one write" concept.

② DAILY JOURNAL
The daily journal (day sheet, daily log of charges and receipts) is a large sheet that is placed over the pegs. The daily journal contains information that identifies all financial transactions that have taken place during the day (or other identified period of time). At the end of the recording period (day), columns are totaled, balanced, and placed in a journal for storage. Information stated in the journal becomes an important document and must be safeguarded against loss or damage.

③ ACCOUNT RECORD
Ledger cards contain individual account information. Information listed on the ledger card identifies the patient, treatment, payment information, and account balance.

Ledger cards are placed alphabetically in trays (Fig. 14-4). The information on the ledger card is considered confidential and is important documentation. The cards are stored in metal boxes which can be tightly closed at the end of the day to protect them from fire and damage.

④ RECEIPT AND CHARGE SLIPS
This portion of the system is used as a communication and audit tool. The clinical assistant or administrative assistant enters transaction information onto the charge slip (communicating with the front office). The information is used to post transactions. The receipt portion of the slip is used to communicate transactions with the patient. Control numbers are printed on each slip, providing a tracking system to ensure that all transactions are posted.

Superbills are used in the same way as receipts. With the addition of insurance coding (CDT Procedure Codes), they can also be used for insurance billing. The completed superbill is given to the patient and it becomes the responsibility of the patient to submit the form to the insurance carrier.

ANATOMY OF DAILY JOURNAL CALCULATIONS

Ⓐ Add each column vertically and place the totals in the corresponding boxes.

Ⓑ Bring previous page totals forward (found in the corresponding box on the previous day's journal).

Ⓒ Add the columns, enter the total in the corresponding box.

Ⓓ Complete "Proof of Posting".

Ⓔ Complete "Accounts Receivable Control".

can be attached to the appropriate section of the daily journal, providing for a "one write" deposit slip.

DAILY ROUTINE FOR MANAGING PATIENT TRANSACTIONS

Steps in Managing Patient Transactions

1. Identify patients.
2. Produce routing slips.
3. Post financial transactions.
4. Document patient treatments.
5. Document payments.
6. Complete end of day procedures.

REMEMBER

All of the following tasks can be performed with use of a manual system, computerized system, or combination of both systems. Although techniques will differ in the completion of tasks, all systems will contain the same types of tasks: identifying patients, producing routing slips, posting transactions, and completing end of day procedures.

Identify Patients

Identify patients who are going to be seen during the day. The day before treatment, pull patients' clinical records, confirm appointments, type daily schedules, and check pending treatments. Members of the dental healthcare team can review the charts before patients arrive. This process allows the team to become aquatinted with the schedule, check for adverse medical conditions, determine what type of anesthetic will be used, acquire information that can be used to personalize a conversation with a patient, check whether laboratory work has been returned, and mentally prepare for the day. It is at this point that the team can have a short meeting to discuss the patients and cases for the day.

Produce Routing Slips

Routing slips are used to communicate treatment information between the treatment area and the business office. Computerized routing slips may contain information about the patient, such as treatment plan, date of last visit, and list of other family members who are patients. Financial information includes previous balance, payment plan, financial arrangements, and insurance balance. Routing slips can be complex, computer-generated forms or simple charge slips. Superbills and encounter forms are frequently used as routing slips.

HIPAA

Privacy Rule

PHI routing slips are attached to all clinical charts and sent to the treatment area. At the conclusion of treatment, the clinical assistant completes the routing slip and returns the slip with the patient to the business office. Treatment information is used to post transactions, and other information is used to schedule patients for their next appointment.

At the end of the day, it is the responsibility of the administrative assistant to account for all routing slips issued during the day. If a slip is missing, it must be located before the audit of daily transactions is completed. All routing slips are placed in numerical order and attached to the audit report. Reports are kept as a backup (when a computerized bookkeeping system is used) for a specified period and then destroyed.

Post Transactions

Posting transactions is accomplished by placing appropriate information on the patient's ledger card, receipt, and daysheet (manual system) or by keying the information into a computerized system, as is discussed in greater detail in Chapter 17.

At the beginning of each day, a new daysheet is placed on the pegboard. Pages are dated and numbered (monthly, quarterly, or annually). A series of **receipts** are aligned on the daysheet (first receipt aligned on the first line of the daysheet).

Ledger cards for each patient can be pulled at the beginning of each day. When the first patient arrives, his or her ledger card is placed under the first receipt. The previous balance is entered, the receipt is dated, and the patient's name is listed. The **charge slip** portion is removed from the receipt and given to the chairside assistant. When treatment is completed and the patient is checking out, the completed charge slip is returned to the administrative

Steps in Managing Patient Transactions

1. At the beginning of the day, set up the pegboard with a daysheet and charge slips.
2. When checking a patient in (or at the beginning of the day), remove the patient's ledger card from the tray (Figure 14-4). Enter the date, patient name, and previous balance on a charge slip. Use a ballpoint pen, and press hard to make sure all copies are legible.
3. Remove the end of the charge slip at the perforation, attach it to the patient's clinical chart (if using the charge slip as a routing slip), and send the chart to the treatment area.
4. Have the clinical assistant complete the charge slip by entering a code for the treatment and the fee.
5. Make sure that you receive the charge slip during the patient's checkout.
6. Return the patient's ledger card to the pegboard, and align it under the correct receipt.
7. Use information communicated on the charge slip to complete the receipt by
   - Placing a code for the professional service.
   - Entering the total charge. Obtain this information from the charge slip, routing slip, superbill, encounter form, or clinical record. Add the figures twice to ensure accuracy.
   - Asking the patient for payment. If a payment is made, enter the amount under the payment. (If using an NCR deposit slip, record the payment in the correct location on the daysheet.) Adjustments are also recorded at this point. The patient may receive a professional courtesy discount, a senior citizen discount, and so forth. Place the amount of the discount in the adjustment column.

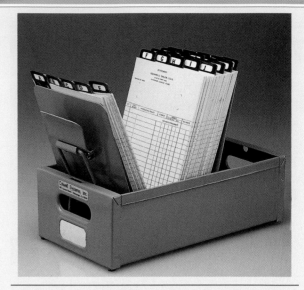

FIGURE 14-4
Ledger tray used for storage of ledger cards. (Courtesy Colwell Systems, Champaign, IL.)

assistant. The administrative assistant returns the patient's ledger card to the correct location under the corresponding receipt and uses the information to complete the transaction. Charges are entered, payments are recorded, and the new balance is calculated. The patient is given the receipt. The charge slip is filed for later use when the audit report is completed.

Several methods can be used to organize the daily posting routine. All methods, although they vary, include the same elements: identify each patient seen during the day, communicate treatment information from the clinical area to the business office, post all transactions (charges, payment, and adjustments), balance the daysheet at the end of the day to ensure accounting accuracy, and complete an audit report to ensure that all transactions have been posted. Missing one or two chargeable transactions daily can cost the dental practice hundreds of dollars.

Complete End of the Day Procedures

At the end of each day, transactions entered on the daysheet must be totaled and balanced. Each column is added vertically and then balanced horizontally. At the bottom of each sheet is a summary section referred to as the **proof of posting.** The function of this section is to double-check all figures for accuracy. When the proof shows an error, it is necessary to go back and re-add all of the columns. The process is not complete until the page balances.

Steps in Managing Patient Transactions—cont'd

8. Calculate the new balance:
   - Enter the previous balance into an adding machine or calculator.
   - Add new charges.
   - Subtract payments.
   - Subtract adjustments.
   - Arrive at new balance.

   Example: Mary Smith is seen for dental treatment (Figure 14-5). Her previous balance was $45.00, and today's treatment was $135.00. She made a payment of $100 and received a 10% senior citizen discount.

   - Previous balance $45.00
     (column D)
   - Today's treatment   +$135.00
     (column A)
   - Payment (column B1)   −$100.00
     $100.00
   - Adjustment   −$13.50
     (column B2) (135.00×.10)
   - Balance (column C) $66.50

9. Remove the receipt from the pegboard and give it to the patient.
10. Keep the charge slip to complete the audit report.

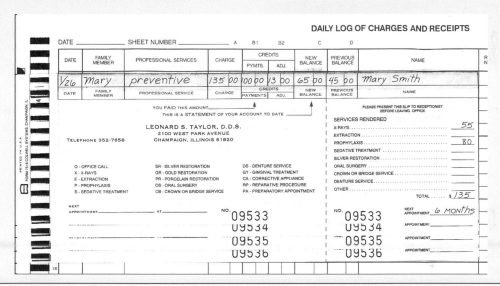

FIGURE 14-5

Illustration calculating patient's balance based on the pegboard system, for Mary Smith. (Courtesy Colwell Systems, Champaign, IL.)

At this point, the administrative dental assistant becomes a detective to determine at what point the error was made. Meticulous tenacity is sometimes needed to discover the error.

Hints for Finding Errors

1. Determine the difference between the answer and the daysheet answer. Check for that amount (it may have been placed in the wrong column).
2. If the difference is a multiple of 3, it may be an error in addition performed with a 10-key adding machine (incorrect finger placement will be off by 3).
3. Re-add all of the vertical columns. If an error in addition is discovered, make the correction and complete the proof of posting procedure.
4. Check horizontal calculations (totals). Recalculate each patient's horizontal figures (previous balance plus charges, less payments, and plus or minus adjustments equals the ending balance). When an error in calculations involves a difference in a patient's balance, correct the ledger card.

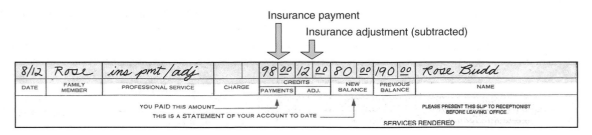

FIGURE 14-6

Example of an insurance payment adjustment. Adjustment information is listed on the Explanation of Benefits form sent with insurance checks. (Form excerpt courtesy Colwell Systems, Champaign, IL.)

REMEMBER

> Corrections are made by drawing a line through the incorrect information and making a new entry. Never use white-out or completely cover an error. Check for incomplete transactions. A common error involves forgetting to enter the previous balance.

5. Sometimes, the adjustment is calculated incorrectly. When a figure is bracketed ($\langle 21.00 \rangle$), the method for calculation is reversed. For example, when a credit balance of $\langle \$22.00 \rangle$ is entered in the new balance column, the figure is subtracted (not added).
6. Sometimes, entries are transposed and numbers are reversed (e.g., instead of 14, 41 has been written).
7. If numbers are poorly written in poor handwriting, they may be interpreted incorrectly.
8. After corrections are made, the proof of posting procedure must be completed and balanced.
9. Complete the other controls (accounts receivable control, accounts receivable proof, cash paid out, and cash control) at the bottom of the daysheet *only after the proof of posting is correctly completed.*

Posting Payments

In addition to receiving payments at the time of service, the practice will receive payments in the mail daily. Checks from patients and insurance companies are posted to accounts receivable in the same manner as daily transactions. The ledger card is pulled for the patient and placed on the daysheet, and payment information is entered.

Most insurance companies do not pay 100% of the amount billed. The balance is therefore billed to the patient as the patient portion. Some contracts with insurance carriers stipulate that a patient cannot be charged a fee higher than the fee allowable by the contract. If a higher fee is charged, the disallowed amount (clearly stated on the Explanation of Benefits form) must be adjusted. The amount is entered in the adjustment column and subtracted from the patient portion (Figure 14-6).

Posting Credit Card Payments

Payment may be made by credit card. In addition to credit cards, there are debit cards. Both cards are processed in the same manner. The card is swiped through an electronic credit card terminal. The terminal electronically sends data to a card center for approval. The credit card terminal also serves as a printer and produces a transaction receipt for the patient and the office. Money is directly deposited into the specified account from the card center. The transaction is recorded on the daysheet the same way that a cash or check payment is recorded.

Adjustments

Adjustments are made to an account for a variety of reasons. Disallowed insurance charges, professional courtesies, senior discounts, and uncollectible fees are all examples of adjustments that reduce the patient's balance (see Figure 14-6).

One adjustment that raises a patient's balance is a returned check. NSF (nonsufficient funds) checks are checks that are not honored by the bank (Figure 14-7). Stop payment checks are another form of returned item from the bank. The amount of the check has already been deducted from the patient's

Charge is added (a returned check fee may be added)

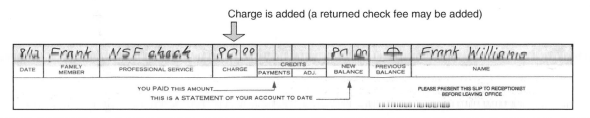

FIGURE 14-7

Example of an entry for recording a check returned for nonsufficient funds (NSF). (Form excerpt courtesy Colwell Systems, Champaign, IL.)

Overpayment creates a credit balance

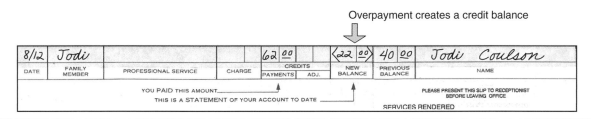

FIGURE 14-8

Example of recording a credit balance. Use brackets to indicate a change in the calculation method. (Form excerpt courtesy Colwell Systems, Champaign, IL.)

Add   Subtract

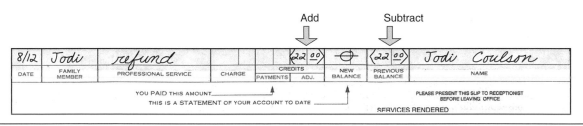

FIGURE 14-9

Example of a refund transaction. Use the opposite function when numbers are bracketed. Add when you usually would subtract, and subtract when you usually would add. (Form excerpt courtesy Colwell Systems, Champaign, IL.)

account balance; therefore, it is necessary to recharge the patient. In addition, most banks add a service charge for returned items, which can be passed on to the patient. Record both transactions in the service column (charge to the account), and clearly identify the source of the charge.

Credit balances are created when there has been a payment that is larger than the balance due (Figure 14-8). This may occur when a patient pays in advance of treatment. When a credit balance remains at the conclusion of treatment, a refund will be made to the patient (Figure 14-9).

It may be necessary to give overdue accounts to an outside agency for collection. This is done after a reasonable attempt has been made to collect payment. The agency charges a commission to collect the amount, and the commission will be adjusted from the patient's balance (Figure 14-10).

Completing the Audit Report

The purpose of an audit report is to track all daily transactions and verify that all transactions were posted correctly. This is an important step and should not be skipped. A simple report walks you

Payment from collection agency

Adjustment for collection agency commission

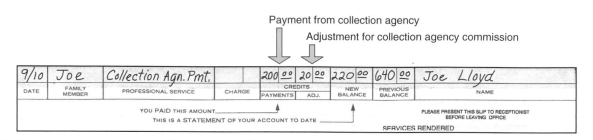

DATE	FAMILY MEMBER	PROFESSIONAL SERVICE	CHARGE	CREDITS PAYMENTS	ADJ.	NEW BALANCE	PREVIOUS BALANCE	NAME
9/10	Joe	Collection Agn. Pmt.		200 00	20 00	220 00	640 00	Joe Lloyd

YOU PAID THIS AMOUNT_____

THIS IS A STATEMENT OF YOUR ACCOUNT TO DATE _____

PLEASE PRESENT THIS SLIP TO RECEPTIONIST BEFORE LEAVING OFFICE

SERVICES RENDERED

FIGURE 14-10

Example of a collection agency payment. (Form excerpt courtesy Colwell Systems, Champaign, IL.)

through all of the steps, is easy to complete, and ensures that every transaction has been recorded.

The audit report is necessary for two reasons: to identify omissions or errors so they can be corrected, and to protect the employer against embezzlement (stealing by an employee).

Steps in Completing an Audit Report

1. Account for all routing slips (or charge slips).
2. Add total charges. The total charges should match the daily production total listed on the daysheet (computerized or manual).
3. Match deposit slips and direct deposits with the reported amounts of money collected.
4. Identify types of payments: mail, insurance, credit card, checks, and cash.
5. Attach documentation (computerized daily journal, copy of proof of posting from daily journal, routing slips, copy of daily schedule, copy of deposit slip).

Petty Cash (Change Fund)

Sometimes, a small amount of cash is kept on hand to make change and to purchase small items. The amount of money placed in the fund varies but must be tracked. When an item is purchased with petty cash, the receipt is placed in the petty cash file and the amount is recorded in the petty cash journal or at the bottom of the daysheet. If the doctor or another staff member requests cash from petty cash, a voucher must be filled out with the amount and date and signed by the person taking the money. When money is replenished, a check is drawn and cashed at the bank, and the new amount is entered

into the journal or onto the daily journal sheet. A check is used for the purpose of tracking the transaction. Cash should not be taken from a deposit because it will change the amount of the deposit so that the deposit total will not match the amount of money collected for the day.

Routine for Managing Financial Transactions

Day Before

- Pull patients' charts and review them.
- Confirm appointments.
- Type a daily schedule and make copies for each treatment room and other areas.
- Check on laboratory work that is due.
- Fill the schedule, if needed, from the call list.

Day of Appointment

- Produce routing slips.
- Check schedule.
- Review charts with office staff (mini-staff meeting).
- When patient arrives, update financial, medical, and insurance information.
- When treatment is completed, proceed with patient checkout, post transactions, and schedule next appointment.
- Process mail payments.

End of Day

- Complete posting of daily transactions.
- Balance daysheet and produce required reports.
- Complete audit report, and account for all charts.
- Complete insurance processing.

REPORTS

Reports are used to summarize and outline various conditions. Reports that are often used in a dental practice identify patients who are due for recall appointments, patients who have not completed treatment plans, and outstanding insurance claims. In addition to the many reports that identify what needs to be done, some reports illustrate the financial status of the dental practice. Reports enable the dental healthcare team to identify strong and weak areas of the practice and to make necessary corrections. Reports are used by accountants and bookkeepers for the purpose of reporting financial information to government agencies and are considered legal documents.

Reports are written with information that is tabulated and collected. Without a computer to organize and store information, report writing can be long and laborious. Reports can be generated in different formats and according to different criteria. Information for financial reports is obtained from check registers, deposit records, and bank statements. Style and criteria are determined by the nature of the report and the needs of the dentist or accountant.

The administrative dental assistant is responsible for collecting and maintaining financial data to help the accountant generate financial reports. Organizing and maintaining financial records that are inaccurate *is not* an option. This information is used to produce legal documents and must be maintained and protected with the utmost care and accuracy.

Types of Reports

Financial reports are used to determine the financial health of a dental practice. Accountants use them to report business, income, and payroll taxes.

Profit and loss statements are used to identify overhead (the cost it takes to operate a business). They also show whether the dental practice is making or losing money.

Accounts receivable reports categorize the monies patients and insurance companies owe the dental practice. When money is slow in being paid to the dental practice, all members of the team are affected. In addition to the amount of money that is owed, the length of time the money is owed is important. **Aging** the accounts receivable reports shows how much of the money that is owed is 30, 60, 90, or 120 days past due. Most dental practices do not charge interest on money owed; therefore, each day money remains unpaid, the value of the money depreciates (loses value). Accounts receivable reports draw attention to the overdue accounts by identifying the amount of money owed, by whom it is owed, and how long it has been since the last payment. With this report, the administrative dental assistant is able to take action in expediting the collection of outstanding accounts.

Production reports identify what type of procedures have been performed and by whom. These reports can be used to determine whether the dental team is productive. Offices with associate dentists and hygienists whose salaries are based on production use these reports to calculate compensation.

Additional Reports

Insurance Reports

- Outstanding insurance claims
- Amount of money owed by insurance companies
- Aging of insurance claims
- Incomplete work
- Work completed but not submitted for payment
- Preauthorized dental treatment

Accounts Payable Reports

- Money owed to others (bills)
- Account balances
- Categories of expenditures (used in financial reports)

Bank Account Reports

- Account balances
- Average daily balance
- Interest
- Credits and debits

Payroll

- Employee accounting (salary, deductions, taxes paid)
- Payment of payroll tax (by the dentist)
- Payment of Workers' Compensation insurance
- Payment to pension and employee benefits funds

KEY POINTS

- **Accounts receivable** is the system by which all financial transactions between the patient and the dental practice are recorded. **Accounts payable** is the system by which money owed by the dental practice to others is recorded. It is the responsibility of the administrative dental assistant to keep accurate records in the management of accounts receivable and accounts payable.
- **Patient financial information** is recorded in a computer system or a manual bookkeeping ledger. The manual system most often used is the pegboard system.
- **Managing financial transactions,** either computerized or manual, includes
  - Posting transactions
  - Balancing day sheets (ensuring factual and accurate reporting)
  - Completing audit reports (ensuring that all transactions have been posted)
  - Billing patients and insurance carriers
- **Reports** are used to illustrate different financial and patient trends. Financial reports are used by accountants and members of the dental health-care team to determine the fiscal health of the dental practice. These reports are also used for mandated documentation and account reporting to government agencies.

 Web Watch

Bookkeeping and Accounting: From Start to Finish

http:www.sba.gov/test/wbc/docs/finance/bkpg_basic1. html

 Log on to Evolve to access additional web links!

http://evolve.elsevier.com

 Critical Thinking Questions

1. List the components of financial records management, and describe how they are used.
2. Design an audit report form, and develop a process for utilization of the form. Identify whether the plan was designed for a manual system or a computerized system. Use information in the text, and consult other resources.

Notes

OUTLINE

KEY TERMS

Accounts Payable
Balance

Invoice
Statement

15

Bookkeeping Procedures: Accounts Payable

LEARNING OBJECTIVES

The student will:

1. Describe the function of accounts payable.
2. Formulate a system to organize accounts payable.
3. Analyze the methods of check writing and state their functions.

4. Discuss steps to reconcile a checking account and list the necessary information.
5. List and discuss the information needed for a payroll record.

INTRODUCTION

Accounts payable is a system by which all dental practice expenditures are organized, verified, and categorized. The system identifies when checks for bills (including payroll) are to be written, verifies charges, and categorizes expenditures. Other elements of the accounts payable system include reconciliation of the checking accounts and preparation of documents for the accountant.

ORGANIZING AN ACCOUNTS PAYABLE SYSTEM

1. Establish set dates each month when checks will be generated. Some payroll checks, payments to government agencies, and other types of payments have a specific date they must be paid on or a penalty will be assessed. Monthly statements include a grace period; when a payment is received after the grace period, additional interest or late fees may be charged. Checks should be mailed 10 days before the due date to allow time for processing.
2. Develop a filing system that categorizes unpaid bills according to the date the checks to pay the bills will be written. When a statement is received, check the due date and file the statement in the correct folder.
3. Before statements are paid, verify postings (charges and payments) by comparing invoices with the statement. If errors are discovered, it is the responsibility of the administrative dental assistant to ensure that corrections are made.
4. Prepare checks using a computer check writing program or a manual check writing system.
5. Stamp the date paid on the statement, and include the check number. File the paid statement in the appropriate file.
6. Categorize expenditures for use in accounting reports.

VERIFICATION OF EXPENDITURES

The accounts payable process begins when an invoice arrives in the office. An **invoice** is a list of purchased items and their charges. The supplier of the goods or service sends a detailed list of the items shipped or the service provided. The assistant who receives the order confirms that the items listed have been included in the shipment. Notations are made if an item has been placed on back order or is not included in the shipment. Invoices are then placed in the appropriate file.

A **statement** is a list of the totals of all invoices. For example, a dental laboratory processes several different cases during the month. Each time a completed case is returned to the dental practice, an invoice is included. At the end of the month, the dental laboratory creates a statement that summarizes all invoices. When a statement arrives from the laboratory for payment, the envelope is opened and the statement removed, along with the return envelope. Invoices received throughout the month are used to verify charges posted on the statement. After all invoices are accounted for, they are stapled to the corresponding statement.

On the day that bills are to be paid, statements are removed from the file. A protocol may be established that outlines a process for paying bills. It may be the responsibility of the administrative dental assistant to organize statements and give them to the dentist or business manager for authorization.

CHECK WRITING

After approval has been received to pay a bill, the next step is to write the checks or authorize payment. An account can be paid in several different ways. Paper checks can be issued in one of several different formats: pegboard (one write) copy, computer printout, or typewritten or handwritten check. Bills can also be paid electronically.

Payment Authorization and Transfer

Checks authorize a bank to transfer funds from a particular account to another person or company. Checks are no longer limited to paper form. They now include digital and electronic authorizations to transfer funds from an account. Check writing, or payment authorization, can be done via telephone, computerized online service, automatic payment, credit card, and debit card. Although methods of authorizing payments vary, the method of documentation, or record keeping, remains the same. Transactions must be recorded, documented, and verified.

Food for Thought

The use of electronic payments raises several questions for the administrative dental assistant. Each question should be addressed with dental personnel, and a proper protocol should be established. How is documentation completed to ensure that all transactions are recorded? Who is authorized to make electronic transfers? Does the vendor accept electronic transfers? What system is in place to check and double-check the activity on an account, to protect the dental practice from fraudulent activity? Before electronic transfers are made, these questions must be answered to protect the integrity of the dental practice and the administrative dental assistant.

Completing a Deposit Slip

When items are taken to the bank to be deposited, a deposit slip must accompany them (Figure 15-1). The deposit slip (usually preprinted) identifies the account and includes the amount of money being deposited into the account. It is necessary to list the types of funds being deposited (coin, cash, or checks) and amounts of each type. When large amounts in coin are being deposited, it is necessary to wrap the coins first. Cash is separated according to denomination. Checks are listed separately. Some banks require that all checks must be listed and ABA numbers (American Bankers Association routing numbers) included for identification; others accept adding machine tapes with individual checks listed. Follow your bank's protocol.

A receipt is given for each deposit. Keep all receipts in a file, and compare them with the bank statement when that is received. This will help with bank account reconciliation and will provide documentation if a deposit is questioned.

Pegboard Check Writing

Components of the pegboard check writing system are similar to those used in bookkeeping: pegboard, check register, and checks. These are lined up to facilitate a one-write system. Information, as it is written, is transferred to the check register, ensuring that all necessary details are transferred: payee, amount, date, and check number. Anatomy of Pegboard Check Writing System (pages 281-284) illustrates how to record information and calculate the bank balance.

DEPOSIT TICKET

FOR CLEAR COPY, PRESS FIRMLY WITH BALL POINT PEN.

BANK OF THE CANYON
1278 Main street
Canyon View, CA 91783

CHECKS AND OTHER ITEMS ARE RECEIVED FOR DEPOSIT SUBJECT TO THE PROVISIONS OF THE UNIFORM COMMERCIAL CODE OR ANY APPLICABLE COLLECTION AGREEMENT

1: 4590277": 6334792445 08" 6221

DATE _____ April 5 _____ 2006

	DOLLARS	CENTS
CURRENCY		00
COIN		00
LIST EACH CHECK		
1. Budd, R	98	00
2. Coulson, J	62	00
3. Gonzales, M	62	00
4. Brown, A	62	00
5. Tracy, L	630	00
6.		
7.		
8.		
9.		
10.		
11.		
12.		
13.		
14.		
15.		
16.		
17.		
18.		
19.		
20.		
PLEASE ENTER TOTAL	914	00

TOTAL DEPOSIT
DEPOSITS MAY NOT BE AVAILABLE FOR IMMEDIATE WITHDRAWAL.

| | 914 | 00 |

PLEASE BE SURE ALL ITEMS ARE PROPERLY ENDORSED

TOTAL ITEMS   4

50-17
223   0107

FIGURE 15-1

Bank deposit slip. (Modified from Chester GA, Dunham PE: Modern Medical Assisting. Philadelphia, WB Saunders, 1998.)

Steps in Writing a Check

1. Use ink that cannot be changed or altered (ink pen, typewriter, or computer). Technology makes it easy to counterfeit checks. The use of special paper and embossing instruments helps eliminate the possibility that a check can be counterfeited or altered.
2. Write neatly, legibly, and accurately.
3. Correctly enter the name of the payee (person or company receiving the check). Write company names as they appear on their statements (check the statement for this information under the heading "Make checks payable to"). When issuing a check to an individual, you need not use titles (e.g., Mr., Mrs.).
4. Clearly write the amount of the check. The amount is written in two different ways, alpha and numeric:
   $346.75
   Three hundred forty-six and 75/100 dollars
5. Transfer information to the check register: check number, payee, and amount. Fill in all spaces on the check so the amount or the payee cannot be altered. Computer-based programs and "one–write" pegboard systems assure that this step is followed.
6. After checks are written, have them signed by an authorized person. Usually, the dentist or the business manager will sign all checks. Some offices require the signatures of two persons; this is referred to as *double custody*. The purpose of double custody is to protect the dental practice from embezzlement of funds. It is not advisable to have the same person write and sign checks without authorization from another person. This protects both the business and the employee from improperly transferred funds.
7. If an error is made in the writing of a check, the check is voided and a new check issued. It is important to keep the voided check for documentation. When voiding a check, write *void* across the face of the check. Other methods include tearing the check in half and then taping it back together, writing *void* in the check signature area, or tearing the signature area from the check.
8. Checks will not be paid if there are insufficient funds in the account. Before mailing checks, balance the account and verify that sufficient funds are available to cover the payments.

RECONCILING A BANK STATEMENT

At the end of each month or banking period, you will receive a bank statement (Figure 15-2). When the bank statement is received, the account should be reconciled. This ensures that your records and the bank records are in agreement.

Information Listed on a Bank Statement

- Date and amount of each deposit. Deposits are identified by type. For example, direct deposits may have been received from insurance companies or credit card companies. In addition to direct deposits, deposits have been made from the office that contain both checks and cash
- Date, check number, and amount of each check processed by the bank
- Debit items and other amounts that have been deducted from the account (i.e., automatic payments, electronic transfers, bank charges, service charges)
- Daily totals of debits and credits
- Beginning and ending balances
- Canceled checks, unless they are kept by the bank, are returned with the bank statement

Items Needed for Reconciling the Account

- Check register (pegboard, checkbook register, or computerized register)
- Deposit records (documentation of all deposits made by the dental practice)
- Bank statement and all documentation sent from the bank (canceled checks and electronic transfer debit and credit slips)

ANATOMY OF A CHECK

FRONT OF CHECK

(1) NAME OF THE PERSON OR COMPANY ISSUING THE CHECK
Can include address and telephone number.
Caution: Do not give more information than necessary. Do not print drivers license number and social security number on the check. This information could be used to counterfeit checks and credit cards.

(2) ABA BANK IDENTIFICATION NUMBER
Number that identifies the name of the bank and the region where it is located.

(3) CHECK NUMBER
Used for documentation and record keeping reference.

(4) DATE
The day the check is authorized to be paid.

(5) PAY TO THE ORDER OF
The name of the individual or company to whom the funds are to be paid (payee).

(6) PAY _____ DOLLARS
The amount of funds to be paid written in words.

(7) AMOUNT
The amount of funds to be paid written in numbers.

(8) NAME AND ADDRESS OF THE BANK ON WHICH THE FUNDS ARE DRAWN
The bank who will authorize payment of the check.

(9) SIGNATURE
Where authorized person who can draw funds from the account signs his or her name.

(10) MEMO LINE
The reason the check was written.

(11) CODES
Codes for electronic identification.

(12) BANK NUMBER CODE

(13) CHECK NUMBER CODE

(14) ACCOUNT NUMBER CODE

Check front showing fields:
MARY A. EDWARDS, D.D.S.
4318 NORTH AVERT WAY
CANYON VIEW, CA 91783
YOUR BANK HERE CITY, STATE ZIP
No. 1854
PAY ___ DOLLARS
TO THE ORDER OF ___
YOUR NAME HERE
"001854" :000000000: 00000000"

BACK OF CHECK

(15) ENDORSEMENT AREA
Signature of payee (stamp or signature) and authorization to deposit funds into an account. Depending on the type of endorsement, different actions may occur. *Restrictive endorsement* contains special instructions (i.e., **For Deposit Only**). *Endorsement in Full* gives authorization for another person to receive funds (i.e., **Pay to the order of ABC Dental Lab** [followed by the signature of the original payee]). *Blank endorsement* contains the **signature of the payee**. When this type of endorsement is used, the check can be cashed by anyone (nonrestrictive). In almost all cases a restrictive signature should be used by a business (For Deposit Only), as this protects the business from unauthorized use.

Steps in Reconciling the Account

Verify Debits

1. Compare each debit document from the bank with the corresponding entry on the check register (these are the items that did not require a paper check: electronic transfer, automatic payment, and returned checks).

2. Mark the item to identify that the item has been verified and processed. Place the mark on the check register, next to the cleared item in the appropriate column.

3. If a debit item has not been entered on the register, enter the item, and recalculate the total.

Text continued on p. 285

Bank of the Canyon
1278 Main Street
Canyon View, CA 91783

PAGE 1

ACCOUNT NO.   518-833-3

STATEMENT PERIOD
07/19/06 TO 08/20/06

Canyon View Dental Associates
4546 North Avery Way
Canyon View, CA 91783

YOUR ACCOUNT SUMMARY

DEPOSIT ACCOUNTS	BALANCE
CHECKING ACCOUNT	2,088.08
SAVINGS ACCOUNT	6.54
TOTAL	2,084.62

CHECKING ACCOUNT

Canyon View Dental Associates

SUMMARY OF ACCOUNT   518-833-3

BEGINNING BALANCE ON 07/18/98	3,055.24
DEPOSITS AND CREDITS	+3,819.02
CHECKS & WITHDRAWALS	-4,786.18
ENDING BALANCE ON 08/20/98	2,088.08

CHECKS PAID: 38

CHECK	AMOUNT	DATE PAID	REFERENCE#	CHECK	AMOUNT	DATE PAID	REFERENCE#
CHECK	450.00	07/19/98	81569110	2226	181.00	08/12/98	05105878
2202	146.23	07/31/98	29521570	2227	24.74	08/19/98	06120827
2203	122.03	07/29/98	29141271	2228	140.00	08/12/98	05022086
2210*	43.00	07/29/98	07046380	2229	148.71	08/16/98	27248941
2211	60.09	08/01/98	04597911	2230	53.16	08/13/98	27852752
2214*	123.59	07/24/98	29470425	2231	50.00	08/14/98	01018325
2215	47.70	07/19/98	12357289	2232	50.00	08/13/98	05080148
2216	9.00	07/22/98	05479786	2233	15.00	08/16/98	04709533
2217	30.00	07/26/98	29841864	2234	13.95	08/19/98	06008593
2218	19.00	07/30/98	04330539	2235	123.59	08/14/98	27050650
2219	12.00	07/24/98	04037820	2236	50.00	08/13/98	05099115
2220	35.93	07/24/98	04068844	2237	50.00	08/15/98	03014667
2221	10.00	08/12/98	05091269	2238	20.00	08/16/98	04675854
2222	23.48	07/24/98	29465653	2239	47.70	08/14/98	06172997
2223	242.43	07/26/98	29804419	2240	24.74	08/19/98	06120925
2224	150.00	07/30/98	29405827	2243*	400.00	08/14/98	29652307
2225	830.00	08/07/98	02242873	2344	400.00	08/14/98	29652306

FIGURE 15-2
Bank statement.

ANATOMY OF PEGBOARD CHECK WRITING SYSTEM

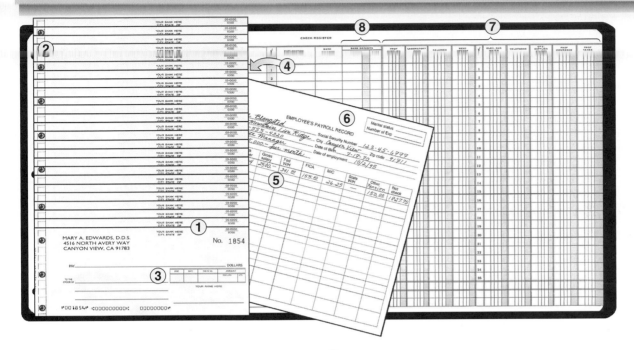

① CHECKS
Checks are supplied in shingles of 25.

② ALIGNMENT
Place the check register over the pegs on the left-hand side of the board. Align the checks with the NCR strip of the first check of the shingle on the first line of the register.

③ TRANSFERRING INFORMATION
Information is entered in the correct space on the check. There is an NCR strip only in the area in which information is needed. When the remainder of the checks are turned under the board, only the information written onto the NCR strip of the current check is transferred to the check register.

④ ELECTRONIC TRANSFERS OR AUTOMATIC PAYMENTS
All authorized electronic transfers and automatic payments are listed directly onto the register. This does not require writing a check unless directed by an accountant. In the check number column, a notation or code is used to identify the type of transaction.

⑤ PAYROLL INFORMATION
Payroll information can be entered by using checks designed for payroll and with the addition of a payroll record card.

⑥ PAYROLL RECORD CARD
This is similar to a patient ledger card (NCR paper). The information is entered on the check and is transferred to the payroll card and the check register.

⑦ EXTENDED CHECK REGISTER
The check register is extended for categorizing expenses. Different headings are entered at the top of the page. These headings can be preprinted or entered manually each time. Remember to use the same headings in the same column of each page to ensure accuracy. The purpose of categorizing expenses is for use in accounting reports. Broad categories are used, allowing for several payees to be entered under a group heading. For example, expenditures such as gas, water, and electricity are grouped together under the heading "Elec.-Gas-Water."

⑧ BANK DEPOSITS
Bank deposit information is entered. The amount of the deposit must match other documentation, deposit receipts, day sheets, credit card deposits, and other electronic deposits.

MONTH _April_

PAGE _1_

PAID TO	DISC.	DATE	CHECK NUMBER	AMOUNT	
BALANCE FORWARDED ⑨					⊖
Smith Labs		4/1	3215	482	31
Diana Blangsted		4/1	3216	1827	75
Deanna Rogers		4/1	3217	331	06
ABC Dental Supplies		4/1	3218	318	00
Edison		4/1	3219	212	46
Phone Company		4/1	3220	281	12
Dental Lab Inc.		4/1	3221	892	00
Payroll Tax		4/1	3222	400	00
Office Rental		4/1	electronic ④	2122	00
Postage		4/1	Phone order debit card	216	00

YOUR BANK HERE CITY STATE ZIP				00-0000 0000	
YOUR BANK HERE CITY STATE ZIP				00-0000 0000	
YOUR BANK HERE CITY STATE ZIP				00-0000 0000	
YOUR BANK HERE CITY, STATE ZIP				00-0000 0000	

MARY A. EDWARDS, D.D.S.
4516 NORTH AVERY WAY
CANYON VIEW, CA 91783

① No. 1854

PAY _____ DOLLARS

	DISC.	DATE	CHECK NO.	AMOUNT	
TO THE ORDER OF _____ ③				DOLLARS	CTS
				YOUR NAME HERE	

⑩

⑩`"001854"` `:0000000000:` `00000000"`

	DISC	DATE	CHECK NO	AMOUNT	
TOTALS (THIS PAGE)				7,082	58
TOTALS MONTH TO DATE ⑭				7,082	58
TOTALS YEAR TO DATE					

ANATOMY OF PEGBOARD CHECK WRITING SYSTEM (cont'd)

√	EXPLANATION	BANK BALANCE	BANK DEPOSITS ⑧		PROF SUPPLIES ⑦	LABORATORY FEES	SALARIES
			AMOUNT	DATE			
	⑨A 5,322.¹³						
1	*lab*					482|31	
2	*payroll* ⑤						1 827|75
3	*payroll*						33 1|06
4	*supplies*				3 1 8|00		
5	*utility*						
6	*utility*					89 2|00	
7	*lab*						
8	*prof. tax*						
9	*rent*						
10	*stamps*						
11			4231|00	4/1			
12			2383|00	4/2			
13			3892|00	4/3			
14			2341|00	electronic 4/8			
15			23|45	Interest 4/10			
16							
17							
18							
19							
20							
21							
22							
23							
24			⑬ ⬇		⑪ ⬇	⑪ ⬇	⑪ ⬇
25		⑮					
		11,110.00	12870|45		3 1 8|00 +	1 3 74|31 +	2 1 58|81 +
		⑩ should equal ⑫ ◄					

ANATOMY OF PEGBOARD CHECK WRITING SYSTEM (cont'd)

Balancing the pegboard check register:

⑨ If more than one ledger page is needed for all the checks written in one month, carry all the column totals forward from the previous page (i.e., on all the pages except the first). Enter them in the "**BALANCE FORWARDED**" row. At the beginning of each month the only total that is entered at the top of the first ledger page is in the "**BANK BALANCE**" column **⑨A**.

(If a different protocol is used, follow the guidelines established by the accountant and system being used at your particular practice).

⑩ Moving down, add the written amounts of each check listed in the "**AMOUNT**" column. Write the total in the "**TOTALS (THIS PAGE)**" row.

⑪ Moving down, add the written amounts in each expense column (that is, those indicated by **⑦**). Write the totals in the "**TOTALS (THIS PAGE)**" row.

⑫ Moving across, add all of the expense column totals together. This sum must equal the total for all the checks written **⑩**. If they do not match, the error must be found and corrected.

⑬ Moving down, add all deposits recorded on the page. Write the total in the "**TOTALS (THIS PAGE)**" row.

⑭ Fill in the "**TOTALS MONTH TO DATE**" row by adding down the "**BALANCE FORWARDED**" and "**TOTALS (THIS PAGE)**" rows.

⑮

DETERMINING ACCOUNT BALANCE

Enter beginning "**BANK BALANCE**" **⑨A** in "**BALANCE FORWARDED**" row	$5,322.13
Add "**BANK DEPOSIT**" total listed in **⑬** "**TOTALS (THIS PAGE)**" row	+12,870.45
	18,192.58
Subtotal	
Subtract total of all checks written in "**AMOUNT**" column listed in **⑩** "**TOTALS (THIS PAGE)**" from subtotal above.	−7,082.58
The result is the new bank balance, which is entered in the "**TOTALS (THIS PAGE)**" row of **⑮** "**BANK BALANCE**" column	$11,110.00

When determining the account balance, do not forget to enter all account transactions, written or electronic, and adjustments.

Verify Deposits

4. Gather all duplicate deposit slips and place them in chronological order.
5. Gather all direct deposit memos and place them in chronological order.
6. Verify deposits with the statement. Record other credits, such as interest earned.

Verify Canceled Checks

7. Arrange the canceled checks in numerical order.
8. Compare the checks with the register.
9. Identify checks that have been cleared the bank by placing a mark on the register.
10. Checks may have been received that were included in a previous reconciliation. Go back and find the check number in the register, and identify the check as cleared.

Verify the Balance

11. The worksheet (Figure 15-3) (included with each monthly bank statement) contains directions for calculating the **balance.** This form provides space for inclusion of outstanding items (checks and deposits that have not been processed by the bank). When the form is completed and the totals checked, they should be the same as the totals on the checkbook register.
12. If the totals are not the same, the error must be located. If the error has been made by the bank, the bank must be notified. If the error is found

---

BALANCING YOUR CHECKBOOK

Worksheet

STEP 1
List all deposits and other credits that do not appear on the bank statement

Date	Amount	
Total	$	

STEP 2
List outstanding checks, withdrawals and other debits that do not appear on the bank statement

Check #	Amount	
Total	$	

Calculation worksheet

CURRENT STATEMENT'S ENDING BALANCE		$	
Add deposits/other credits not yet credited on this statement (Step 1)	+	$	
SUBTOTAL	=	$	
Subtract checks/other debits not listed on this statement (Step 2)	−	$	
CURRENT CHECKBOOK BALANCE	=	$	

FIGURE 15-3
Worksheet to help with reconciliation of a checking account.

in calculations on the checkbook register, corrections must be made there and the totals recalculated. The error could also be seen in the calculations on the worksheet; double-check all calculations.

Making Corrections to the Register

13. Make all necessary adjustments to the account, and clearly identify the source of these adjustments.
14. Recalculate the totals of all columns on the register (if changes or additions have been made). Corrections are made by drawing a line through the figure and entering the correct figure. Never totally cover an entry by crossing it out or using white-out.
15. You are finished when the adjusted balance in the check register matches the ending balance on the monthly bank statement worksheet.

Steps to Take When the Account Does Not Balance

1. Check to see that all checks were properly entered on the check register (the same totals are listed on the check and recorded on the bank statement).
2. Check to see whether all totals on the deposits are the same as those listed on the bank statement.
3. Make sure that all checks are accounted for: Either verify that they have been cleared by the bank, or list them on the worksheet as outstanding checks. Do not forget to check previous statements for outstanding checks.
4. Make sure all electronic debits and credits are accounted for. Have they been entered on the check register?
5. Make sure all service charges are accounted for. Have they been entered on the check register?
6. Check to see that worksheet calculations are correct.
7. Double-check all addition and subtraction entries in the checkbook. Are they listed in the correct column? Were the debits (service charges, electronic payments, canceled checks, returned checks, corrections in deposits) subtracted from the balance? Were the credits (deposits, direct deposits, interest) added to the balance?
8. If the checkbook still does not balance, you may wish to request help from a coworker, bank worker, or accountant.

COMPUTERIZED CHECK WRITING

Check writing software has eased the processes of writing, recording, categorizing, and reconciling checking accounts. These software programs will perform the functions required by the pegboard check writing system, such as producing a check register or deposit slip and generating numerous reports (Figures 15-4 and 15-5). When it is time to write checks, the program can fill in such information as payee, amount of payment, and code for category. Payments can be identified as paper checks or electronic checks. Deposit and payment information is used to calculate the account balance. When a statement is returned from the bank, it is reconciled in a manner similar to that used for the manual reconciliation. Verification is made on the electronic check register. Outstanding checks and deposits are identified. The computer program will use the information to compare balances. If the balances do not match, you will be directed to locate the error and make corrections. When all information has been corrected, the program will recalculate the information on the worksheet and will determine whether you are in balance.

PAYROLL

Creating and maintaining payroll records, calculating payroll, producing payroll reports, and depositing payroll taxes may be duties assigned to the administrative dental assistant. The Internal Revenue Service (IRS) Publication 15, Circular E, *Employer's Tax Guide,* outlines important information on this topic. This circular is updated annually and can be obtained from the IRS or from the Internet (http://www.irs.gov/pub/irs-pdf/p15.pdf).

Creating the Payroll Record

Each employee must have a separate payroll record with proper documentation. New employees must complete the Immigration and Naturalization Service (INS) Form I-9, Employment Eligibility Verification (Figure 15-6). You can obtain this form from the INS. After the form has been completed, it is the responsibility of the employer to check approved documentation (see the list of approved documentation in Figure 15-6).

Banking Summary: Mary A. Edwards DDS
4/1/2006 Through 4/30/2006

Canyon View Dental	Page 1
Category Description	4/1/2006- 4/30/2006
INCOME	
Credit Card	2,341.00
Interest Inc	23.45
Mary Edwards DDS Production	10,506.00
TOTAL INCOME	12,870.45
EXPENSES	
Laboratory	1,374.31
Payroll	2,158.81
Postage	216.00
Rent	2,122.00
Supplies	318.00
Tax, Business	
Fed	400.00
TOTAL Tax, Business	400.00
Utilities	
Gas & Electric	212.46
Telephone	281.00
TOTAL Utilities	493.46
TOTAL EXPENSES	7,082.58
Balance Forward	
Bal Fwd Canyon View Dental	5,322.13
TOTAL BALANCE FORWARD	5,322.13
OVERALL TOTAL	11,110.00

FIGURE 15-4

Example of a computer-generated report in which income and expenses are categorized.

Office Equipment

Social Security number (SSN) must be recorded with the employee's name and address. If an employee does not have an SSN, he or she must contact the Social Security Administration (SSA) and apply for a card. If the name on the card is different from the name provided by the employee (because of marriage or divorce), instruct the employee to contact the SSA and request a name change. For government reporting, the name as it appears on the card should be used until an official change has been documented. All employees must have a card because the SSN is needed for tax reports and W-2 forms (reports of wages earned). A copy of the card can be kept in the employee's payroll record.

Employees must also complete a W-4 form (Figure 15-7), Employee's Withholding Allowance

Publication 15, Cirular E, Employer's Tax Guide

What's New
Calendar
Reminders
Introduction
1. Employer Identification Number (EIN)
2. Who Are Employees?
3. Family Employees
4. Employee's Social Security Number (SSN)
5. Wages and Other Compensation
6. Tips
7. Supplemental Wages
8. Payroll Period
9. Withholding From Employees' Wages
10. Advance Earned Income Credit (EIC) Payment
11. Depositing Taxes
12. Filing Form 941
13. Reporting Adjustments on Form 941
14. Federal Unemployment (FUTA) Tax
15. Special Rules for Various Types of Services and Payments
16. How To Use the Income Tax Withholding and Advance Earned Income Credit (EIC) Payment Tables
Tables:
    2006 Income Tax Withholding Tables:
        Percentage Method
        Wage Bracket Method
    2006 Advance EIC Payment Tables:
        Percentage Method
        Wage Bracket Method
Index
Form 7018-A (order blank)
Quick and Easy Access to IRS Tax Help and Tax Products

Revised January 2006.

Certificate (Internal Revenue Service). The withholding allowance and filing status are used to calculate the amount of income tax that should be withheld from the employee's wages. Employees must complete a new W-4 when a change has occurred in filing status, number of deductions, or name. When employees file for an exempt withholding allowance, they must complete the form annually (see the IRS calendar for the correct dates).

Form W-5 is used for those who qualify for an advance earned income credit (EIC). To obtain these payments, the employee must complete and sign the form (contact the IRS for additional help).

Mary A. Edwards, D.D.S.

Canyon View Dental						**Page 1**
Date	**Num**	**Transaction**	**Payment**	**C**	**Deposit**	**Balance**
4/1/2006		Opening Balance cat: [Canyon View Dental]		R	5,322.13	5,322.13
4/1/2006		 cat: Mary Edwards DDS Production			4,231.00	9,553.13
4/1/2006	EFT	Office Rental cat: Rent	2,122.00			7,431.13
4/1/2006	ATM	Postage cat: Postage	216.00			7,215.13
4/1/2006	3215	Smith Labs cat: Laboratory	482.31			6,732.82
4/1/2006	3216	Diane Blangsted cat: Payroll	1,827.75			4,905.07
4/1/2006	3217	Deanna Rogers cat: Payroll	331.06			4,574.01
4/1/2006	3218	ABC Dental Supplies cat: Supplies	318.00			4,256.01
4/1/2006	3219	Edision cat: Utilities : Gas & Electric	212.46			4,043.55
4/1/2006	3220	Phone Company cat: Utilities : Telephone	281.00			3,762.55
4/1/2006	3221	Dental Lab Inc. cat: Labortory	892.00			2,870.55
4/1/2006	3222	Payroll Tax cat: Tax, Business : Fed	400.00			2,470.55
4/2/2006		 cat: Mary Edwards DDS Production			2,383.00	4,853.55
4/3/2006		 cat: Mary Edwards DDS Production			3,892.00	8,745.55
4/8/2006		 cat: Credit Card			2,314.00	11,086.55
4/10/2006		 cat: Interest Inc.			23.45	11,110.00

FIGURE 15-5

Example of a computer-generated check register.

Department of Homeland Security
U.S. Citizenship and Immigration Services

OMB No. 1615-0047; Expires 03/31/07

Employment Eligibility Verification

INSTRUCTIONS
PLEASE READ ALL INSTRUCTIONS CAREFULLY BEFORE COMPLETING THIS FORM.

Anti-Discrimination Notice. It is illegal to discriminate against any individual (other than an alien not authorized to work in the U.S.) in hiring, discharging, or recruiting or referring for a fee because of that individual's national origin or citizenship status. It is illegal to discriminate against work eligible individuals. Employers **CANNOT** specify which document(s) they will accept from an employee. The refusal to hire an individual because of a future expiration date may also constitute illegal discrimination.

Section 1- Employee. All employees, citizens and noncitizens, hired after November 6, 1986, must complete Section 1 of this form at the time of hire, which is the actual beginning of employment. **The employer is responsible for ensuring that Section 1 is timely and properly completed.**

Preparer/Translator Certification. The Certification must be completed if Section 1 other than the employee. A preparer/translator when the employee is unable to complete Section However, the employee must still sign Section

Section 2 - Employer. For the purpose form, the term "employer" includes those re fee who are agricultural associations, agricu labor contractors.

Employers must complete Section 2 by exa identity and employment eligibility within thr the date employment begins. If employees but are unable to present the required docu business days, they must present a receipt document(s) within three business days and within ninety (90) days. However, if employ duration of less than three business days, S completed at the time employment begins. 1) document title; 2) issuing authority; 3) do expiration date, if any; and 5) the date empl Employers must sign and date the certificat present original documents. Employers may photocopy the document(s) presented. The However, employers are still responsible

Section 3 - Updating and Reve must complete Section 3 when updating an Employers must reverify employment eligibi or before the expiration date recorded in Se **CANNOT** specify which document(s) they w employee.

- If an employee's name has change being updated/reverified, complete
- If an employee is rehired within thr this form was originally completed eligible to be employed on the sam indicated on this form (updating), signature block.
- If an employee is rehired within th this form was originally completed authorization has expired **or** if a c authorization is about to expire (re Block B and:

EMP
PLEASE D

— examine any document that reflects that the employee is authorized to work in the U.S. (see List A or C),

— record the document title, document number and expiration date (if any) in Block C, and

---

Department of Homeland Security
U.S. Citizenship and Immigration Services

OMB No. 1615-0047; Expires 03/31/07

Employment Eligibility Verification

Please read instructions carefully before completing this form. The instructions must be available during completion of this form. ANTI-DISCRIMINATION NOTICE: It is illegal to discriminate against work eligible individuals. Employers CANNOT specify which document(s) they will accept from an employee. The refusal to hire an individual because of a future expiration date may also constitute illegal discrimination.

Section 1. Employee Information and Verification. To be completed and signed by employee at the time employment begins.

Print Name: Last	First	Middle Initial	Maiden Name
Address (Street Name and Number)		Apt. #	Date of Birth (month/day/year)
City	State	Zip Code	Social Security #

I am aware that federal law provides for imprisonment and/or fines for false statements or use of false documents in connection completion of this form.

I attest, under penalty of perjury, that I am (check one of the following):
☐ A citizen or national of the United States

Employee's Signature

Preparer and/or Translator other than the employee.) I attest, un of my knowledge the information is tr

Preparer's/Translator's Signature

Address (Street Name and Number,

Section 2. Employer Review and Ver examine one document from List B and one fr any, of the document(s).

List A
Document title:
Issuing authority:
Document #:
Expiration Date (if any):
Document #:
Expiration Date (if any):

CERTIFICATION - I attest, under penalty employee, that the above-listed docume employee began employment on (month is eligible to work in the United States. (S

Signature of Employer or Authorized Representa

Business or Organization Name   Add

Section 3. Updating and Reverificati
A. New Name (if applicable)

C. If employee's previous grant of work authoriza eligibility.   Document Title:

I attest, under penalty of perjury, that to the b presented document(s), the document(s) I ha
Signature of Employer or Authorized Representa

NOTE: This is th
current printing
components.

LISTS OF ACCEPTABLE DOCUMENTS

LIST A		**LIST B**		**LIST C**
Documents that Establish Both Identity and Employment Eligibility	**OR**	Documents that Establish Identity	**AND**	Documents that Establish Employment Eligibility

LIST A — Documents that Establish Both Identity and Employment Eligibility

1. U.S. Passport (unexpired or expired)

2. Certificate of U.S. Citizenship (Form N-560 or N-561)

3. Certificate of Naturalization (Form N-550 or N-570)

4. Unexpired foreign passport, with I-551 stamp or attached Form I-94 indicating unexpired employment authorization

5. Permanent Resident Card or Alien Registration Receipt Card with photograph (Form I-151 or I-551)

6. Unexpired Temporary Resident Card (Form I-688)

7. Unexpired Employment Authorization Card (Form I-688A)

8. Unexpired Reentry Permit (Form I-327)

9. Unexpired Refugee Travel Document (Form I-571)

10. Unexpired Employment Authorization Document issued by DHS that contains a photograph (Form I-688B)

LIST B — Documents that Establish Identity

1. Driver's license or ID card issued by a state or outlying possession of the United States provided it contains a photograph or information such as name, date of birth, gender, height, eye color and address

2. ID card issued by federal, state or local government agencies or entities, provided it contains a photograph or information such as name, date of birth, gender, height, eye color and address

3. School ID card with a photograph

4. Voter's registration card

5. U.S. Military card or draft record

6. Military dependent's ID card

7. U.S. Coast Guard Merchant Mariner Card

8. Native American tribal document

9. Driver's license issued by a Canadian government authority

For persons under age 18 who are unable to present a document listed above:

10. School record or report card

11. Clinic, doctor or hospital record

12. Day-care or nursery school record

LIST C — Documents that Establish Employment Eligibility

1. U.S. social security card issued by the Social Security Administration (other than a card stating it is not valid for employment)

2. Certification of Birth Abroad issued by the Department of State (Form FS-545 or Form DS-1350)

3. Original or certified copy of a birth certificate issued by a state, county, municipal authority or outlying possession of the United States bearing an official seal

4. Native American tribal document

5. U.S. Citizen ID Card (Form I-197)

6. ID Card for use of Resident Citizen in the United States (Form I-179)

7. Unexpired employment authorization document issued by DHS (other than those listed under List A)

Illustrations of many of these documents appear in Part 8 of the Handbook for Employers (M-274)

Form I-9 (Rev. 05/31/05)Y Page 3

FIGURE 15-6

US Department of Justice, Immigration and Naturalization Service: List of Acceptable Documents, Employment Eligibility Verification, and Instructions.

Form W-4 (2006)

Purpose. Complete Form W-4 so that your employer can withhold the correct federal income tax from your pay. Because your tax situation may change, you may want to refigure your withholding each year.

Exemption from withholding. If you are exempt, complete only lines 1, 2, 3, 4, and 7 and sign the form to validate it. Your exemption for 2006 expires February 16, 2007. See Pub. 505, Tax Withholding and Estimated Tax.

Note. You cannot claim exemption from withholding if (a) your income exceeds $850 and includes more than $300 of unearned income (for example, interest and dividends) and (b) another person can claim you as a dependent on their tax return.

Basic instructions. If you are not exempt, complete the **Personal Allowances Worksheet** below. The worksheets on page 2 adjust your withholding allowances based on itemized deductions, certain credits, adjustments to income, or two-earner/two-job situations. Complete all worksheets that apply. However, you may claim fewer (or zero) allowances.

Head of household. Generally, you may claim head of household filing status on your tax return only if you are unmarried and pay more than 50% of the costs of keeping up a home for yourself and your dependent(s) or other qualifying individuals. See line **E** below.

Tax credits. You can take projected tax credits into account in figuring your allowable number of withholding allowances. Credits for child or dependent care expenses and the child tax credit may be claimed using the **Personal Allowances Worksheet** below. See Pub. 919, How Do I Adjust My Tax Withholding, for information on converting your other credits into withholding allowances.

Nonwage income. If you have a large amount of nonwage income, such as interest or dividends, consider making estimated tax payments using Form 1040-ES, Estimated Tax for Individuals. Otherwise, you may owe additional tax.

Two earners/two jobs. If you have a working spouse or more than one job, figure the total number of allowances you are entitled to claim on all jobs using worksheets from only one Form W-4. Your withholding usually will be most accurate when all allowances are claimed on the Form W-4 for the highest paying job and zero allowances are claimed on the others.

Nonresident alien. If you are a nonresident alien, see the Instructions for Form 8233 before completing this Form W-4.

Check your withholding. After your Form W-4 takes effect, use Pub. 919 to see how the dollar amount you are having withheld compares to your projected total tax for 2006. See Pub. 919, especially if your earnings exceed $130,000 (Single) or $180,000 (Married).

Recent name change? If your name on line 1 differs from that shown on your social security card, call 1-800-772-1213 to initiate a name change and obtain a social security card showing your correct name.

Personal Allowances Worksheet (Keep for your records.)

A Enter "1" for **yourself** if no one else can claim you as a dependent . . . . A ______

B Enter "1" if: { • You are single and have only one job; or • You are married, have only one job, and your spouse does not work; or • Your wages from a second job or your spouse's wages (or the total of both) are $1,000 or less. } . . B ______

C Enter "1" for your **spouse.** But, you may choose to enter "-0-" if you are married and have either a working spouse or more than one job. (Entering "-0-" may help you avoid having too little tax withheld.) . . . . C ______

D Enter number of **dependents** (other than your spouse or yourself) you will claim on your tax return . . . . . . D ______

E Enter "1" if you will file as **head of household** on your tax return (see conditions under **Head of household** above) . E ______

F Enter "1" if you have at least $1,500 of **child or dependent care expenses** for which you plan to claim a credit . . F ______

(**Note.** Do **not** include child support payments. See **Pub. 503,** Child and Dependent Care Expenses, for details.)

G **Child Tax Credit** (including additional child tax credit):

- If your total income will be less than $55,000 ($82,000 if married), enter "2" for each eligible child.
- If your total income will be between $55,000 and $84,000 ($82,000 and $119,000 if married), enter "1" for each eligible child plus "1" **additional** if you have four or more eligible children. G ______

H Add lines A through G and enter total here. (**Note.** This may be different from the number of exemptions you claim on your tax return.) ▶ H ______

For accuracy, complete all worksheets that apply.
- If you plan to **itemize or claim adjustments to income** and want to reduce your withholding, see the **Deductions and Adjustments Worksheet** on page 2.
- If you have **more than one job** or are **married and you and your spouse both work** and the combined earnings from all jobs exceed $35,000 ($25,000 if married) see the **Two-Earner/Two-Job Worksheet** on page 2 to avoid having too little tax withheld.
- If **neither** of the above situations applies, **stop here** and enter the number from line H on line 5 of Form W-4 below.

Cut here and give Form W-4 to your employer. Keep the top part for your records.

Form **W-4** — Department of the Treasury, Internal Revenue Service

Employee's Withholding Allowance Certificate

▶ **Whether you are entitled to claim a certain number of allowances or exemption from withholding is subject to review by the IRS. Your employer may be required to send a copy of this form to the IRS.**

OMB No. 1545-0074 — **2006**

1 Type or print your first name and middle initial. | Last name | 2 Your social security number

Home address (number and street or rural route) | 3 ☐ Single ☐ Married ☐ Married, but withhold at higher Single rate. **Note.** If married, but legally separated, or spouse is a nonresident alien, check the "Single" box.

City or town, state, and ZIP code | 4 **If your last name differs from that shown on your social security card, check here. You must call 1-800-772-1213 for a new card.** ▶ ☐

5 Total number of allowances you are claiming (from line **H** above **or** from the applicable worksheet on page 2) 5 ______

6 Additional amount, if any, you want withheld from each paycheck . . . . 6 $ ______

7 I claim exemption from withholding for 2006, and I certify that I meet **both** of the following conditions for exemption.
- Last year I had a right to a refund of **all** federal income tax withheld because I had **no** tax liability **and**
- This year I expect a refund of **all** federal income tax withheld because I expect to have **no** tax liability.

If you meet both conditions, write "Exempt" here . . . . ▶ 7 ______

Under penalties of perjury, I declare that I have examined this certificate and to the best of my knowledge and belief, it is true, correct, and complete.

Employee's signature
(Form is not valid unless you sign it.) ▶ **Date** ▶

8 Employer's name and address (Employer: Complete lines 8 and 10 only if sending to the IRS.) | 9 Office code (optional) | 10 Employer identification number (EIN)

For Privacy Act and Paperwork Reduction Act Notice, see page 2. Cat. No. 10220Q Form **W-4** (2006)

Page **2**

Deductions and Adjustments Worksheet

n to itemize deductions, claim certain credits, or claim adjustments to income on your 2006 tax return.

temized deductions. These include qualifying home mortgage interest,
d local taxes, medical expenses in excess of 7.5% of your income, and
006, you may have to reduce your itemized deductions if your income
ied filing separately). See *Worksheet 3* in Pub. 919 for details.) . . . 1 $ ______

ng jointly or qualifying widow(er)
usehold . . . . 2 $ ______
arried filing separately

2 is greater than line 1, enter "-0-" . . . . 3 $ ______

nts to income, including alimony, deductible IRA contributions, and student loan interest 4 $ ______

total. (Include any amount for credits from *Worksheet 7* in Pub. 919) . 5 $ ______

onwage income (such as dividends or interest) . . . . 6 $ ______

the result, but not less than "-0-" . . . . 7 $ ______

3,300 and enter the result here. Drop any fraction . . . . 8 ______

nal Allowances Worksheet, line H, page 1 . . . . 9 ______

otal here. If you plan to use the **Two-Earner/Two-Job Worksheet,** also
Otherwise, **stop here** and enter this total on Form W-4, line 5, page 1 . 10

/Two-Job Worksheet (See *Two earners/two jobs* on page 1.)

structions under line H on page 1 direct you here.

(or from line 10 above if you used the **Deductions and Adjustments Worksheet**) 1 ______

w that applies to the **LOWEST** paying job and enter it here . . . . 2 ______

o line 2, subtract line 2 from line 1. Enter the result here (if zero, enter
page 1. **Do not** use the rest of this worksheet . . . . 3 ______

r "-0-" on Form W-4, line 5, page 1. Complete lines 4–9 below to calculate the additional
o avoid a year-end tax bill.

his worksheet . . . . 4 ______

his worksheet . . . . 5 ______

. . . . 6 ______

w that applies to the **HIGHEST** paying job and enter it here . . . . 7 $ ______

r the result here. This is the additional annual withholding needed . . 8 $ ______

ay periods remaining in 2006. For example, divide by 26 if you are paid
ete this form in December 2005. Enter the result here and on Form W-4,
nal amount to be withheld from each paycheck . . . . 9 $

Table 1: Two-Earner/Two-Job Worksheet

Married Filing Jointly				All Others	
Enter on line 2 above	If wages from **HIGHEST** paying job are—	AND, wages from **LOWEST** paying job are—	Enter on line 2 above	If wages from **LOWEST** paying job are—	Enter on line 2 above
0	$42,001 and over	32,001 - 38,000	6	$0 - $6,000	0
1		38,001 - 46,000	7	6,001 - 12,000	1
2		46,001 - 55,000	8	12,001 - 19,000	2
3		55,001 - 60,000	9	19,001 - 26,000	3
		60,001 - 65,000	10	26,001 - 35,000	4
0		65,001 - 75,000	11	35,001 - 50,000	5
1		75,001 - 95,000	12	50,001 - 65,000	6
2		95,001 - 105,000	13	65,001 - 80,000	7
3		105,001 - 120,000	14	80,001 - 90,000	8
4		120,001 and over	15	90,001 - 120,000	9
5				120,001 and over	10

Table 2: Two-Earner/Two-Job Worksheet

…ointly		All Others	
If wages from **HIGHEST** paying job are—	Enter on line 7 above	If wages from **HIGHEST** paying job are—	Enter on line 7 above
$0 - $60,000	$500	$0 - $30,000	$500
60,001 - 115,000	830	30,001 - 75,000	830
115,001 - 165,000	920	75,001 - 145,000	920
165,001 - 290,000	1,090	145,001 - 330,000	1,090
290,001 and over	1,160	330,001 and over	1,160

Privacy Act and Paperwork Reduction Act Notice. We ask for the information on this form to carry out the Internal Revenue laws of the United States. The Internal Revenue Code requires this information under sections 3402(f)(2)(A) and 6109 and their regulations. Failure to provide a properly completed form will result in your being treated as a single person who claims no withholding allowances; providing fraudulent information may also subject you to penalties. Routine uses of this information include giving it to the Department of Justice for civil and criminal litigation, to cities, states, and the District of Columbia for use in administering their tax laws, and using it in the National Directory of New Hires. We may also disclose this information to other countries under a tax treaty, to federal and state agencies to enforce federal nontax criminal laws, or to federal law enforcement and intelligence agencies to combat terrorism.

You are not required to provide the information requested on a form that is subject to the Paperwork Reduction Act unless the form displays a valid OMB control number. Books or records relating to a form or its instructions must be retained as long as their contents may become material in the administration of any Internal Revenue law. Generally, tax returns and return information are confidential, as required by Code section 6103.

The average time and expenses required to complete and file this form will vary depending on individual circumstances. For estimated averages, see the instructions for your income tax return.

If you have suggestions for making this form simpler, we would be happy to hear from you. See the instructions for your income tax return.

Printed on recycled paper

FIGURE 15-7
Employment Form, W-4.

REMEMBER

It is your responsibility to follow the guidelines. Read the publications offered by the Internal Revenue Service (IRS), and seek the advice of the dental practice accountant.

Payroll Records

Each employee must have a separate payroll record. This record can be a form that is filled in by the payroll clerk, a computer printout, or a payroll card that is used in a one-write system. Each record must include the same type of information (see Anatomy of a Payroll Record).

REMEMBER

Payroll records are important documents that must be kept for a period of 4 years (check current government regulations). Personnel records are different from payroll records. Personnel records contain information regarding performance reviews and contracts. These are confidential and must be kept separate from payroll records.

Calculating Payroll

Before payroll checks can be written, the amount due must be calculated through determination of taxes and other deductions. Gross salary is the amount of pay given before any deductions have been taken out. Deductions are subtracted from the gross salary to calculate the net salary or "take home" salary (the amount the check is written for).

Employment Tax Rates

Federal tax deductions include withholding taxes, social security tax (FICA), and Medicare taxes. Federal unemployment (FUTA) taxes are paid by the employer on behalf of an employee. In addition to federal taxes, individual state taxes may be collected. Other deductions include contributions to a pension fund, a health insurance plan, a life and disability insurance program, and a savings program.

Employment tax rates and wage bases in 2005

Social Security tax
- Tax rate: 6.2% for each employer and employee
- Wage base: $72,000

Medicare tax
- Tax rate: 1.45% for each employer and employee
- All wages are subject to Medicare tax

Federal unemployment tax
- Tax rate: 6.2% before state credits (employers only)
- Wage base: $7,000

Calculating Net Salary

With the help of tax tables and percentage calculation guides, the administrative dental assistant must calculate the various taxes that are deducted from each employee's pay. Several steps are followed in determining the net salary of each employee.

Salary can be calculated in various ways. Hourly employees are paid according to the number of hours worked during a pay period. Salaried employees have a set amount they are paid each month, regardless of the number of hours worked. Contract employees may be paid according to the amount of work they produce or the amount of money they collect, or by a daily rate. Some employees may be paid a base salary with incentives added on the basis of different conditions, such as amount of money collected or the level of treatment produced. It is important to understand the different pay levels and how the salaries should be calculated.

Withholding tax is determined by the filing status (married or single) and the number of deductions stated on the employee's W-4 form. Withholding tax can be calculated in two ways. The first is with the use of a tax table. These tables are provided in IRS Publication 15 (see earlier). Locate the table that describes the pay period: daily, weekly, biweekly, semimonthly, or monthly. Then, select the table for the correct filing status (single or married), and locate the gross salary and number of deductions (see tax tables used in Scenario 1, p 293).

A Percentage Method of Withholding formula can be used to calculate the amount of withholding tax. The correct table is identified by the payroll period and filing status (see Scenario 2, p 294).

ANATOMY OF A PAYROLL RECORD

Marital status	④
Number of Exp	④

EMPLOYEE'S PAYROLL RECORD

Name: ① _____ Social Security Number ③ _____
Address ① _____ City _____ Zip code _____
Telephone _____ Date of Birth ② _____
Occupation: _____ Date of employment ② _____
Pay rate: ⑤ _____

Date	Check number	Gross salary	Fed W/H	FICA	M/C	State W/H	Other	Net check
1/ / ⑥		⑦	⑧	⑧	⑧	⑧	⑧	⑨
1/ /								
1/ /								
1/ /								
JAN TOTAL		⑩	⑩	⑩	⑩	⑩	⑩	⑩
2/ /								
2/ /								
2/ /								
2/ /								
FEB TOTAL								
3/ /								
3/ /								
3/ /								
MAR TOTAL								
FIRST QT. TOTALS		⑪	⑪	⑪	⑪	⑪	⑪	⑪

① **NAME AND ADDRESS OF EMPLOYEE**

② **PERSONAL DATA**
Date of birth, date of employment, and home telephone number.

③ **SOCIAL SECURITY NUMBER**
Mandated by law.

④ **NUMBER OF DEDUCTIONS AND FILING STATUS**
Information taken from W-4.

⑤ **PAY RATE**
How much the employee is being paid, and how it is calculated (hourly, weekly, monthly).

⑥ **DATE CHECK IS ISSUED**

⑦ **GROSS PAY**
The total amount earned before deductions.

⑧ **DEDUCTIONS**
These are amounts that are subtracted from the gross pay. They include income tax withholdings (federal and state if applicable), FICA (Federal Insurance Contributions Act [social security]), and Medicare. In some states, other taxes may be withheld. In addition to taxes, deductions may include insurance, pension fund contributions, and savings deposits.

⑨ **NET SALARY**
The amount remaining after all deductions have been subtracted.

⑩ **MONTHLY TOTALS**
The total gross salary, total deductions for each category, and total net salary.

⑪ **QUARTERLY TOTALS**
These are the totals of the three monthly totals. This information is used by the accountant when completing the quarterly government payroll reports. At the end of the year, these totals are added up to make the "Year End Total," which is then used to complete the year end reports for government agencies. Each employee is given a copy of this report (W-2 form). This information is used by the employees when calculating their tax liability for the year and must be attached to their tax form.

EXAMPLES OF PAYROLL CALCULATIONS

MARRIED Persons—SEMIMONTHLY Payroll Period
(For Wages Paid in 2005)

If the wages are—		And the number of withholding allowances claimed is—										
At least	But less than	0	1	2	3	4	5	6	7	8	9	10
		The amount of income tax to be withheld is—										
$1,420	$1,440	$134	$114	$94	$74	$56	$43	$30	$16	$3	$0	$0
1,440	1,460	137	117	97	77	58	45	32	18	5	0	0
1,460	1,480	140	120	100	80	60	47	34	20	7	0	0
1,480	1,500	143	123	103	83	63	49	36	22	9	0	0
1,500	1,520	146	126	106	86	66	51	38	24	11	0	0
1,520	1,540	149	129	109	89	69	53	40	26	13	0	0
1,540	1,560	152	132	112	92	72	55	42	28	15	2	0
1,560	1,580	155	135	115	95	75	57	44	30	17	4	0
1,580	1,600	158	138	118	98	78	59	46	32	19	6	0
1,600	1,620	161	141	121	101	81	61	48	34	21	8	0
1,620	1,640	164	144	124	104	84	64	50	36	23	10	0
1,640	1,660	167	147	127	107	87	67	52	38	25	12	0
1,660	1,680	170	150	130	110	90	70	54	40	27	14	0
1,680	1,700	173	153	133	113	93						
1,700	1,720	176	156	136	116	96						
1,720	1,740	179	159	139	119	99						
1,740	1,760	182	162	142	122	102						
1,760	1,780	185	165	145	125	105						
1,780	1,800	188	168	148	128	108						
1,800	1,820	191	171	151	131	111						
1,820	1,840	194	174	154	134	114						
1,840	1,860	197	177	157	137	117						
1,860	1,880	200	180	160	140	120						
1,880	1,900	203	183	163	143	123						
1,900	1,920	206	186	166	146	126						
1,920	1,940	209	189	169	149	129						
1,940	1,960	212	192	172	152	132						
1,960	1,980	215	195	175	155	135						
1,980	2,000	218	198	178	158	138						
2,000	2,020	221	201	181	161	141						
2,020	2,040	224	204	184	164	144						
2,040	2,060	227	207	187	167	147						
2,060	2,080	230	210	190	170	150						
2,080	2,100	233	213	193	173	153						
2,100	2,120	236	216	196	176	156						
2,120	2,140	239	219	199	179	159						
2,140	2,160	242	222	202	182	162						
2,160	2,180	245	225	205	185	165						
2,180	2,200	248	228	208	188	168						
2,200	2,220	251	231	211	191	171						
2,220	2,240	254	234	214	194	174						
2,240	2,260	257	237	217	197	177						
2,260	2,280	260	240	220	200	180						
2,280	2,300	263	243	223	203	183						
2,300	2,320	266	246	226	206	186						
2,320	2,340	269	249	229	209	189						
2,340	2,360	272	252	232	212	192						
2,360	2,380	275	255	235	215	195						
2,380	2,400	278	258	238	218	198						
2,400	2,420	281	261	241	221	201						
2,420	2,440	284	264	244	224	204						
2,440	2,460	287	267	247	227	207						
2,460	2,480	290	270	250	230	210						
2,480	2,500	293	273	253	233	213						
2,500	2,520	296	276	256	236	216						
2,520	2,540	299	279	259	239	219						
2,540	2,560	302	282	262	242	222						
2,560	2,580	305	285	265	245	225						
2,580	2,600	308	288	268	248	228						
2,600	2,620	311	291	271	251	231						
2,620	2,640	314	294	274	254	234						
2,640	2,660	317	297	277	257	237						
2,660	2,680	320	300	280	260	240						
2,680	2,700	323	303	283	263	243						
2,700	2,720	326	306	286	266	246						
2,720	2,740	329	309	289	269	249						

$2,740 and over — Use Table 3(b) for a **MARRIED person** on pa

Scenario #1.
Diana Blangsted is the office manager. Her monthly salary is five thousand dollars (gross salary). She is paid semi-monthly on the 1st and 15th of each month. In addition to the normal deductions, she has 6% of her salary deducted for her pension plan.

EMPLOYEE'S PAYROLL RECORD

Marital status ___M___
Number of Exp ___2___

Name: *Diane Blangsted*   Social Security Number: *123-45-6777*
Address: *264 Mountain Lion Ridge*   City: *Canyon View*   Zip code: *91711*
Telephone: *626-555-4320*   Date of Birth: *7-17-70*
Occupation: *Office Manager*   Date of employment: *10/2/95*
Pay rate: *$5,000.— per month*

Date	Check number	Gross salary	Fed W/H	FICA	M/C	State W/H	Other Pension	Net check
1/15/05	2684	2500,—	256.00	155.00	26.25	—	150.00	1912.75
1/ /								
1/ /								
1/ /								
JAN TOTAL								
2/ /								
2/ /								
2/ /								
2/ /								
FEB TOTAL								
3/ /								
3/ /								
3/ /								
MAR TOTAL								
FIRST QT. TOTALS								

Page 49

Steps to determine her semimonthly take home salary

1. Determine semimonthly salary ....$5,000 ÷ 2 = $2,500
2. Determine federal withholding.........Use tax table on left or calculate percentage amount from tax table, married, 2 deductions: $256.00
3. Determine FICA..............................$2,500 x .062 (6.2%) = $155.00
4. Determine Medicare........................$2,500 x .0145 (1.45%) = $36.25
5. Determine pension..........................$2,500 x .06 (6%) = $150.00

EXAMPLES OF PAYROLL CALCULATIONS (continued)

Tables for Percentage Method of Withholding
(For Wages Paid in 2005)

TABLE 1—WEEKLY Payroll Period

(a) SINGLE person (including head of household)—

If the amount of wages (after subtracting withholding allowances) is:		The amount of income tax to withhold is:	
Not over $51		$0	
Over—	But not over—		of excess over—
$51	—$188 . .	10%	—$51
$188	—$606 . .	$13.70 plus 15%	—$188
$606	—$1,341 . .	$76.40 plus 25%	—$606
$1,341	—$2,922 . .	$260.15 plus 28%	—$1,341
$2,922	—$6,313 . .	$702.83 plus 33%	—$2,922
$6,313	. . . . . .	$1,821.86 plus 35%	—$6,313

(b) MARRIED person—

If the amount of wages (after subtracting withholding allowances) is:		The amount of income tax to withhold is:	
Not over $154		$0	
Over—	But not over—		of excess over—
$154	—$435 . .	10%	—$154
$435	—$1,273 . .	$28.10 plus 15%	—$435
$1,273	—$2,322 . .	$153.80 plus 25%	—$1,273
$2,322	—$3,646 . .	$416.05 plus 28%	—$2,322
$3,646	—$6,409 . .	$786.77 plus 33%	—$3,646
$6,409	. . . . . .	$1,698.56 plus 35%	—$6,409

TABLE 2—BIWEEKLY P...

(a) SINGLE person (including head of household)—

If the amount of wages (after subtracting withholding allowances) is:		The amount of income tax to withhold is:	
Not over $102		$0	
Over—	But not over—		of excess over—
$102	—$377 . .	10%	—$102
$377	—$1,212 . .	$27.50 plus 15%	—$377
$1,212	—$2,683 . .	$152.75 plus 25%	—$1,212
$2,683	—$5,844 . .	$520.50 plus 28%	—$2,683
$5,844	—$12,625 . .	$1,405.58 plus 33%	—$5,844
$12,625	. . . . . .	$3,643.31 plus 35%	—$12,625

TABLE 3—SEMIMONTHLY

(a) SINGLE person (including head of household)—

If the amount of wages (after subtracting withholding allowances) is:		The amount of income tax to withhold is:	
Not over $110		$0	
Over—	But not over—		of excess over—
$110	—$408 . .	10%	—$110
$408	—$1,313 . .	$29.80 plus 15%	—$408
$1,313	—$2,906 . .	$165.55 plus 25%	—$1,313
$2,906	—$6,331 . .	$563.80 plus 28%	—$2,906
$6,331	—$13,677 . .	$1,522.80 plus 33%	—$6,331
$13,677	. . . . . .	$3,946.98 plus 35%	—$13,677

TABLE 4—MONTHLY P...

(a) SINGLE person (including head of household)—

If the amount of wages (after subtracting withholding allowances) is:		The amount of income tax to withhold is:	
Not over $221		$0	
Over—	But not over—		of excess over—
$221	—$817 . .	10%	—$221
$817	—$2,625 . .	$59.60 plus 15%	—$817
$2,625	—$5,813 . .	$330.80 plus 25%	—$2,625
$5,813	—$12,663 . .	$1,127.80 plus 28%	—$5,813
$12,663	—$27,354 . .	$3,045.80 plus 33%	—$12,663
$27,354	. . . . . .	$7,893.83 plus 35%	—$27,354

Page 36

Scenario #2.

Deanna Rogers is a part-time hourly employee. She has worked a total of 32.5 hours for this pay period. Her hourly wage is $12.50. She has a filing status of single and is claiming 0 deductions.

EMPLOYEE'S PAYROLL RECORD

Marital status _S_
Number of Exp _O_

Name: _Deanna Rogers_   Social Security Number _123-45-6778_
Address _42 S. Eagle Nest_   City _Canyon View_   Zip code _91711_
Telephone _626-555-4664_   Date of Birth _11/24/80_
Occupation: _Part time chairside asst._   Date of employment _9/12/98_
Pay rate: _$12.50 per hour_

Date	Check number	Gross salary	Fed W/H	FICA	M/C	State W/H	Other	Net check
1/15/05	2683	406.25	40.62	25.19	5.60	—	—	334.84
1/ /								
1/ /								
1/ /								
JAN TOTAL								
2/ /								
2/ /								
2/ /								
2/ /								
FEB TOTAL								
3/ /								
3/ /								
3/ /								
MAR TOTAL								
FIRST QT. TOTALS								

Steps to determine her semimonthly take home salary

1. Determine semimonthly salary .... $12.50 x 32.5 = $406.25

2. Determine federal withholding using Percentage Method of Withholding .... $406.00 − $110.00 = $296.00 (see table 3 on the left)
$296.00 x .10 (10%) = $40.62

3. Determine FICA .... $406.25 x .062 (6.2%) = $25.19

4. Determine Medicare .... $406.25 x .0145 (1.45%) = $5.60

Payroll Taxes: Reports and Deposits

After taxes have been calculated, they are reported to the IRS and deposited. Taxes to be reported include Federal Income, Social Security, and Medicare taxes. In addition to these taxes, the employer must pay FUTA taxes.

Federal Income, Social Security, and Medicare taxes are reported on Form 941, Employer's Quarterly Federal Tax Return (Figure 15-8). This form, which is filed with the IRS on a quarterly basis (every 3 months beginning in January), is completed by the bookkeeper, accountant, or payroll service with the use of information documented in the payroll records.

The employer's FUTA tax is calculated quarterly. To determine tax liability, total payroll wages paid during the quarter are multiplied by 0.008 (0.8%).

This amount is deposited along with Form 8109, Federal Tax Deposit Coupon. Once an employee has received $7,000 in wages for the year, wages are no longer subject to FUTA deposits. FUTA taxes are also reported annually with Form 940 or 940-EZ, Employer's Annual Federal Unemployment Tax Return.

Before forms are filed with the IRS, the money collected for taxes must be deposited. When depositing taxes, use Form 8109, Federal Tax Deposit Coupon (Figure 15-9). Each coupon must show the deposit amount, the type of tax, the period for which you are making a deposit, and your telephone number. Use a separate coupon for each tax and filing period. On each check or money order, include the Employer Identification Number (EIN), the type of tax, and the tax period for the payment. The deposit must be made at an authorized financial

Employer Responsibilities

The following list provides a brief summary of your basic responsibilities. Because the individual circumstances for each employer can vary greatly, their responsibilities for withholding, depositing, and reporting employment taxes can differ.

New Employees

- Verify work eligibility of employees
- Record employees' names and SSNs from social security cards
- Ask employees for 2005 Form W-4

Each Payday

- Withhold federal income tax based on each employee's Form W-4
- Withhold employee's share of social security and Medicare taxes
- Include advanced earned income credit payment in paycheck if employee requested it on Form W-5
- Deposit:
- Withheld income tax
- Withheld and employer social security taxes
- Withheld and employee Medicare taxes

  NOTE: *Due date of deposit generally depends on your deposit schedule (monthly or semiweekly).*

Quarterly (By April 30, July 31, October 31, and January 31)

- Deposit FUTA tax in an authorized financial institution if undeposited amount is over $500
- File form 941 (pay tax with return if not required to deposit)

Annually (See Calendar for Due Dates)

- Remind employees to submit a new Form W-4 if they need to change their withholding
- Ask for a new Form W-4 from employees claiming exemption from income tax withholding
- Reconcile Forms 941 with Forms W-2 and W-3
- Furnish each employee with a Form W-2
- File Copy A of Forms W-2 and the transmittal Form W-3 with the SSA
- Furnish each other payee a Form 1099 (for example, Forms 1099-R and 1099-MISC)
- File forms 1099 and the transmittal Form 1096
- File Form 940 or Form 940-EZ
- File Form 945 for any nonpayroll income tax withholding

Modified from Publication 15 (Circular E), Employer's Tax Guide (Rev. Jan 2006, page 3). Courtesy Internal Revenue Service.

Form **941 for 2006:** Employer's QUARTERLY Federal Tax Return   990106
(Rev. January 2006)   Department of the Treasury — Internal Revenue Service

(EIN)
Employer identification number ☐☐ — ☐☐☐☐☐☐☐   OMB No. 1545-0029

Name (not your trade name)

Trade name (if any)

Address
    Number   Street   Suite or room number
    City   State   ZIP code

Report for this Quarter ...
(Check one.)

☐ 1: January, February, March
☐ 2: April, May, June
☐ 3: July, August, September
☐ 4: October, November, December

Read the separate instructions before you fill out this form. Please type or print within the boxes.

Part 1: Answer these questions for this quarter.

1 Number of employees who received wages, tips, or other compensation for the pay period
  including: Mar. 12 (Quarter 1), June 12 (Quarter 2), Sept. 12 (Quarter 3), Dec. 12 (Quarter 4) . . .   1

2 Wages, tips, and other compensation   2   .

3 Total income tax withheld from wages, tips, and other compensation   3

4 If no wages, tips, and other compensation are subject to social security or Medicare tax .

5 Taxable social security and Medicare wages and tips:

	Column 1		Column 2
5a Taxable social security wages		× .124 =	.
5b Taxable social security tips		× .124 =	.
5c Taxable Medicare wages & tips		× .029 =	.

5d Total social security and Medicare taxes (Column 2, lines 5a + 5b + 5c = line 5d) . .   5

6 Total taxes before adjustments (lines 3 + 5d = line 6) . . . .
7 TAX ADJUSTMENTS (Read the instructions for line 7 before completing lines 7a through 7h.):

  7a Current quarter's fractions of cents . . . .
  7b Current quarter's sick pay . . . .
  7c Current quarter's adjustments for tips and group-term life insurance .
  7d Current year's income tax withholding (attach Form 941c) . .
  7e Prior quarters' social security and Medicare taxes (attach Form 941c) .
  7f Special additions to federal income tax (attach Form 941c) . . .
  7g Special additions to social security and Medicare (attach Form 941c) .

  7h TOTAL ADJUSTMENTS (Combine all amounts: lines 7a through 7g.)   7

8 Total taxes after adjustments (Combine lines 6 and 7h.) . . . .

9 Advance earned income credit (EIC) payments made to employees . . . .

10 Total taxes after adjustment for advance EIC (line 8 – line 9 = line 10) . . . . . .

11 Total deposits for this quarter, including overpayment applied from a prior quarter .

12 Balance due (If line 10 is more than line 11, write the difference here.) . . . .
   Make checks payable to United States Treasury.

13 Overpayment (If line 11 is more than line 10, write the difference here.) . . . . . .
▶ You **MUST** fill out both pages of this form and **SIGN** it.

For Privacy Act and Paperwork Reduction Act Notice, see the back of the Payment Voucher.

990206

Name (not your trade name)   Employer identification number (EIN)

Part 2: Tell us about your deposit schedule and tax liability for this quarter.

If you are unsure about whether you are a monthly schedule depositor or a semiweekly schedule depositor, see Pub. 15
(Circular E), section 11.

14 ☐☐ Write the state abbreviation for the state where you made your deposits OR write "MU" if you made your
        deposits in multiple states.

15 Check one: ☐ Line 10 is less than $2,500. Go to Part 3.

            ☐ You were a monthly schedule depositor for the entire quarter. Fill out your tax
              liability for each month. Then go to Part 3.

            Tax liability: Month 1 _____ .
                            Month 2 _____ .
                            Month 3 _____ .

            Total liability for quarter _____ . Total must equal line 10.

            ☐ You were a semiweekly schedule depositor for any part of this quarter. Fill out Schedule B (Form 941):
              Report of Tax Liability for Semiweekly Schedule Depositors, and attach it to this form.

Part 3: Tell us about your business. If a question does NOT apply to your business, leave it blank.

16 If your business has closed or you stopped paying wages . . . . ☐ Check here, and

   enter the final date you paid wages __/__/__

17 If you are a seasonal employer and you do not have to file a return for every quarter of the year . ☐ Check here.

Part 4: May we speak with your third-party designee?

Do you want to allow an employee, a paid tax preparer, or another person to discuss this return with the IRS? See the
instructions for details.

☐ Yes. Designee's name

     Phone ( ) —   Personal Identification Number (PIN) ☐☐☐☐☐

☐ No.

Part 5: Sign here. You MUST fill out both sides of this form and SIGN it.

Under penalties of perjury, I declare that I have examined this return, including accompanying schedules and statements, and to
the best of my knowledge and belief, it is true, correct, and complete.

X Sign your name here

   Print name and title

   Date __/__/__   Phone ( ) —

Part 6: For PAID preparers only (optional)

Paid Preparer's
Signature

Firm's name

Address   EIN

                                               ZIP code

Date __/__/__ Phone ( ) —   SSN/PTIN

☐ Check if you are self-employed.

Page **2**   Form **941** (Rev. 1-2006)

FIGURE 15-8
Employer's Quarterly Federal Tax Return Form and Form 941, Payment Voucher.

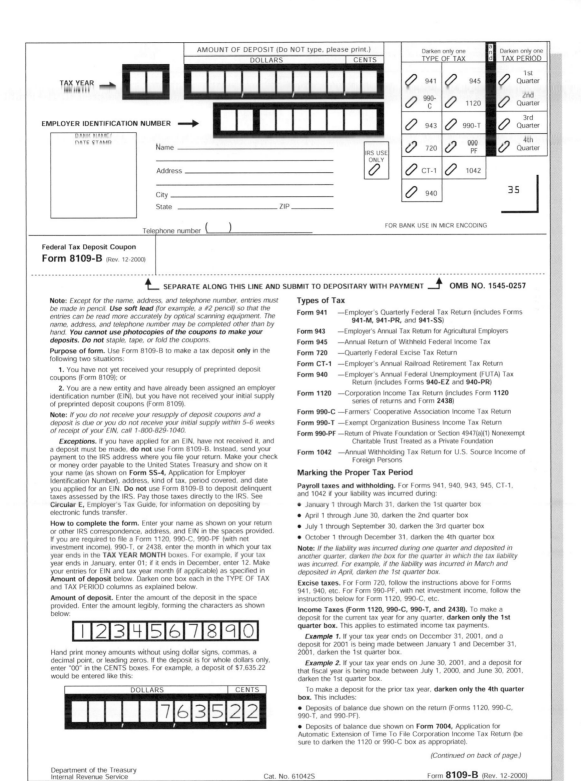

Note: *Except for the name, address, and telephone number, entries must be made in pencil.* **Use soft lead** *(for example, a #2 pencil) so that the entries can be read more accurately by optical scanning equipment. The name, address, and telephone number may be completed other than by hand.* **You cannot use photocopies of the coupons to make your deposits.** *Do not* staple, tape, or fold the coupons.

Purpose of form. Use Form 8109-B to make a tax deposit **only** in the following two situations:

1. You have not yet received your resupply of preprinted deposit coupons (Form 8109); or

2. You are a new entity and have already been assigned an employer identification number (EIN), but you have not received your initial supply of preprinted deposit coupons (Form 8109).

Note: *If you do not receive your resupply of deposit coupons and a deposit is due or you do not receive your initial supply within 5–6 weeks of receipt of your EIN, call 1-800-829-1040.*

Exceptions. If you have applied for an EIN, have not received it, and a deposit must be made, **do not** use Form 8109-B. Instead, send your payment to the IRS address where you file your return. Make your check or money order payable to the United States Treasury and show on it your name (as shown on **Form SS-4,** Application for Employer Identification Number), address, kind of tax, period covered, and date you applied for an EIN. **Do not** use Form 8109-B to deposit delinquent taxes assessed by the IRS. Pay those taxes directly to the IRS. See **Circular E,** Employer's Tax Guide, for information on depositing by electronic funds transfer.

How to complete the form. Enter your name as shown on your return or other IRS correspondence, address, and EIN in the spaces provided. If you are required to file a Form 1120, 990-C, 990-PF (with net investment income), 990-T, or 2438, enter the month in which your tax year ends in the **TAX YEAR MONTH** boxes. For example, if your tax year ends in January, enter 01; if it ends in December, enter 12. Make your entries for EIN and tax year month (if applicable) as specified in **Amount of deposit** below. Darken one box each in the TYPE OF TAX and TAX PERIOD columns as explained below.

Amount of deposit. Enter the amount of the deposit in the space provided. Enter the amount legibly, forming the characters as shown below:

Hand print money amounts without using dollar signs, commas, a decimal point, or leading zeros. If the deposit is for whole dollars only, enter "00" in the CENTS boxes. For example, a deposit of $7,635.22 would be entered like this:

Types of Tax

Form 941 —Employer's Quarterly Federal Tax Return (includes Forms **941-M, 941-PR,** and **941-SS**)

Form 943 —Employer's Annual Tax Return for Agricultural Employers

Form 945 —Annual Return of Withheld Federal Income Tax

Form 720 —Quarterly Federal Excise Tax Return

Form CT-1 —Employer's Annual Railroad Retirement Tax Return

Form 940 —Employer's Annual Federal Unemployment (FUTA) Tax Return (includes Forms **940-EZ** and **940-PR**)

Form 1120 —Corporation Income Tax Return (includes Form **1120** series of returns and Form **2438**)

Form 990-C —Farmers' Cooperative Association Income Tax Return

Form 990-T —Exempt Organization Business Income Tax Return

Form 990-PF —Return of Private Foundation or Section 4947(a)(1) Nonexempt Charitable Trust Treated as a Private Foundation

Form 1042 —Annual Withholding Tax Return for U.S. Source Income of Foreign Persons

Marking the Proper Tax Period

Payroll taxes and withholding. For Forms 941, 940, 943, 945, CT-1, and 1042 if your liability was incurred during:

• January 1 through March 31, darken the 1st quarter box

• April 1 through June 30, darken the 2nd quarter box

• July 1 through September 30, darken the 3rd quarter box

• October 1 through December 31, darken the 4th quarter box

Note: *If the liability was incurred during one quarter and deposited in another quarter, darken the box for the quarter in which the tax liability was incurred. For example, if the liability was incurred in March and deposited in April, darken the 1st quarter box.*

Excise taxes. For Form 720, follow the instructions above for Forms 941, 940, etc. For Form 990-PF, with net investment income, follow the instructions below for Form 1120, 990-C, etc.

Income Taxes (Form 1120, 990-C, 990-T, and 2438). To make a deposit for the current tax year for any quarter, **darken only the 1st quarter box.** This applies to estimated income tax payments.

Example 1. If your tax year ends on December 31, 2001, and a deposit for 2001 is being made between January 1 and December 31, 2001, darken the 1st quarter box.

Example 2. If your tax year ends on June 30, 2001, and a deposit for that fiscal year is being made between July 1, 2000, and June 30, 2001, darken the 1st quarter box.

To make a deposit for the prior tax year, **darken only the 4th quarter box.** This includes:

• Deposits of balance due shown on the return (Forms 1120, 990-C, 990-T, and 990-PF).

• Deposits of balance due shown on **Form 7004,** Application for Automatic Extension of Time To File Corporation Income Tax Return (be sure to darken the 1120 or 990-C box as appropriate).

(Continued on back of page.)

Department of the Treasury
Internal Revenue Service

Cat. No. 61042S

Form **8109-B** (Rev. 12-2000)

FIGURE 15-9
Form 8109, Federal Tax Deposit Coupon.

Record Keeping

A record of all employment taxes must be kept for at least 4 years. These records must be available for Internal Revenue Service (IRS) review and must contain the following information:

- Employer identification number
- Amounts and dates of all wage, annuity, and pension payments
- Amount of tips reported
- Fair market value of in-kind wages paid
- Names, addresses, social security numbers, and occupations of employees and recipients
- Employee copies of Form W-2 that were returned as undeliverable
- Dates of employment
- Periods for which employees and recipients were paid while absent because of sickness or injury, and the amount and weekly rate of payments you or third party payers made to them
- Copies of employees' and recipients' income tax withholding allowance certificates (Forms W-4, W4P, W-S, and W-4V)
- Dates and amounts of tax deposits made
- Copies of returns filed
- Records of fringe benefits provided, including substantiation

institution or a Federal Reserve Bank in the area. If the deposit is mailed, it must *arrive by the due date*. If deposits are late, a penalty will be added to the amount. Review the IRS calendar annually for important dates.

Employer Identification Number

All employers who report employment taxes or provide tax statements to employees will need an employer identification number (EIN). The EIN is a nine-digit number that is issued by the IRS. Digits are arranged as follows: 00-0000000. The EIN is used to identify tax accounts of employers. The EIN must be placed on all items sent to the IRS or the SSA.

Computerized Payroll

Computer programs are available that calculate and record all payroll information. These programs use the information kept in a payroll record. After the account has been established, payroll information is entered, and the program determines the amount of tax and other deductions. Reports are generated on the basis of information stored in the employee database.

PAYROLL SERVICES

Payroll services are provided by banks and outside contractors who calculate payroll. Such services maintain records, generate payroll checks, provide reports, and complete government forms. In addition, they arrange for direct deposit of payroll into employees' personal accounts, thereby eliminating the need for paper checks.

KEY POINTS

- Accounts payable is a system by which all dental practice expenditures are organized, verified, and categorized. Organization of these accounts is necessary to ensure that timely payments are made.
- Check writing has been expanded to include paper instruments, electronic transfers, and the use of credit and debit cards. Checks can be generated with the use of computers, one-write systems, and outside services. Accountants use information from the check register to categorize expenditures and create reports.
- A bank statement must be reconciled to ensure that all records are in agreement. Steps in reconciling include verifying debits, deposits, and canceled checks and comparing balances.
- Payroll functions include calculating payroll, deducting taxes, writing checks, and filing tax reports. These functions can be performed manually, with the use of a computer software package, or by an outside agency.

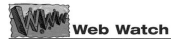 **Web Watch**

Bookkeeping and Accounting: From Start to Finish

http://www.sba.gov/test/wbc/docs/finance/bkpg_basic1.html

  Log on to Evolve to access additional
http://evolve.elsevier.com web links!

Critical Thinking Questions

1. With the use of information provided in this chapter, how would you organize the accounts payable system for a small dental office?

2. You have been assigned the task of reconciling a checkbook. List the materials you will need to complete the task.

3. Your job description includes writing checks, making deposits, and signing checks. Explain how you will perform these tasks (manually or with a computer), and identify safeguards that should be in place to protect your employer and yourself from unauthorized use of funds. Use information given in this chapter as well as outside resources to support your plan.

OUTLINE

Introduction

Electronic Business Equipment
- Hardware
- Software
- Data
- Personnel
- Procedures

Telecommunication
- Telephone Systems
- Electronic Communication Devices

Intraoffice Communications
- Manual Systems
- Electronic Systems

Office Machines

Business Office Environment
- Questions to Consider When Organizing a Business Office
- Safety

KEY TERMS AND CONCEPTS

Americans With Disabilities Act
Application Software
Background Noise
Central Processing Unit (CPU)
Data
Ergonomics

Hardware
Information System
Input Devices
Keyboard
Lighting
Modem

Mouse
Operating System Software
Output Devices
Scanner
Software
Telecommunication

16

Office Equipment

LEARNING OBJECTIVES

The student will:

1. List the components of a dental practice information system and explain the function of each component.

2. Categorize the various functions of a dental practice telecommunication system.

3. Describe the features of a telephone system and explain how they can be used in a modern dental practice.

4. Design an ergonomic workstation. Identify important elements and state their purpose.

INTRODUCTION

Office equipment helps the administrative dental assistant organize and perform tasks and saves time by integrating different types of procedures. Equipment is selected according to the needs of the staff. Equipment can be divided into two broad categories: equipment used to gather, transfer, and store information, and equipment used to create a working environment that is safe, organized, and functional.

ELECTRONIC BUSINESS EQUIPMENT

The primary functions of the dental business office are collection, transmission, management, and storage of information. In a manual dental practice, the collection and processing of information require a variety of manual skills and tasks. Most dental practices in the 21st century gather similar information, and the information is organized, processed, and stored with electronic technology supported by a computerized information system. An **information system** is a combination of equipment, **software,** data, personnel, and procedures for processing information. The functions of a computerized system are discussed in Chapter 17.

Components of an Information System
• Hardware
• Software
• Data
• Personnel
• Procedures

Hardware

Computer **hardware** is the physical part of the computer system. The hardware in a simple computer system includes the **central processing unit** (CPU), monitor, keyboard, mouse, and printer (Figure 16-1). Additional hardware may include peripherals such as scanners, modems, and external drives.

Central Processing Unit

The **CPU** is the main operating component of the hardware. After data are entered through an input

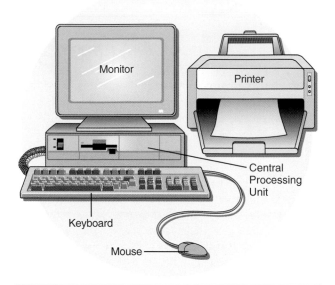

FIGURE 16-1

Computer system: CPU, monitor, keyboard, mouse, and printer.

device, the CPU processes the data and stores the information. When a command is given, the information can be transferred via an output device and a copy can be printed.

Common Input Devices

Input devices are peripheral pieces of hardware that transfer data into a computer system. Common input devices include the keyboard and the mouse. The **keyboard,** which is the most common type of input device, is similar in configuration to a typewriter. In addition, the keyboard may have a variety of function keys. These function keys are located at the top of the keyboard and are used to activate various functions of software applications. On the right side of many keyboards is a number pad that is configured in the same manner as a calculator. The number pad facilitates quick entry of numeric information. Directional arrows (right, left, up, or down) may also be located on the keyboard to permit scrolling (moving through information on the screen). In addition to the keyboard commands, a **mouse** can be used to activate commands. The mouse comes in a variety of styles.

Data can be transferred into a computer via a scanner or modem. Patient forms, radiographs, and intraoral images can be transferred to a patient's electronic record through a scanner. A **scanner** takes a picture of the information on a piece of paper and digitizes it. If the digitized image contains text, it can then be converted with special software into electronic text. This eliminates the need for typing the information into the computer.

Information can also be transferred by way of a modem. A **modem** electronically transfers information from the CPU through a transmission line (commonly a telephone line) to another location. The primary advantages of electronic transfer are its speed and the elimination of a hard copy (paper).

Data entry operations can vary widely. Newer input devices include touch screens (monitors) that are activated when the operator touches the screen. Some systems are designed to receive data via voice command. The computer learns commands and activates functions when the voice message is received. These types of input devices are extremely helpful in the clinical area for management of infection control. Other input devices include joysticks, microphones, and digitizing tablets.

Common Output Devices

Several **output devices** are common to most computer systems: monitors, printers, and storage devices. These devices are used to transfer data out of the computer.

Monitors are designed for viewing information. A monitor is similar to a television screen. The sizes and shapes of monitors, as well as their resolutions, vary. High-quality monitors have a high level of color resolution (clear bright picture) and may have a flat screen (a screen that is only a few inches thick). Monitor screens can, with special software, be activated by touch with a finger or a special wand. Touch screens enable the monitor to act as an input device and as an output device.

A printer is used to produce a hard copy of information stored in the CPU. In a dental practice, a printer is used to print reports, letters, and forms (insurance and statements).

Printers produce black ink printouts, and some can print color as well. Ink jet and laser printers are the most common types of printers. They use plain paper, produce a document of high visual quality,

and can accommodate different sizes and weights of paper. The same printer can be used for insurance claims, billing statements, business letters, and envelopes, as well as for recall cards.

Storage devices (disk drives and tape drives) are similar to monitors in that they can act as both input and output devices. Information can be moved from one computer to another via storage devices. One of their most important uses as an output device is for backing up information. Storage devices allow users to keep additional copies of information in case the computer system fails.

Software

Operating System Software

Programs that allow the user to perform specialized tasks on the computer are called software. **Operating system software** provides the information needed for the computer to be able to function at any level and to run other programs or applications. Examples of operating systems are MS Windows, DOS, and Unix.

Application Software

Application software is designed for specific tasks. Application software tasks include word processing, spreadsheets, databases, and graphics. Dental practice management software packages are combinations of various application softwares and are designed to perform specific dental-related procedures (see Chapter 17 for more detailed information on dental-related procedures performed with a computer).

Data

Data are pieces of information. Both manual and computerized systems use the same information. For example, when new patients arrive at the dental practice, they are asked to complete several forms. Patient financial information is used to establish an account and process insurance. Medical alerts are identified and noted on the patient's clinical record (paper and electronic). Clinical information is used to establish a treatment plan. The manner in which the information is processed, organized, transmitted, and stored varies greatly between manual and electronic systems. A manual system relies on personnel to initiate and complete procedures. Throughout this book, you have learned different ways that information can be processed in a manual system.

An electronic system has the capability of sharing data, which results in the completion of functions and procedures automatically. These functions are discussed in Chapter 17.

Personnel

The number of people who will operate the information system will vary depending on the size of the dental practice and the type of computer system used. Personnel who enter data are responsible for the accurate transfer of information. In a dental practice, the administrative dental assistant performs most of the information processing. In a large dental practice, networked computers (computers that share programs and information) may require a network manager. The duties of the manager are to maintain the system and to provide support for those who operate the system.

Procedures

For optimal use of an information system, it is necessary for personnel to know how to operate the equipment. This knowledge can be obtained from training sessions, from the vendor's technicians, and from the user's manual. Office procedural manuals should outline the procedures and functions that are unique to the dental practice.

TELECOMMUNICATION

Telecommunication is the use of equipment to transfer information or to communicate among people over a distance. In a dental practice, telecommunication methods include the telephone system and intraoffice communications.

Telephone Systems

Business telephone systems can be designed and customized to meet the needs of the individual business (Figure 16-2). A typical dental practice will have a multiline service. This service allows the dental practice to receive several calls at the same time. In addition to receiving and sending telephone calls, telephone lines are used for computer transmissions. Once the desired parts of the system are identified, the appropriate equipment can be selected.

The most visible component of a telephone system is the telephone unit. Basic components include the base unit and the handset. Located on the base unit are the keys used to activate the various functions. The handset contains the receiver and the transmitter. On cordless telephones, the handset is not connected to the base unit and will contain the same keys and functions as the base unit. Telephone units can be desk mounted or wall mounted.

Telephones are designed and programmed for several different tasks. A multiline telephone allows the user to access various lines by simply pressing a button. When a multiline telephone is used, it is very important to know how to answer, transfer, and place telephone calls (review the information in Chapter 3). The design of the system allows more than one call to be received or placed at the same time. In addition to multiple telephone lines, several telephone units can be placed conveniently throughout the dental practice.

Features and Functions of Telephone Systems

- *Answering machines* automatically answer the telephone and deliver a message when an assistant is not available (during lunch hours or when the office is closed). Incoming callers are given information in the message. The system can be designed to be a message-only center or to accept incoming messages.
- *Voice mail* is a form of electronic message center. It is a method used to direct calls to individuals or departments. If the party is unavailable to answer the call, a message can be left in the voice mailbox. For example, a patient calls and has a question concerning insurance. The patient's call is forwarded to the insurance clerk. The insurance clerk has a message on her voice mail asking the patient to leave a message and saying that the call will be returned as soon as possible. Questions can be researched before the call is returned, which saves the insurance clerk and the patient time.
- A *headset* is a lightweight plastic earphone and microphone. When wearing a headset, the operator is able to move freely without the constraint of a handset. Headsets are attached to the base of

Computer Terminology

Address: See URL.

Bit: A unit of information.

Browser: A program used to view hypertext (World Wide Web) pages, such as Netscape or Internet Explorer.

Byte: Small unit of storage; 8 bits; usually holds one character.

CD-ROM: Compact disk read-only memory (CD-ROM) storage medium that can hold 640 megabytes of information; usually used for large software programs.

CPU: Central processing unit (CPU); the brain of the computer; controls the other elements of the computer.

Database: A large, structured set of data; a file that contains numerous records with numerous fields.

Domain Name: The last component of a computer address, that is, com = commercial; edu = educational, gov = government.

Download: Transferring data from one computer to another.

e-mail: Electronic mail (e-mail); messages passed from one computer to another over a network.

Field: One part of a record; several fields become a record; several records become a database.

File: An element of data storage; a single sequence of bytes.

Floppy Disk: A small flexible disk used for storing computer data.

Floppy Drive: A peripheral device that reads or writes information on a floppy disk.

FTP: File transfer protocol (FTP); a protocol used to move software or data from one computer to another over a network.

Function Key: Special key on the keyboard that is programmed to perform certain actions.

GUI: Graphical user interface (GUI); uses pictures and words to represent ideas.

Hard Drive: A device (usually within the CPU) that reads and writes information.

Hardware: Physical parts of a computer; a fixed part of a computer.

Hypertext: Cross-reference or link; permits easy movement from one document to another.

Icon: A small picture used to represent a file or program in a GUI interface.

Internet: A network of computer networks encompassing the World Wide Web, FTP, telnet, and many other protocols.

Internet Explorer: One of the two most recognized World Wide Web browsers.

Intranet: A network, similar to the Internet, used within an organization with links to company information.

Keyboard: A hardware peripheral used to input data with the pressing of keys.

Kilobyte: 1,024 bytes.

LAN: Local area network (LAN); a network of computers that are geographically close (e.g., in separate buildings) and can share information.

Listserv: An automatic mailing list; e-mail messages are automatically mailed to every subscriber.

Login: Procedure necessary to begin a computer session; usually requires an identification name or number and a password.

Megabyte: 1,048,576 bytes *or* 1,024 kilobytes; enough storage to approximately equal a 600-page paperback book.

Modem: A hardware peripheral device used to connect one computer to another over a telephone line.

Monitor: A hardware device used to display information visually.

Mouse: A hardware peripheral device used to point to items on a monitor.

Netscape: One of the two most recognized World Wide Web browsers.

Network: A collection of computers that are connected.

Operating System: The most basic level of software that interfaces with peripherals.

Password: A string of characters, usually chosen by the user, that must be entered before certain information can be accessed; provides a layer of security; often used to log in to a computer.

Peripheral: Any of a number of hardware devices connected to the CPU.

Protocol: A set of rules governing the transmission of data.

RAM: Random access memory (RAM); the type of storage that changes; when the computer is turned off, the RAM memory is erased.

Record: One part of a database; a collection of fields.

Continued

Computer Terminology—cont'd

ROM: Read-only memory (ROM); the type of storage that cannot be changed, even when the computer is turned off.

Software: Instructions executed by a computer.

Spreadsheet: A program of rows and columns in which data can be manipulated.

Telnet: A protocol that enables your computer to act like a computer at another site.

Toolbar: A graphical representation of program activities; a row of icons used to perform tasks in a program.

URL: Uniform resource locator (URL); the address of a site on the World Wide Web; a standard way of locating objects on the Internet.

WAN: Wide area network (WAN); a network of computers that is geographically diverse (i.e., in different states or countries) and permits the sharing of information.

Window: A screen in a software program that permits the user to view several programs at one time.

World Wide Web: A network of hypertext pages that are viewable by browsers.

Zip Drive: A peripheral device that reads or writes information on 100-megabyte disks.

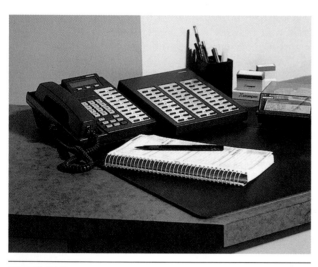

FIGURE 16-2

Multiline business telephone. (From Young AP: Kinn's The Administrative Medical Assistant. 5th edition. Philadelphia, WB Saunders, 2003.)

the telephone with a long cord (typically 10 feet long); more advanced headsets are wireless. Having both hands free enables the operator to move to different locations, retrieve files, record information, use the computer, or make entries in the appointment book while talking on the telephone. An additional benefit is that the operator does not strain neck muscles by cradling the headset between the ear and the shoulder.

- *Speaker phones* can be used when a hands-free environment is needed, or if a conference call is being conducted. During a conference call, a speaker phone is used so that everyone can hear and contribute to the conversation. Caution should be exercised if the conversation is confidential.

- *Speed dialing* is a method of programming the telephone to automatically dial telephone numbers when a simple numeric code or telephone key is pressed. This feature is used to quickly access frequently called telephone numbers.

- *Call forwarding* allows the user to forward incoming telephone calls to another number or station.

- *Intercom paging* allows communication between different stations within the telephone system. For example, when the administrative dental assistant needs to speak to the assistant in the treatment area, the intercom is activated and communications are established.

- *Call management* is that feature of the telephone system that monitors and routes telephone calls. Incoming calls can be answered by a preprogrammed message that welcomes callers to the dental practice and gives them a selection of options. Callers can be transferred to different extensions or placed on hold to listen to music or recorded educational messages.

- *Computer integration* allows communication between a computer and a telephone. Telephone numbers can be automatically dialed by computer with the use of information in the computer database. The computer can initiate audio messages. These features can be part of an automated calling system to remind patients of appointments, overdue accounts, and so forth.

Other individual features vary depending on the type of system and equipment used. These features include remote access to messages, programming features, security codes, voice mailboxes, and enhanced keypad functions.

Electronic Communication Devices

Cellular Telephones

Cellular telephones are wireless telephone systems that permit the receiving and sending of calls anywhere a signal can be received (transmission areas are referred to as *cells*). Cell phones are extremely popular for both business and private use because they are small, can be easily carried in a pocket, and are always available. Use of a cell phone in a dental practice depends on the practice's needs.

Pagers

Pagers are activated by signals and notify a person when a message comes in. When a message is received and the pager responds, the user knows to make a call and retrieve the message. In a dental practice, staff members may use pagers to monitor emergency calls. If a patient calls after hours with an emergency, the answering service or telephone system pages the staff member. The staff member can then respond to the emergency call.

Fax Machines

Facsimile (fax) machines are used to transmit information quickly (Figure 16-3). A document can be sent and received in a matter of seconds over a telephone line and printed out. In a dental practice, a fax can be used to send patient information to insurance companies or to another professional. Care should be taken to ensure the confidentiality of the information being sent. If security cannot be confirmed, it is best to send confidential documents via regular mail.

A fax machine may use plain paper, produce color copies, double as a printer, or integrate with a computer system. A fax machine is an essential piece of

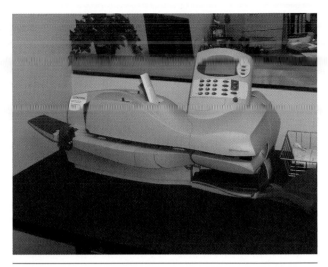

FIGURE 16-3
Postage meter.

office equipment in the dental practice of the 21st century.

INTRAOFFICE COMMUNICATIONS

Communication between members of the dental healthcare team is essential to the smooth operation of the practice. It is necessary for staff to send and receive messages during the day. For example, the administrative dental assistant may need to communicate with the clinical assistant when a patient arrives for treatment. Again, these communications can be manual or electronic or a combination of the two.

Manual Systems

Manual communication systems include intraoffice memos, voice mail, coded light systems (Figure 16-4), and intercoms. Paper intraoffice memos are a frequently used method of communication between departments. They enable team members who are not in the same place at the same time to communicate. Voice mail is another form of communication. It is often easier and faster to leave a voice mail message than to send a memo. Voice mail is also a more private method of conveying information. Coded light systems can be used to inform members of the team of basic information such as when a patient is ready for treatment or when additional

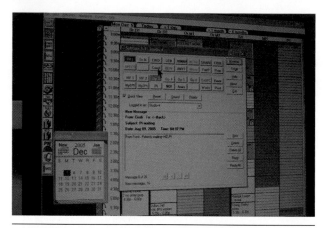

FIGURE 16-4

Staff members in the front office can communicate with back office staff via an integrated practice management system. (Courtesy William C. Domb, DMD, Upland, CA.)

help is needed. Complex communication cannot take place with coded lights. Intercoms provide an alternative form of communication whereby two-way conversations can take place. Remember to respect your patient's privacy. Intercoms should not be used to relay private information if someone else can overhear the conversation.

Electronic Systems

Electronic communication systems include intraoffice memos in electronic form. Electronic memos are usually more secure than their paper counterparts because most computer systems require passwords before they can be accessed. Other forms of electronic communication systems are electronic schedulers, e-mail, and intranets. Electronic schedulers provide a simple method of communication for the dental team. Members can tell, very quickly, where other members are and what they are doing. This enables someone to determine which of the other communication systems should be used to contact someone else. For example, if the hygienist is busy with a patient, the administrative dental assistant can use a system that provides one-way contact. If, however, the hygienist is just in another part of the office, the administrative assistant can initiate two-way contact.

E-mail is becoming a more frequent tool for communicating internally, within the practice, and externally, with other companies or patients. E-mail

is the most frequently used tool on the Internet because it provides a fast, simple form of communication from one person to another, who may or may not be at the computer when the message arrives. E-mail will sit in storage until the receiver is available. Intranets are becoming a more popular way to communicate information among entire staffs or companies. Intranets are similar to the Internet but are not accessible by people outside of an office. They provide a place for frequently needed information or for information needed by several people. Instead of sending everyone in the office a memo, users can place the memo on the intranet for everyone to view.

Unfortunately, no intraoffice communication system can work without the full support of all members of the team. If one person forgets to check his or her mailbox, voice mailbox, or e-mail, communication will not take place efficiently.

OFFICE MACHINES

Copiers can perform tasks of varying complexity depending on the model selected. A basic model is small enough to fit on a tabletop and can copy one document at a time in black ink. A more advanced copier can print multiple documents, collate and staple, print in color, and, in some cases, incorporate fax and e-mail functions.

Postage meters are used to weigh and calculate the correct postage for outgoing mail. These machines can process several pieces of mail quickly. Envelopes are run through the machine, and the correct postage and a postmark are stamped onto the envelope (Figure 16-5). Postage and postmarks can also be printed on labels and the labels applied to oversized envelopes and packages.

Credit card terminals are used to process credit card payments. A credit card is processed by being swiped through the terminal; information contained in the magnetic strip on the back of the credit card is read (Figure 16-6). The amount of the charge is keyed into the terminal's keypad, and other information may be coded (according to the correct protocol). Data are electronically transmitted to the credit card company. After the company authorizes the transaction, a receipt is printed by the terminal and the money is deposited into the dental practice's account.

Typewriters and *word processors* may still be used in some dental practices, although most of their

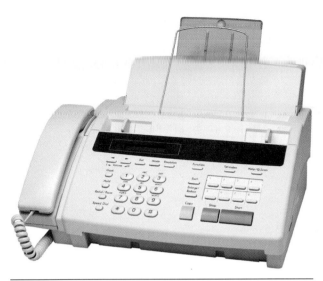

FIGURE 16-5
Facsimile (Fax) machine.

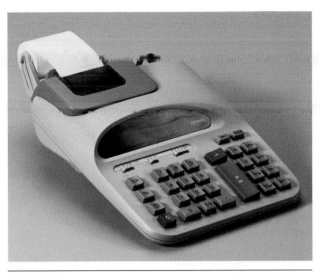

FIGURE 16-7
Printing calculator.

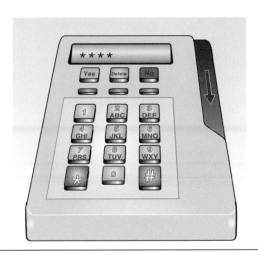

FIGURE 16-6
Credit card terminal.

functions can be accomplished with a computerized system.

Calculators used in a dental practice should be printing calculators (Figure 16-7). These are larger than nonprinting ones, and they provide a printout of all calculations. This type of calculator has a keypad with numbers and function keys (for adding, subtracting, multiplying, and so forth).

BUSINESS OFFICE ENVIRONMENT

The dental practice environment should be organized, safe, and pleasant for those who work in the office and those who patronize it. The organization of a dental practice business office is based on several factors, including the size of the business area, the number of rooms, the function of each area, the accessibility of the area by patients, the number of personnel working in the area, and the equipment used in the office.

Questions to Consider When Organizing a Business Office

How many workstations will be needed? It is necessary to know how many people are going to be working at one time. Workstations should be designed to accommodate the type of equipment (computer, telephone, and so forth) that will be housed there. For example, expanded counter space is needed when an appointment book is used instead of a computer scheduler. Assistants who complete forms and balance daysheets will need extra space to accommodate the size of these papers.

What type of equipment will be used? Types and specifications of equipment will determine how many electrical outlets and telephone lines are

ANATOMY OF AN ERGONOMIC WORK STATION

WORKPLACE ENVIRONMENT
- Most important consideration is working comfortably and efficiently
- Sufficient desk area for keyboard, monitor, mouse, document holder, telephone, etc.
- Organize the area so that it reflects the way you use equipment
- Things you use most often should be within easiest reach
- Vary your tasks
- Take frequent breaks
- If area is shared, be sure all who use it can adjust everything to their needs
- Document holders same height and distance from monitor
- Adequate leg room
- Unobscured line of sight

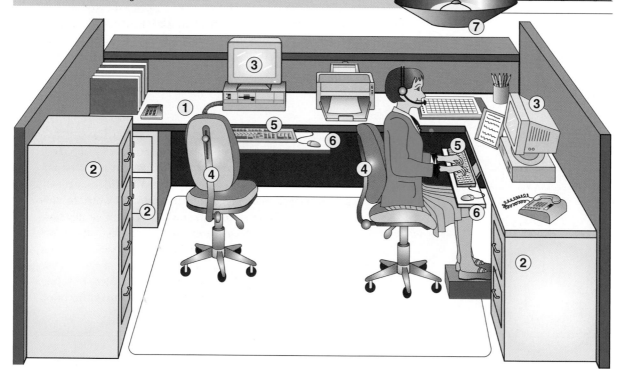

① WORK SURFACE
- Proper height and angle
- Neutral postures
- Adjustable
- Standing—prevent slipping, adequate traction
- Sit/stand stools
- Anti-fatigue floor mats
- Darker, matte finishes are best

② STORAGE AREAS
- Good body positions
- Reduce muscular forces
- Avoid excessive reach
- Heavy items between knee and shoulder height
- Frequently used storage closest to worker

③ VIDEO DISPLAY TERMINAL (VDT) [MONITOR]
- Position to minimize glare and reflections
- Top of screen is slightly below eye level
- Tilted slightly backward (less than 15 degrees)
- Distance from display 18-30 inches
- Perpendicular to windows
- Keep your head upright
- Set contrast and brightness
- Clean the screen (and your glasses)
- Anti-glare filters
- Adjustable monitor arm

④ CHAIRS
- Comfortable (padded seats that swivel)
- Back and seat are adjustable while seated
- Provide good back support (can add additional cushion if necessary)
- Adjustable arm support
- Back straight
- Knees slightly higher than chair bottom
- Thighs are horizontal
- Feet flat on the floor (use a footrest if necessary)
- Change positions occasionally

⑤ KEYBOARD
- Back should be lower than the front
- Rounded edges
- Wrist rests (sharp edges, neutral position) same height as front of keyboard
- Type properly; don't force your fingers to stretch to incorrect keystrokes

⑥ MOUSE
- Keep it on the same level as the keyboard or slightly above
- Keep wrist straight
- Do not stretch your arm; keep mouse within immediate reach
- Use the whole arm to move the mouse...not just the forearm

⑦ LIGHTING
- Less illumination for computer work
- Indirect lighting is best

AVOID THE FOLLOWING

- **Awkward posture**
  Can include reaching behind, twisting, working overhead, kneeling, bending and squatting. Deviation from ideal working posture can lead to fatigue, muscle tension and headaches. **Correct working posture**—arms at sides, elbows bent at approximately 90 degrees, forearms parallel to floor, wrists straight.

- **Repetitiveness**
  Judgment is based on frequency, speed, number of muscle groups used, required force. Not all people react to the same conditions, so carefully monitor your personal physical response to repetitiveness.

needed. Sizes and heights of counters should be configured to meet the specifications of the equipment.

What are the storage requirements? Storage equipment includes cabinets for supplies and filing cabinets for patient and business files. Workstations should include conveniently located drawers and cubicles for storage of items used often during the day.

What types of business office personnel will be hired? The types of business personnel (e.g., business manager, office manager, insurance clerk, bookkeeper, receptionist) to be hired will determine the number of rooms or cubicles needed and the type of space they will require. Some areas will have to be more private than others.

Safety

The Occupational Safety and Health Administration is concerned with safety in the workplace. Safety concerns in a dental practice business office primarily involve equipment and ergonomics. Other considerations include background noise, lighting, temperature, and humidity.

Ergonomics

Ergonomics is the science of fitting the job to the worker. When the job does not match the physical capacity of the worker, work-related musculoskeletal disorders (WMSDs) can result. These injuries usually occur over a prolonged time. Research has revealed that all workers are at risk for WMSDs. In the business office, repeated movement (e.g., when one is using a computer keyboard or typewriter) may place the operator at risk for carpal tunnel syndrome. Placement of the keyboard, height of the chair, and other factors play an important role in the comfort and health of the operator.

Background Noise

In a dental practice, **background noise** can come from a number of different sources and may vary in intensity. The ambient sound level should not be higher than 55 decibels.

Lighting

It is crucial for a comfortable and productive workstation to have the correct type and amount of **lighting.** The optimal light level depends on the task at hand. The best level of illumination for people who use video display terminals (VDTs) as well as paper documents is 300 to 400 lux (30 to 40 foot-candles). If paper documents are not used, the level can be reduced to 200 lux.

To minimize screen glare, light from windows should be controlled by drapes, dark film, blinds, or louvers. Intense overhead lighting may also produce glare. In this case, louvers or screens for overhead lights may help. Filters for monitor screens may help reduce reflections.

Temperature and Humidity

Most workers in an office environment find that they are comfortable when the relative humidity level is between 40% and 60%. Stable temperatures are important for computer systems as well as for people. Major temperature fluctuations can damage a computer.

The Americans With Disabilities Act

The **Americans With Disabilities Act,** signed into law on July 26, 1990, prohibits discrimination on the basis of disability in employment, programs, and services provided by state and local governments and goods and services provided by private companies, and in commercial facilities. Access to buildings and public offices must be easy and safe for all people. Dental offices must provide access for patients in wheelchairs, as well as for employees with disabilities. When designing a new dental office or remodeling an old one, one should keep in mind that these regulations must be met.

KEY POINTS

- Office equipment helps the administrative dental assistant to organize tasks, and it saves time by integrating different types of procedures. Equipment can be divided into two broad categories: equipment used to gather, transfer, and store information, and equipment used to create a work environment that is safe, organized, and functional.

- A computerized information system is a composite of equipment (hardware), software, data, personnel, and procedures for processing information.
- Telecommunication is the use of equipment to transfer information to or communicate with someone over a distance. In a dental practice, telecommunication includes the telephone system and intraoffice communications.
- The work environment should be organized, safe, and pleasant for those who work in the office and those who patronize it.

 Web Watch

ADA Guide for Small Businesses

http://www.usdoj.gov/crt/ada/publicat.htm#Anchor-ADA-35326

Business Owner's Toolkit: Your Office and Equipment

http://www.toolkit.cch.com/text/P040000.asp

 Log on to Evolve to access additional web links!

http://evolve.elsevier.com

 Critical Thinking Questions

1. How would you classify the different types of business equipment? Explain the function of each type.
2. What is the function of a dental practice electronic information system?
3. What can be done to enhance the work environment according to recommended ergonomic design?

Notes

OUTLINE

KEY TERMS

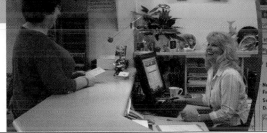

17

Computerized Dental Practice

LEARNING OBJECTIVES

The student will:

1. Compare the three levels of function of dental practice management software and discuss their application.
2. List the functions to consider when selecting dental practice management software.
3. Discuss the role of the administrative dental assistant in the operation of a computerized dental practice.
4. Identify the different computer tasks performed by the administrative dental assistant.
5. Compare the daily routines performed with a computer system and a manual system, and discuss their differences and similarities.
6. Describe the importance of a computer system backup routine.

INTRODUCTION

The use of computers in a dental practice is becoming standard. Computers help staff to manage office functions, submit insurance claims, track patients, schedule appointments, and record treatments. It is the duty of an administrative dental assistant to become familiar with and capable of using a computer system.

LEVELS OF FUNCTION OF DENTAL PRACTICE MANAGEMENT SOFTWARE

Dental practice management software combines several aspects of word processing, spreadsheet, and database functions. It is this design that allows the dental practice to perform several functions at one time. As you have learned by reading this text, each step and function, when performed manually, is time consuming. For example, bookkeeping tasks require several steps to be followed by the administrative dental assistant before the daily process is completed. Financial data must be correctly placed on the daysheet, columns added, and reports calculated. When errors are committed, it is the responsibility of the assistant to locate and correct them all before proceeding. A computerized system completes several of these steps for the assistant, correctly calculating totals, adding columns, and alerting the assistant when erroneous information is entered.

Software programs are of three levels of complexity: level one—basic; level two—intermediate; and level three—advanced. Several functions can be performed more efficiently and in less time with a computer than manually. The software design will determine at what level the software can function. A level three system can be used at level two or level one, but a level one system cannot perform advanced tasks. The desire, level of training, and cooperation of the dental healthcare team will determine at which level the software is used.

Various tasks, common to most systems, are described in the following classification of basic systems, intermediate systems, and advanced systems.

Basic Systems

A level one system, or **basic system,** can organize and create a database and perform spreadsheet and word processing tasks. These functions represent basic paperwork handled in the dental practice.

Retain Demographic and Financial Information

- Names, addresses, and telephone numbers.
- Employer identification numbers, social security numbers.
- Insurance information: primary (guarantor 1) and secondary (guarantor 2).
- New patients and referral sources.
- Medical alerts.

Create Accounts (Multiple Patients)

- Categorize individual items of patient information within an account.
- Print treatment plans.
- Generate statements.

Process Insurance Information

- Generate insurance claims (printed and electronic).
- Categorize insurance information, including group plans, deductibles, and benefits.
- Print claims for preauthorization.
- Track unpaid insurance claims and unobtained preauthorizations.
- List insurance carriers.

Perform Accounting Tasks

- Post transactions (payments, charges, and adjustments).
- Use a coding system for insurance processing and accounting reports.
- Print daily routing forms.

Perform Recall and Reactivation Procedures

- List patients who are due for recall.
- Generate notices.
- Track overdue recalls.
- Identify patients who have not completed treatment plans.

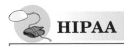
Practice management software programs provide the data fields needed to enter information that will be needed for compliance with HIPAA standards. The following screen shots are examples of how a program may address the four different HIPAA standards.

Security Rule

Password protection is one method of securing electronic protected health information (EPHI).

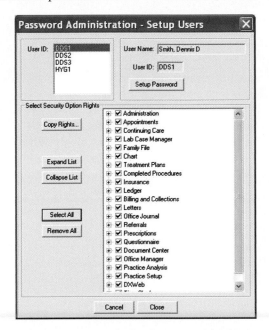

(Courtesy Dentrix Dental Systems, American Fork, UT.)

National Provider Identifier Standard

The National Provider Identifier Standard (NPI) is required on all electronic transactions as of later than May 23, 2007.

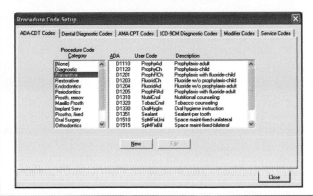

Electronic Transactions and Code Sets

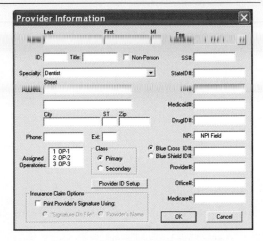

Examples of Code on Dental Procedures and Nomenclature; includes procedure code category (standardized), ADA or CDT code (standardized), User Code (unique to software program), and Description (unique to software program).

Provider Specialties

Provider Specialties are listed in the Provider Information window for selection. DENTRIX comes with the following specialties:

1. 122300000X Dentist
2. 126800000X Dental Assistant
3. 124Q0000X Dental Hygienist
4. 1223D0001X Dental Public Health
5. 1223E0200X Endodontics
6. 1223X0400X Orthodontics
7. 1223P0106X Pathology, Oral and Maxillofacial
8. 1223P0221X Pediatric Dentistry
9. 1223P0300X Periodontics
10. 1223P0700X Prosthodontics
11. 1223S0112X Surgery, Oral and Maxillofacial
12. 126900000X Dental Laboratory Technician
13. 1223G0001X General Practice
14. 1223X0008X Oral and Maxillofacial Radiology

Examples of the Healthcare Providers Taxonomy Code list used in HIPAA transactions.

(Courtesy Dentrix Dental Systems, American Fork, Utah.)

Maintain an Audit Trail

- Mark entries with the following information: date of entry, time, and employee identification (hidden information).
- List scheduled patients (daily).
- Identify patients scheduled without a charge or entry.
- Identify patients with incomplete transactions.

Provide Software Security

- Prevent unauthorized entry into the system.

Allow Multitasking

- Perform more than one task at a time from one terminal.
- Use more than one terminal at a time.

Perform Basic Word Processing Tasks

- Create letters.
- Merge patient data into letters.

Allow Use of a Modem

- Share information with vendors.
- Submit insurance claims electronically.
- Access the Internet.

Intermediate Systems

A level two system, or **intermediate system,** has the same basic functions as a level one system along with the following additional functions.

Allow Interoffice Communications

- Send messages between terminals.
- Communicate with computers in other office sites.

Add Flexibility

- Accommodate options in treatment planning.
- Accommodate budget plans.
- Charge interest to specified accounts.
- Customize reports.
- Customize statements: use different styles and messages depending on the intended need (reminders, collection notes, or recall information).

Process Insurance Information

- Batch claims for group submission.
- Print individual claims.
- Determine patient portion based on information stored in the database.

Perform Word Processing Tasks

- Batch print.
- Record letters sent in the patient record and print lists.
- Write prescriptions.

Generate Automatic Reminders

- Staff task reminders.
- Notes.
- Tickler files for patient scheduling.

Perform Electronic Scheduling

- Schedule and track appointments.
- Set production goals.
- Schedule by treatment room.
- Color code types of treatment.
- Produce electronic reminders for patients.
- Customize matrixing of the scheduler.
- Produce patient call lists identifying patients who missed or canceled appointments.

Support Group Practices

- Allow use by several providers.
- Accommodate different fee schedules.
- Generate reports according to provider.

Personalize Recall and Reactivation Procedures

- Attach personal reasons (incomplete treatment, preventive or restorative treatment) for recall or reactivation.
- Generate reports with notes.

Advanced Systems

Dental practices that use an **advanced system** integrate the business office with the clinical practice. The dental healthcare team is responsible for entering information and accessing the system. Terminals are located in treatment areas, allowing chairside assistants to complete charting procedures. Digitized radiographs are taken and stored within the computer system. The dream of a paperless dental practice moves closer with integrated software. In addition to level one and level two functions, the following level three functions may be performed.

Maintain Clinical Information

- Progress notes.
- Treatment and tooth charting.
- Periodontal charting.
- Medical and dental histories.
- Legal paperless clinical record.

Accommodate Integrated Clinical Workstations

- Intraoral imaging.
- Digital radiographs.
- Orthodontic case presentations.

The level of operation of a dental practice management software program depends on the scope of the software and the commitment of the dental healthcare team. The success of the software program directly depends on the operator.

SELECTING A SOFTWARE PACKAGE

Before a software package is selected, it is necessary to assess the need for a system. Questions should be asked and careful consideration should be given before a package is selected. One way to accomplish this is to meet with all of those who will have a stake in the system: dentist, business manager, accountant, associate dentists, hygienist, and administrative dental assistants. These people will provide feedback on what they consider important. Accountants and dentists may be interested in the types of reports generated. Hygienists will want to look at the recall function, and administrative dental assistants will want to know how the system will help them with paperwork: maintaining patient records, posting transactions, sending statements, and completing insurance claims. Each individual will provide valuable information and will identify different needs of the dental practice.

After basic needs have been determined, the next step is to assess level two and then level three functions. Most software vendors provide complex questionnaires to help dental personnel identify what they want and what they will need in a package. Not all packages offer the same features. It is necessary for dental personnel to select a package that will meet their needs and provide them with the support they need to run the software.

FUNCTIONS TO CONSIDER WHEN SELECTING A SOFTWARE PACKAGE

Many different functions should be considered when a software package is selected: general requirements, patient information, patient billing, treatment planning, insurance processing, recall and reactivation, practice management reports, electronic scheduling, database management and word processing, clinical integration, and HIPAA (Health Insurance Portability and Accountability Act) requirements for system security. Not all functions will be important to all dental practices. The following discussion can be used to identify what may or may not be important functions. Once target functions have been identified, the next step is to compare the functions of software packages and select the one that will meet the needs of the practice. Although this process is time consuming, it is essential.

General Requirements

General requirements are those elements of the software program that permit it to perform different functions.

- Security systems protect the integrity of the information stored. Those who operate the software are given passwords and must follow established HIPAA protocol to ensure the integrity of electronic protected health information (EPHI).
- Audit trails identify who entered or edited information. This is important for a paperless dental practice because it records all changes to information and identifies who made the changes and on what date; it also meets the mandates of the HIPAA Security Rule.
- Those with access to the software may be assigned different levels of access. This protects the system from unauthorized changes to system functions.
- The system can purge inactive accounts automatically.
- Some systems support clinical applications: tooth charting, periodontal charting, digital radiographs, and imaging.
- Context-sensitive help screens are useful.
- The system permits error checking to correct erroneous dates and tooth numbers, thereby preventing incorrect tooth surfaces from being entered.

- The system allows you to move between screens without returning to the main menu.
- The system allows print options, such as starting from where you left off, using preprinted forms, and creating documents with a laser printer.
- The system can track more than one provider and provide multiple fee schedules.

Patient Information

Functions that help the administrative dental assistant to organize patient information include the following:

Locate a Patient by Name or Number

- Scan information into the system, such as patient history, medical and dental histories, laboratory reports, insurance correspondence, and referral letters.
- Use two different addresses for each patient, such as home address and billing address.
- Correct errors within fields without retyping the complete field.
- Automatically capitalize names, addresses, cities, and so forth.
- Use coded information for repeated information, such as ZIP codes matched with cities, insurance carrier information for common carriers, and group and employer information for patients with common employers.
- Integrate patient clinical records, treatment notes, medical history, and registration information into the system to create a paperless dental practice.

Patient Billing

Patient billing should be flexible and should offer the dental practice more than one way to produce statements. Statements include monthly billing statements, budget plan statements, and walkout statements.

Walkout Statements

- Contain posttreatment instructions, such as information on care after extractions.
- Separate insurance and patient portions.
- State minimum amount due.
- List the next appointment or series of appointments and state what treatments will be provided.

Patient Statements

- Produce one for each patient.
- Customize patient messages, such as collection notes and recall notices.
- Customize for different providers within the same dental practice.
- Print budget plans, interest charges, and truth in lending statements.
- Itemize insurance payments, patient portions, and calculated adjustments.

Billing Statements in Cycles

- Produce billing statements for accounts that are overdue at specific times, such as every 30 days.

Year-End Summaries

- List all treatments.
- List all payments made by the patient for tax reporting.

Treatment Planning

Treatment planning is an important component of the computerized system. With several options available, the administrative dental assistant is able to develop quickly and efficiently a clear and concise plan for patients.

Print treatment plans and options.
- Prioritize treatments for long-range planning.
- Integrate treatment plan with insurance information to show all treatments for the year, deductibles, and patient portion.

Insurance Processing

The system allows the administrative dental assistant to submit claims daily, track all claims, and print reports for follow-up.

The program knows what additional information, such as a radiograph or a report, is needed for a specific procedure and prompts the user for that additional information.

- Claims can be printed a second time so lost claims are replaced.
- The system prompts the user to submit insurance claims.
- The system prompts the user to submit secondary insurance claims after the primary insurance company pays.

- The system can separate treatment dates if the patient changes insurance carriers midway through treatment.
- The complete insurance form is filled out, including the charting of missing teeth.
- Insurance forms can be printed on a form or from a laser printer without preprinted forms.
- Orthodontic treatments can be billed cyclically.
- The system can generate medical claims, including correct International Classification of Diseases (ICD)-9 and diagnostic codes.
- When a procedure code is entered, the system automatically files the correct dental or medical claim form using the appropriate HIPAA Transactions and Code Sets.
- The system stores fees reported on paid insurance claims, creating a database that is accurate when estimating the insurance company's portion.
- The system can estimate the insurance company's portion by considering deductibles and remaining insurance or unused benefits and coordinating benefits for primary and secondary insurance companies.
- Notations and procedures can be printed on the patient insurance form but not on the patient statement.
- Narratives can be added to both printed and electronic insurance forms.
- In group practices, the provider of the service can be identified on the individual claim form, even if the provider changes from visit to visit.
- The system can track patients who have not completed preauthorized dental treatment plans.
- The system can submit claims electronically.

Recall and Reactivation

In a computerized system, information stored in the database is used to automatically generate notices and produce reports that identify patients who are scheduled for recall and reactivation.

- Recall dates for an entire family are easily identified in account and patient records.
- Recall dates can be customized at various monthly intervals (1 month, 2 months, 3 months, 4 months, 5 months, 6 months, or longer).
- The system alerts the user if the recall does not meet the insurance company's standard.
- Recall notices for all patients due in a month are automatically produced.

- Selected recall letters or cards are automatically produced.
- Appointment notices for patients who are scheduled with the electronic scheduler are automatically produced.
- Patients are tracked for recall compliance, and tracking reports and notices to patients who do not keep appointments are generated.
- The type of recall is identified, and notices are customized to match the type of recall.
- Patients with incomplete treatment are tracked with lists, and letters to gain compliance are generated.
- Patients who are due for recall are listed until they schedule and keep an appointment or wish to be removed from the list.

Management Reports

A number of reports can be generated, depending on the needs of the practice.

- Produce age accounts, which are customized reports showing the oldest account, past due budget plans, and the largest amount past due.
- Produce production reports according to provider (dentist, associate dentist, hygienist), and categorize by hour, day, week, and month.
- Generate reports by transaction code.
- Produce insurance reports that show the amounts billed to different carriers, and then age the amount due.
- Customize reports for staff incentive programs (new patients, production, collections).
- Be flexible in generating the types and designs of reports required to meet the individual needs of the practice.

Electronic Scheduler

The electronic scheduler is the digital version of the appointment book. An electronic scheduler aids the administrative dental assistant in organizing and maximizing the schedule for efficiency.

- Allows the scheduling of patients 1 year in advance.
- Allows the scheduler to leave one screen and schedule an appointment for another patient on another screen.
- Keeps a list of patients who wish to come in earlier than their scheduled appointment, including their telephone numbers, the time they wish to come in, and the last time you contacted them.

- Allows the user to matrix the appointment scheduler according to production goals, preferred time of day for emergencies, and high and low production procedures.
- Customizes according to dental healthcare provider.
- Schedules by treatment room.
- Generates outside reminders such as meeting notices, to-do lists, and staff reminders.
- Tracks laboratory cases and alerts the staff if the patient is scheduled before the laboratory work will be returned.
- Alerts the scheduling staff if sufficient time is not scheduled between appointments.
- Prints a report of all patients due the next day.
- Runs an audit report to ensure that a charge or entry is made for every patient scheduled.
- Allows the addition of emergency and walk-in patients to the schedule (ensuring that all patients are part of the audit trail).
- Allows daily reports that will age accounts and shows outstanding treatments and medical alerts (for patients with scheduled appointments).
- Alerts the staff in a group practice if appointments are scheduled with the hygienist when the dentist of record is not scheduled.
- Coordinates schedules when the patient sees more than one provider in the same day.
- Has a find feature for easy access to a patient's record.
- Tracks patients from the time they enter the dental practice until they have completed the checkout process.
- Prints routing slips for all scheduled patients, listing scheduled treatment, recall information, insurance information, and medical alerts.
- Allows the user to customize the routing slip to meet the needs of individual practices.

Database Management and Word Processing

Information stored in the database can be merged into word processing software to create a variety of letters, referrals, and marketing tools.
- The system, under designed conditions, automatically generates letters without staff direction.
- The system keeps track of letters sent to patients and others.

- The system automatically accesses a database to merge letters, reports, and statements by such criteria as past due account information, incomplete dentistry, and scheduling information.
- Word processing programs can be accessed without exit from the dental software.
- The word processor interacts with the scheduler so it can automatically generate confirmation letters, such as notes confirming preappointed recall visits.
- The system stores commonly used letters and forms and merges information such as name and address to personalize each letter.

Clinical Integration

- A fully integrated system.
- Alerts clinical staff when patients enter the practice, what treatment room they are assigned to, and what treatment is scheduled for the day.
- Integrates into the patient's digital record information recorded via an intraoral camera.
- Records digital radiographs into the digital record.
- Allows scanning of traditional radiographs into the digital record.
- Uses strategically located monitors in treatment areas to directly record patient information such as clinical findings, periodontal examination results, and treatment notes.
- Allows scheduling from any monitor.
- Integrates with other digital devices such as periodontal probes to record the findings.
- Creates a legal paperless clinical record.
- Applies HIPAA Security Standards.

BASIC OPERATION OF A SOFTWARE PACKAGE

Although many software packages are available, most offer similar basic features and operations. Most updated and revised editions use a Windows format. Windows offers the ability to complete more than one task at a time. The various screens of these programs have the same basic elements: **title bars, menu bars, tool bars, power bars,** and **status bars.**

ROLE OF THE ADMINISTRATIVE DENTAL ASSISTANT

The roles of the administrative dental assistant vary, depending on the software program used by the dental practice. All programs have some common functions. These common functions include recording patient demographics, posting transactions, using a general database, processing insurance claims, scheduling electronically, and producing reports.

Recording Patient Demographics

Patient demographic information is provided by patients on their registration forms. This information is taken from the registration form and entered into the software database. This process is accomplished by keying the information into the correct field.

Creating an Account

A computerized account is the same as a manual account; it identifies the person who is financially responsible for paying the account (Figure 17-1). When all fields are filled in, the system stores this information in its database and uses it to bill patients and complete insurance claim forms. The system assigns an account number that is unique to this account and is used to locate the account in the computer database.

Maintaining Patient Records

After an account has been established, patient information is entered (Figure 17-2). All information entered, such as address (if different from the account address), date of birth, Social Security number, medical alert information, student status, and relationship to insurer (this information will be used to complete insurance claims), is directly related to the patient. After the patient information section has been completed, the computer assigns the patient another number (different from the account number). The administrative dental assistant records the patient number on the patient's clinical chart. This number is used to locate the patient in the computer database.

More than one patient can be assigned to an account (Figure 17-3). This often occurs in families whose members all go to the same dentist. For

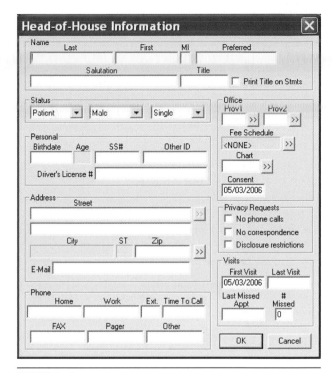

FIGURE 17-1

Head of House Information Window. This window shows basic information that is used to create a family account. The information entered on this screen pertains to the person who is financially responsible for the account (may or may not be the patient and may not be a patient of the dental practice). (Courtesy Dentrix Dental Systems, American Fork, UT.)

example, the account number assigned to the Abbott family is ABB 100. When the computer is asked to locate account number ABB 100, it lists all members of the Abbott family who are patients. Each patient is assigned a corresponding patient number: Kim Abbott (father) ABB 101; Patricia Abbott ABB 102; and Timothy Abbott ABB 103.

Posting Transactions

In a manual system, records of charges and payments are posted to the account according to a bookkeeping system (pegboard or "one-write" system). The same functions are available in computerized and manual systems. After treatment has been provided, charges are posted to the patient's computer record (Figure 17-4).

ANATOMY OF COMPUTER SCREEN ELEMENTS

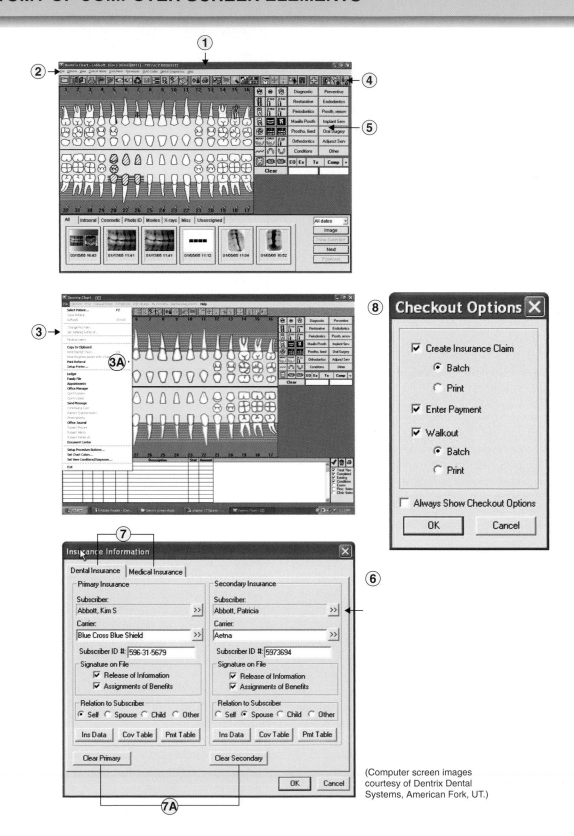

(Computer screen images courtesy of Dentrix Dental Systems, American Fork, UT.)

① **TITLE BAR**

The title bar identifies the software being used and the mode that is currently active.

② **MENU BAR**

The menu bar lists the categories of options available to the user. There are two ways to reach the list of options for each category. With the mouse, place the pointer on the category title and click once on the left mouse button. Alternatively, you can use the function keys. While holding down the ALT key, press the key that matches the underlined letter of the option. Either of these operations will produce a **drop-down menu**.

③ **DROP-DOWN MENU**

A list of options available under each category on the menu bar is given in the drop-down menu. An option can be selected using the mouse or the keystroke selection method (using the key that matches the underlined letter). Options available will be in bold print. Options not available in the current mode will be gray. ③A A **next arrow** after the option indicates that there is a sub-menu present. To view the sub-menu, place the pointer on the function. The sub-menu will drop down.

④ **TOOL BAR**

The tool bar shows a group of icons configured as buttons that identify commonly used functions. Clicking on a button is a shortcut toward accessing these functions. Which functions are available will vary depending on the operation that is currently active. For example, if you are using a word-processing operation the buttons will be common for that operation, while the buttons for a spreadsheet operation will be different. Many programs offer an identification mode, which will allow you to identify the function of each button by placing the pointer on the button. A text box will appear to identify the function.

⑤ **POWER BAR**

The power bar provides quick access to selected features and reports. They normally are composed of customized icons that are unique to a particular software program. The user may have the option of activating or closing the power bar.

⑥ **SEARCH BUTTON**

This will give you information about the screen you are currently working in. It may identify the user who has logged on, date, time, and the current operating mode. Choose this button to open or reveal additional options.

⑦ **TABBED SCREENS**

Tabs are used to arrange the parts of a screen into a logical order. There may be a common area to all screens; this information will be displayed with each tab. Tabbed screens are commonly used to enter information. There will be several different fields, and you will move from field to field by using the tab key or arrows (depending on the software being used). ⑦A Buttons are also used to take the user from one screen to the next.

⑧ **DIALOG WINDOWS OR BOXES**

A dialog window will appear when additional input is needed, effectively asking you a question. To answer the question it will be necessary to activate the correct button. Common responses to dialog windows are yes, no, OK and cancel.

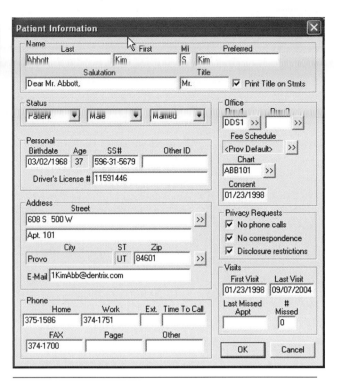

FIGURE 17-2

Patient Information Window. This window is used to enter patient information. The screen also allows the user to assign a provider, fee schedule, chart number, privacy request, and visit history. (Courtesy Dentrix Dental Systems, American Fork, UT.)

The administrative dental assistant receives information from the treatment area via several different types of communications: patient routing slips, patients' clinical charts, or charge slips. The assistant will use this information during the check-out procedure.

Using a General Database

One advantage of the computerized system is common information may be shared. Information that will be common with all accounts includes insurance carrier identification (Figure 17-5), transaction codes (Figure 17-6), and provider demographics (Figure 17-7). This information is entered only once into the system. A series of codes are assigned to the pieces of information. When it is necessary to enter information that is stored in the common database, coding is used to simplify this procedure.

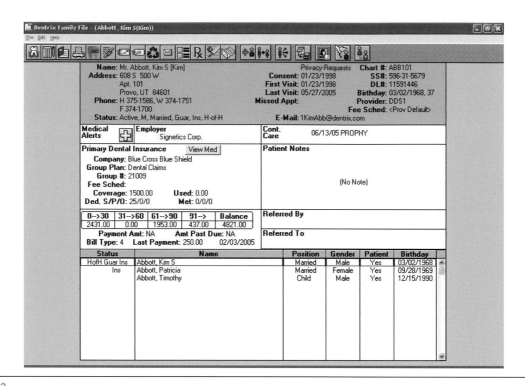

FIGURE 17-3

Family File Screen. This window identifies the head of household and all patients listed under the account. (Courtesy Dentrix Dental Systems, American Fork, UT.)

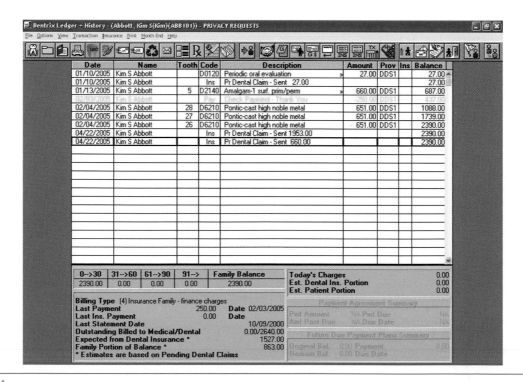

FIGURE 17-4

Ledger and History Window. This window displays individual patient history and transactions. (Courtesy Dentrix Dental Systems, American Fork, UT.)

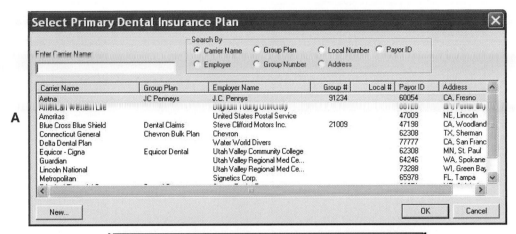

FIGURE 17-5
A, Select Primary Dental Insurance Plan. This window lists all dental plans currently stored in the software database.
B, Dental Insurance Plan Information Window. This window is used to add a new dental plan to the software database.
(Courtesy Dentrix Dental Systems, American Fork, UT.)

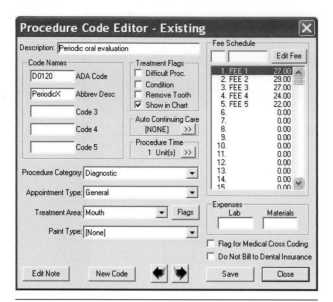

FIGURE 17-6

Procedure Code Editor Window. This window is used to add information and descriptions to a CDT code. The user is able to add information for appointment scheduling, procedure time, charting, insurance billing, fee schedules, laboratory results, and medical cross coding. (Courtesy Dentrix Dental Systems, American Fork, UT.)

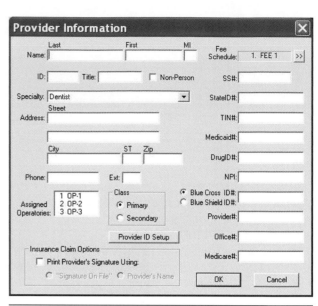

FIGURE 17-7

Provider Information Window. This window is used to enter information about each provider that will be used to complete and file insurance claim forms. (Courtesy Dentrix Dental Systems, American Fork, UT.)

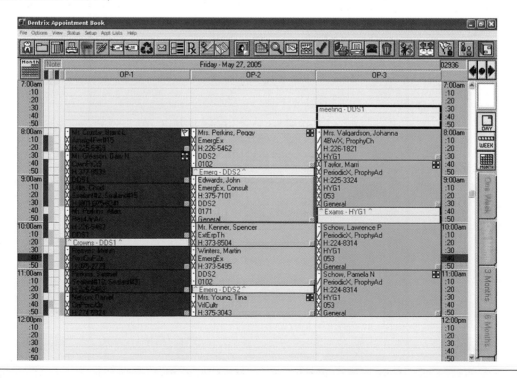

FIGURE 17-8

Appointment Book (daily). This window is an example of a filled appointment book page. The page shows dates, operatories, and color-coded providers. Each patient listed is coded to include contact information, procedure, and provider. (Courtesy Dentrix Dental Systems, American Fork, UT.)

Processing Insurance Claims

Insurance processing is simplified with the use of a computer. The computer system allows the user to link several different codes to complete claim forms. For example, insurance CPT (current procedural terminology) codes are entered once. When it is necessary to enter information in the transaction mode, a code is entered and all pertinent information stored in the database is entered into the patient account. This code identifies the service and asks for details such as tooth number and surface. The code is linked to a fee schedule, and the system automatically selects the correct fee. The provider of the service can also be linked to the code. When the corresponding code is entered, all pertinent provider demographic information is entered.

When an insurance claim is requested, the system links all codes and correctly places information in the appropriate fields of the insurance claim form (patient demographics, insurance carrier information, provider demographics, and CPT codes and fees). When information is shared, several tasks can be completed through the simple linking of needed information through a coding system. This process ensures accuracy and improves efficiency by saving time for the administrative dental assistant.

Claims can be coded for electronic submission or batched for printing. Most systems can also print the information on a preprinted form or on plain paper. With the use of information in the system, reports can be generated that will track the location and amount of the claim and will alert the administrative dental assistant when the claim has not been paid in a timely manner. The system converts all elements of an efficient manual tracking system into a highly effective computer system, providing the necessary tools for successful management of insurance claims.

Scheduling Electronically

The system allows the scheduler to be matrixed in the same way that an appointment book is matrixed. The user identifies what days of the week and what hours patients can be scheduled and customizes the schedule for each provider (dentist, assistant dentist, and hygienist). Users can also program the system to automatically schedule according to procedure and can enter patient options such as time and provider (Figure 17-8).

Tabbed screens allow users to scan the appointment book in several different modes. They can automatically schedule appointments or can check week at a glance and month at a glance modes to find open time slots (Figure 17-9). Appointments can be scheduled with production goals in mind or color coded to identify time slots for designated procedures, meetings, lunches, and emergencies. The scheduler is matrixed according to specific requirements of the individual dental practice.

Producing Reports

Reports can be customized to meet the needs of each office. Large dental practices with more than one provider will want the capability of generating reports unique to each provider. Reports identify production, collections, and adjustments, calculate the amount of time used to complete procedures, and track production goals. Insurance and recall tracking can be accomplished with the use of monthly reports that identify current statuses. Reports, including accounting reports, patient reports, recall/appointment reports, provider/referring doctor reports, insurance reports, American Dental Association (ADA)/transaction/diagnosis code reports, prescription/pharmacy/laboratory reports, and practice management reports, can be customized to meet almost any need of the dental practice.

DAILY PROCEDURES WITH A COMPUTERIZED SYSTEM

One advantage of a computerized system is that it allows the administrative dental assistant and other members of the dental healthcare team to complete several functions by maximizing the computerized database, spreadsheet, and word processing functions. When these tasks are completed before the patient leaves the office, the dental practice is assured that all necessary transactions have been posted, the insurance process has been completed, and the next appointment has been scheduled. These steps improve communications with the patient by providing detailed information and help the assistant become more organized in the completion of required tasks.

The type of computer system used determines the exact order and characteristics of the start-up procedures. Each system offers different options, and it

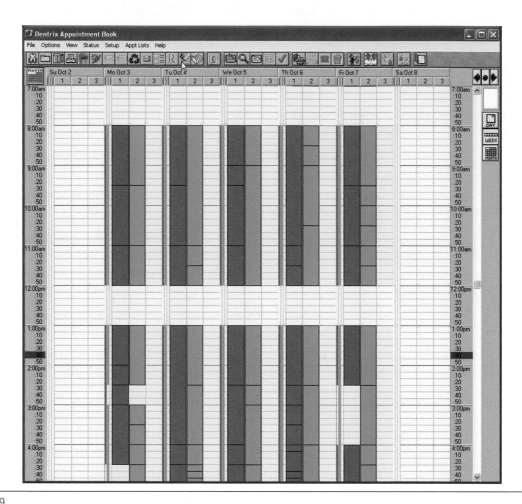

FIGURE 17-9

Appointment Book (week at a glance). This window is color-coded (matrixed) and is used to show the full week at a glance. The window identifies openings in the schedule, providers, and operatories. (Courtesy Dentrix Dental Systems, American Fork, UT.)

is the responsibility of the administrative dental assistant to become familiar with these options. Following are examples of daily procedures performed with a basic computer system.

Opening Procedure

1. A password is entered to access the system.
2. Information is entered that brings up a screen that lists all patients scheduled for the day. This may be done with the help of a **status window** that directs the user to enter the date and to print routing slips for the day (Figure 17-10).

3. A screen appears that lists all patients scheduled for the day. This screen gives the following information: appointment time, name of patient, insurance status, current balance, estimated patient payment for the scheduled procedure, provider name, treatment room, and a code for the first treatment to be performed (much of the information on the screen will appear in code).
4. When patients arrive for their appointments, the administrative dental assistant has the necessary information available. The assistant can check the financial status of the patient and ask whether there has been any change in address,

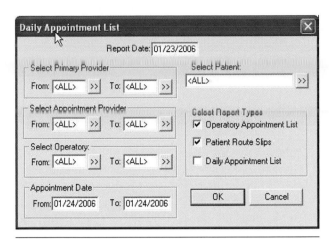

FIGURE 17-10

Daily Appointment List Window. This window is used each day during the opening procedure. From this screen, the administrative dental assistant is able to print an appointment list for each provider, a list for each operatory, and a route slip for each patient. (Courtesy Dentrix Dental Systems, American Fork, UT.)

employer, or insurance. When changes must be made, the assistant can easily access the patient's record.

5. After patients have entered the office, the assistant can track their location from reception room to treatment area and finally to checkout. The names on the screen will change colors to indicate the patient's location, draw attention to medical alerts, and notify the clinical staff when patients are added to the daily schedule. When the system is optimized, it provides information for all members of the dental healthcare team.

6. When an integrated system is used, the clinical assistant can view on the monitor in the treatment area information from the database. When information, such as changes in medical status, addition of digital images, and new treatment records, is added to the patient's clinical record, notes can be generated from the treatment area terminal. In some systems, the complete checkout process can be completed from the treatment area monitor.

7. When patients are finished with their treatment, they return to the business office to complete the checkout procedure.

Checkout Procedure

1. The administrative dental assistant checks the patient's clinical record and routing slip. The routing slip communicates treatment that was completed during this appointment, the treatment to be performed at the next appointment, and how much time is needed for the next appointment.

2. The administrative dental assistant uses the patient's number to open the correct window in the computer. Following the protocol for the software package, the assistant enters the appropriate code for the treatment performed. This code gives a description of the treatment provided and prompts the assistant to enter additional information such as tooth number, surface, or quantity. If a payment is received, the code that corresponds to the type of payment is entered. The assistant is prompted to enter information such as bank number, check number, and amount.

3. When an electronic scheduler is used, the assistant is prompted to schedule the next appointment or recall (Figure 17-11).

4. When the patient has insurance, the assistant is prompted to request an insurance claim form.

5. At the completion of the posting, the assistant generates a walkout statement to be given to the patient. The function of the walkout statement is to communicate to the patient the services rendered, the account balance, and the time of the next appointment.

Posting Mail Payments Procedure

During the day, payments from insurance companies and patients arrive. These must be processed.

1. Patient payments are posted to patients' accounts in the same way that transactions are posted during the day.

2. The account is accessed by name or by account number (if the payment includes a payment coupon, the number will be listed on the coupon; otherwise, the patient's account can be located by name and checked for correctness).

3. The account is posted with the correct code for the type of payment: personal check, insurance check, cash, or budget plan. The system may ask for additional information, such as bank number and check number, to be used on the deposit slip.

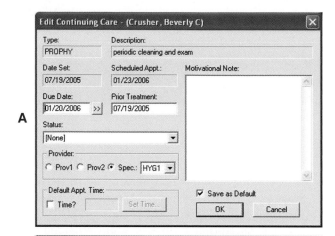

FIGURE 17-11

A, Edit Continuing Care Window. This window is used to identify procedures, time intervals, and providers for continuing care such as prophy, radiography, periodontal care, and periodic screenings. **B,** Continuing Care Window. This window identifies which procedures the patient will require in the future. This prompts the scheduler to schedule such procedures as prophy, radiographs, and screenings. (Courtesy Dentrix Dental Systems, American Fork, UT.)

4. Insurance checks require additional information. The system prompts the user to enter information that identifies what treatment the payment represents. If an amount is not allowable under the provisions of the insurance contract, an adjustment must be made to the account. If this information is not correctly entered, it is very difficult to identify the correct patient portion, and billing problems may ensue.

End of the Day Procedure

After all daily transactions (charges, payments, and adjustments) have been posted, several reports must be generated.

1. Audit report.
2. Daily production report or daysheet. (This is similar to the pegboard daysheet. The system correctly totals all transactions for the day and calculates accounts receivable.)
3. Customized reports requested by the dental practice (production report by producer, transaction report, recall and insurance reports).
4. Bank deposit slips. (These are printed, and information is listed when payment transactions are posted. The report identifies cash, checks, and credit card transactions.)
5. The next day's schedule. (Routing slips can give the administrative assistant time to pull charts, confirm appointments, and prepare for the next day.)
6. A list of patients who require a follow-up telephone call, including the names of patients, their telephone numbers, and the treatments they have been given.
7. Lists of insurance payments submitted for the day, either electronically or manually.

The final procedure for the day is to back up all of the information stored in the computer.

Backup System

It is necessary to have a system in place that backs up information stored in the computer. The purpose of the backup is to protect the information stored on the hard drive. Information can be lost because of hard drive failure, power surges, power losses, and misdirected system commands. If information is lost and there is no backup, countless days and hours are necessary to restore the lost information. In some cases, the information is never recovered. The only way to protect stored information is to consistently back up the system.

The computer vendor will recommend an appropriate method for backup. Some common ways include the use of internal and external tape cartridges or removable hard disks. Some vendors offer a backup service via a modem. Whatever the process, it must be used.

As an administrative dental assistant, you may experience a time when the computer system is down (inaccessible) and you must continue with the daily operation of the dental practice. If an electronic scheduler is used, it is prudent to print the weekly appointment book at the end of each day. This will provide a backup appointment book for a few days in the event that the system is down.

During system down time, you can use a manual system. Record transactions in a daily journal, and enter data when the system is up and running. Keep track of patients who need appointments, and contact them as soon as possible to schedule their next appointment. In most cases, a system will be down for only a few hours.

 REMEMBER

You never know when a computer system may fail. All members of the dental healthcare team must be prepared with a back-up plan. This plan includes having an administrative dental assistant who can perform the basic skills manually (posting transactions, scheduling patients, processing insurance information, and performing basic bookkeeping tasks). These skills are important to safeguard the practice from a loss of time and valuable information.

KEY POINTS

- Dental practice management software is available in three levels. Level one, basic, primarily deals with the paperwork functions of the dental practice. Level two, intermediate, has the same basic functions but adds greater flexibility and options. Level three, advanced, integrates business office functions with clinical functions. Use of an integrated system requires the cooperation of all members of the dental healthcare team and may lead to a paperless dental practice.

- **Selecting a software package** requires that the dental healthcare team must identify its needs and express its desire to use a particular system. The team should consider different functions: general requirements, patient information, patient billing, treatment planning, insurance processing, recall/reactivation, practice management reports, electronic scheduling, database and word processing capabilities, and clinical integration.

- **The role of the administrative dental assistant** varies, depending on the software used. Some functions are common to all software programs. These include maintaining patient demographics, posting transactions, storing information in a general database, processing insurance claims, using an electronic scheduler, and producing reports.

- **Daily procedures with a computerized system** are performed by the administrative dental assistant and other members of the dental healthcare team. These procedures rely on the computerized database and the spreadsheet and word processing functions. Daily procedures include opening, checkout, mail posting, and end of day.

- **Backup** procedures are vital in protecting a dental practice's information. A backup system is routinely used to protect the integrity of the computer system. The dental practice should have a plan in place that will allow the dental practice to function without the computer system for a period of several days. This plan requires that the administrative dental assistant must be trained in manually posting transactions, scheduling patients, processing insurance, and performing basic bookkeeping tasks.

 Web Watch

ADA Guide to Dental Practice Management System

http://www.ada.org/prof/prac/tools/software/index.asp

 Log on to Evolve to access additional web links!

Critical Thinking Questions

1. Suppose you could select a dental practice management software package. How would you go about making the selection? Use information learned in this chapter and from outside resources.
   - Identify the stakeholders (dentist, accountant, hygienist, and assistants), and list information that they consider important.
   - Using the information given by the stakeholders, select the functions needed to accommodate their requests.
   - Compare the functions you have selected with information in this chapter; identify the level of function (level one, two, or three) and justify.
2. Describe how an administrative dental assistant would use a computer software system to complete daily tasks.

Notes

OUTLINE

KEY TERMS

Benefits

Chronological Resumes

Cover Letter

Educational Institutes

Employment Agency

Employment Agreement

Functional Resumes

Hybrid Resumes

Job Search Log

Newspaper Advertisements

Objective

Online Resume

Personal Career Portfolio

Professional Networking

Professional Organizations

Resumes

Temporary Agencies

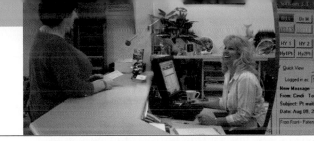

18

Employment Strategies

LEARNING OBJECTIVES

The student will:

1. List career opportunities for administrative dental assistants.
2. Identify the steps to be followed in developing an employment strategy. Discuss the function of each step.
3. Produce a high-quality resume.
4. Write a cover letter.
5. Explain the function of a personal career portfolio, and discuss its advantages.
6. Plan a personal employment strategy.

INTRODUCTION

Hundreds of jobs are waiting for the right person to fill them. The hiring decision is based on the ability of the prospective employee to successfully present himself or herself. Convincing the employer that you are the best person for the job is not easy. The process begins with a self-study and ends with a personal interview. Along the way, you will identify career options, answer questions about yourself, research possible employment opportunities, produce a quality resume, construct a letter of introduction, complete an application, and prepare mentally and physically for an oral interview.

CAREER OPPORTUNITIES FOR ADMINISTRATIVE DENTAL ASSISTANTS

While completing your training as a dental assistant, you have learned about available career options in dentistry. During your on-the-job training, you may have had the opportunity to experience different avenues of dental assisting in different settings.

Private Practice

Private practice offers the dental assistant a variety of job opportunities, depending on the size and specialty of the practice.

Small Practice

A small practice with one or two dentists and a hygienist can offer an assistant the opportunity to use multiple skills. For example, administrative dental assistants may be responsible for most of the business office tasks. In addition, they may be cross-trained in clinical assisting to help in the clinical area when needed.

Benefits of working in a small dental practice
- The assistant may have the opportunity to be cross-trained in business office skills and clinical area skills. This becomes necessary when few people are available to perform many tasks.
- A family atmosphere develops because all members of the dental healthcare team work closely together on a daily basis. Patients are familiar with all team members because they see the same members at each visit. This relationship can also extend into the community when patients and team members meet at the supermarket, work together on other projects, and attend social functions.
- Loyalty toward the dental practice seems to be stronger because of the close relationship between team members.

Large Practice

Larger dental practices, or corporate practices with several locations, need assistants who have specialized skills. For example, in a large practice, the administrative dental assistant may be responsible only for insurance billing. This type of setting provides the assistant with the opportunity to become specialized or expert in a single area of the business office.

Benefits of working in a large dental practice
- The administrative dental assistant will have the opportunity to become specialized in a single area.
- Professional interaction is greater because of the ability to draw from several different types of professional experiences.
- Advancement opportunities are greater.
- Employee benefits packages will have a greater number of choices.
- Networking within a large organization is possible.

Insurance Companies

Insurance companies use trained administrative dental assistants for a variety of jobs. Insurance processing trainers hold workshops on how to correctly complete insurance claim forms. Assistants familiar with dental terminology and procedures are assigned to claims processing. The environment of an insurance company provides an opportunity for dental assistants to expand their business and administrative skills.

Management and Consulting Firms

Administrative dental assistants who gain experience and develop management skills may consider a position with a management and consulting firm. These firms specialize in consulting and training for individual and group dental practices. They make recommendations based on the needs of the dental practice. Dental practices may use consultants to improve patient relations, enhance productivity, develop efficient computer systems, or build a professional healthcare team. In addition to large firms that specialize in these services, individuals and small groups may provide management services.

Teaching

Working as a dental assisting educator is a rewarding career choice because it enables you to share with others the knowledge and experience you have acquired in the dental profession. Settings in which dental assisting educators are used include high school programs, community colleges, adult education programs, and proprietary schools.

Qualifications and credentials vary according to educational system and state requirements. Typically, a school requires an applicant to have acquired a set number of years of work experience, to have completed teaching methodology course work (or to be working toward completion), and to have earned dental assisting certification (CDA [certified dental assistant]) or appropriate state licensure. Additional requirements may include a bachelor's degree and graduation from an accredited dental assisting program.

Future Career Opportunities

As computers become more advanced, additional career opportunities will be created. Within a dental practice, computer skills will be applied to a greater number of functions, and well-trained staff will be required. Distributors of software packages will need the skills of experienced administrative dental assistants for their sales force and training staffs.

Technology will also open doors to new avenues for administrative and clinical dental assistants. The ability of the dental assistant to acquire new skills and perform increasingly challenging tasks will result in the creation of a dental healthcare team of life-long learners.

STEPS FOR DEVELOPING EMPLOYMENT STRATEGIES

You have already taken the first step toward exploring dental career opportunities by enrolling in a dental assisting program. As you prepare for completion of this course, you may be given the oppor-

tunity to train in a dental practice setting. This experience will give you the opportunity to acquire work experience in a dental practice, ask questions, and work side by side with a dental professional. Additional career exploration opportunities may include job shadowing, career research, networking, and career fairs.

Assessing Yourself and Your Career Options

As you go through the job seeking process, you will proceed through a series of steps:
- Assessing yourself and your career options
- Gathering information
- Producing a resume
- Looking for a job
- Completing an application
- Going on an interview
- Accepting a job offer

The first step is to assess yourself and identify what you are looking for in a job. What are the things that are important to you? Formulate a list. Consider the number of hours per week that you can or want to work. What is the distance you are willing to travel? Do you prefer to work in a large or a small dental practice? What position do you want (administrative or clinical assistant)? Identify your personal philosophy, and describe the type of dentist you would like to work for. Complete a budget, and decide how much salary you have to make to survive. Rate your findings. Finally, are you willing to compromise?

Gathering Information

To fill out an application, compose a resume, prepare for an interview, and complete an employment record, you will need to gather specific pieces of information. These include the following:
- **Social Security card.** You must enter your Social Security number onto an application, and a copy of your Social Security card will be required when you are hired.
- **Driver's license, resident card, or picture identification card.** These documents are required when you are hired.
- **Diplomas, certificates, and licenses.** These documents are used to verify education, certification, and licensure.

- **Master application information.** A master application is a form that organizes information that will be used to complete applications and employment records. Not all of this information will be used on every document, but by gathering this information and recording it on a master form, you will be able to complete applications and answer questions quickly and efficiently.
  - Name, address, telephone number
  - Date and place of birth, US citizenship, resident card number, passport/visa
  - Details of any conviction for a crime, and whether you are bondable
  - *Emergency information:* Name and address of a physician who should be contacted in case of an emergency, insurance information; list of disabilities, medications, or allergies
  - *Education:* Names, dates, and locations of schools attended and your grade point averages
  - *Additional information:* Special training received, skills attained, machines/equipment you can operate, extracurricular activities in which you participated, hobbies/outside interests, professional organizations to which you belong, and honors/awards received
  - *Availability:* Date available to start, days and times of day (shift) that you are available to work
  - Salary requirements
  - *US military service:* Branch of service in which you worked, date entered, date discharged, rank, special training and duties
  - *Employment records (paid and nonpaid):* Company name, address, telephone number, dates of employment, rate of pay, name of supervisor, duties of the job, reason for leaving
  - *References:* Name, address, telephone number, occupation, number of years acquainted (References are people who know you personally and are willing to verify your abilities, skills, and attitudes. References should be former employers, teachers, counselors, coaches, neighbors, or clergy. Before using a person as a reference, you should first ask his or her permission.)

Composing a Resume

The most important tool of the job search process is the resume. **Resumes** are personal marketing tools created with one goal—to get a job interview. A strong resume will give you a competitive advantage, help you organize your thoughts, and help you make a good impression.

Applicants and employers use resumes in various ways. Resumes may be used to reach a large number of prospective employers in a mass mailing or to contact a dentist individually in person. The objective is to gain the attention of a prospective employer and be granted an interview. Employers use resumes as the first step in the screening process. They review resumes and select for an interview those persons who seem to meet the qualifications required for the job.

Organizing Information

Before you start writing your resume, take some time to organize your information and to complete a few simple worksheets. You will need your master application information and five pieces of paper with the following headings: Objective, Education, Work Experience, Skills and Abilities, and Miscellaneous (for professional affiliations, certifications, and so forth).

Objective

The **objective** is an important component of your resume. It identifies the position for which you are applying and is supported by information listed in the body of your resume. The objective is written to meet the employer's needs, outline the job you are seeking, and identify skills that you have to offer the employer. This is accomplished in a brief statement of one or two sentences. The following list of questions and answers will help you formulate the job objective:

- *What job do you want?* Identify the job for which you are applying, for example, dental assistant, administrative dental assistant, office manager, business manager, insurance clerk, or chairside dental assistant. Try to be specific, and use actual job titles. With the use of a computer, it is easy to change a few key words in a resume to customize it for a specific job title.
- *For whom do you prefer to work?* Identify the setting for the job you would like to have. If you are using a generic job title like business manager, insurance clerk, or office manager, add for whom you would like to work, for example, business manager in a progressive dental

ANATOMY OF A RESUME

1234 Valley Boulevard
Canyon View, CA 12345
Phone (123) 555-7890

Ima Graduate ①

Objective ② Interested in obtaining a position as an administrative dental assistant. Offering excellent skills in patient communication, appointment scheduling, and computer applications. Enjoy working as a member of a professional healthcare team.

Education ③

1998–1999	Canyon View Junior College	Canyon View, CA
	Administrative Dental Assistant	
	Certification of Completion	
1994-1998	Canyon View High School	Canyon View, CA
	Diploma	

Work Experience ④

January–September 1999   Canyon View Dentistry
                          Canyon View, CA
Administrative Dental Assistant
• Patient scheduling
• Computer data entry and management
• Patient relations

Skills and Abilities ⑤
• Computer skills
• Telephone procedures
• Patient communications
• Enthusiastic team member
• Organized
• Able to work unsupervised

Professional Affiliations and Certification ⑥
• ADAA, American Dental Assistants Association
• CDPMA, Certified Dental Practice Management Assistant
• American Heart Association, CPR–Healthcare Provider
• Radiology Certification

References ⑦   Available upon request

A resume is a summary of your skills, abilities, education, and work experience. The completed resume serves as an introduction; depending upon your resume you may or may not obtain an interview.

① HEADING
The heading will include full name, address and telephone number. Additional information such as fax number or e-mail address may be added to the heading if appropriate.

② JOB OBJECTIVE
A job objective focuses on the type of job you are seeking and what you can offer the prospective employer. The statements made should be specific and concise. Information listed in the objective will be supported in the body of the resume. **The objective** is considered one of the most important sections of the resume.

③ EDUCATION
Information included in your education statement: dates attended, diplomas, degrees, awards and certificates earned. Workshops and seminars that contribute to your qualifications should also be included in this section. List the information in chronological order (start with the most recent date and work back in time).

④ WORK HISTORY
This section can also come under the heading **Work Experience, Employment History, Professional Experience, or Experience**. In this section you will list the name and location of each company or organization, starting and ending dates, and a brief description of your duties. You can also list volunteer work experience, especially if it demonstrates skills and abilities that will enhance your job qualifications (non-paid training can also be listed). List the experience in chronological order.

⑤ Skills and Abilities
Use this section to highlight skills, abilities, and strengths that are pertinent to the job you are applying for. Statements should be action-oriented, begin with verbs, and be concise.

⑥ MISCELLANEOUS
Headings and information include such items as extracurricular activities, clubs, memberships in professional organizations, certification, volunteer activities, awards, and achievements.

⑦ REFERENCES
You can include two professional references or state: Reference furnished upon request. The use of references is optional. When listing references state the name, title or occupation, address, and telephone number.

ORDER OF INFORMATION
Prime space is the top one-third of the page, so list the most important sections first.

MECHANICS
Typed on one page, easy to read, with correct spelling, grammar, and punctuation. Eliminate unessential words or phrases.

MARGINS
The finished resume should appear balanced, centered from top to bottom and left to right.

PAPER
Use heavy stock standard size (8.5" x 11") resume paper of good quality (white, cream, or light gray). Print on high quality setting or have professionally printed. Pages should be free of streaks, fading, or correction fluid.

practice, or insurance clerk for a large dental practice.

- *Where would you like to work?* Identify the setting in which you would like to work, for example, corporate dental practice, solo dental practice, management firm, insurance company, or school.
- *What level of responsibility do you prefer to assume?* Identify your level of training or certification, for example, entry level, Certified Dental Practice Management Assistant, Certified Dental Assistant, or Registered Dental Assistant.
- *What skills or abilities do you have?* Brainstorm and think of all the duties you perform during the day and the skills and abilities they require. Make a long list, and then select three or four of the most important skills and abilities.

After you have completed your worksheets, review your answers and formulate your objective. It may not be necessary to list all information as long as the objective is clear and concise and can be supported by information you list in the body of the resume. Following are examples of well-worded objectives:

- Seeking a position with a group dental practice that would provide an opportunity to demonstrate my experience as a Certified Dental Practice Management Assistant. Skilled in patient communications, computer applications, and team building.
- Seeking a position with a dental practice as an entry level administrative dental assistant. Offering excellent skills in telephone techniques, computer applications, and filing. Cheerful outlook and a positive attitude.
- Offering dental management, communication, and insurance processing skills. Seeking to apply these skills as an administrative assistant in a dental insurance company.

Identification of an objective followed by a bulleted list of highlights (under the heading Highlights of Qualifications) is an effective format that you may wish to use. This method provides a very short, concise objective supported by qualifications. The highlights of qualifications are written with action verbs (see Resume Action Verbs box) that describe your relevant skills, experiences, credentials, and accomplishments. For example:

- Collaborated in the successful design of a computerized recall system
- Developed a system for tracking and monitoring electronically submitted dental claims
- Managed a dental office for 3 years
- Certified as a Dental Practice Management Assistant
- Skilled in the use of computer applications (add a list of specific applications)
- Able to work with a dental practice with professionalism and confidence

Education

Using the information you listed on your master application sheet, list the schools you attended, the dates you attended, and the diplomas, certificates, and degrees that you earned.

Work Experience

List paid and unpaid job positions, start and end dates, and employers and their locations. It is important to include all work experience that relates to the job for which you are applying (if you have had several jobs that do not apply to the new position, they will be listed on your application).

Skills and Abilities

Be sure to list unpaid or volunteer positions that demonstrate responsibility, specific job skills, and work habits.

Miscellaneous

List all activities that you have been involved in, including clubs, memberships in professional organizations, and volunteer activities. Keep a list of all of your certificates, licenses, and awards.

Constructing the Resume

After you have gathered all the information and completed the worksheets, organize the information and put it into a resume format. Resumes are individual works that represent the writer. Be creative and gain the attention of the reader. It has been noted that the most important part of the resume is the top one third of the page. Information that you want noticed should go in this area. Resumes can be prepared with three basic formats: chronological, functional, and hybrid.

Chronological resumes arrange information in order of occurrence, with the most recent information presented first. The objective is presented, followed by work experience, education background (order can be reversed depending on the importance), skills and abilities acquired, and miscellaneous information.

Functional resumes place skills and abilities first, according to importance, regardless of the time of occurrence. After objective statements are listed, skills and abilities are highlighted, followed by information on work experiences, educational background, and miscellaneous information.

Hybrid resumes combine the best features of chronological and functional resumes with information rearranged and with focus only on information that is relevant to the current job objective. The hybrid resume begins with a job objective that is followed by highlights of qualifications, relevant skills and experiences, chronological work history, and a listing of relevant education and training.

Online resumes are posted on Web sites for perspective employers to review. Before posting your resume, you *must* take precautions to protect yourself and preserve your personal identity. To better understand how posting your resume works, you first must understand the "business" side of the process. A job placement Web site will not charge you a fee to post your resume; they generate revenue by selling to employers access to their resume database. The database is typically sold to anyone who is willing to pay the fee; this means that they do not filter who will receive your information. Because of the lack of security involved in posting a resume, it is recommended that you follow some simple precautions before you do so.

1. Remove your standard contact information
   - Name
   - Address
   - Phone numbers
   - Business e-mail
   - Personal e-mail
   - Add a new personal e-mail address that is located on a large Web-based service, for example, Yahoo or Hotmail. When you select your new e-mail address, use a name that is general in nature and reflects the "professional" you. Cute e-mail addresses are fine for your friends, but they will not impress a prospective employer.
2. Do not use names of companies in your work history. You can change the wording to say the same thing, but leave out who you worked for. For example, instead of stating that you worked for Dr. Mary Edwards, DDS, you could say, "Worked in single doctor dental office; my duties included . . . ."
3. Review privacy statements of the Web site.

Resume Services

Some businesses and organizations write resumes. They charge a fee and use information given to them by the applicant. Such a service may be expensive, but these companies do create resumes of professional quality.

Electronic resumes are resumes that are available through the Internet. Resume services will scan your resume or transfer it to a digitized copy. Prospective employers contact the service and request copies of resumes. The service does not charge the employee for this service. The prospective employer pays for a copy of your resume. Cover letters and resumes can be directed to prospective employers by way of e-mail (without use of a service). This method is relatively new to the dental profession. This may eventually become the way that all cover letters and resumes are submitted.

Cover letters and resumes can also be faxed to prospective employers. Unfortunately, you will lose the ability to place your resume on quality paper. If this method is used, care should be taken to create a resume that will transfer easily and maintain a professional appearance.

Writing Cover Letters

The purpose of a **cover letter** (letter of introduction or application) is to introduce yourself to a prospective employer. Cover letters should accompany all resumes sent by mail (including those sent via electronic transfer and fax). They can also be used as an introduction during an informational interview. Cover letters are personalized and addressed to a specific individual. They express an interest in working with a specific employer or company. They should convey enthusiasm and commitment. Cover letters balance professionalism with personal warmth and friendship and outline specifically what you are seeking and offering.

Looking for a Job

With proper marketing tools (resume and cover letter), you are ready to begin seriously looking for

Resume Action Verbs

Management Skills

- Administered
- Analyzed
- Assigned
- Attained
- Chaired
- Consolidated
- Contracted
- Coordinated
- Delegated
- Developed
- Directed
- Evaluated
- Executed
- Improved
- Increased
- Organized
- Oversaw
- Planned
- Prioritized
- Produced
- Recommended
- Reviewed
- Scheduled
- Straightened
- Supervised

Communication Skills

- Addressed
- Arbitrated
- Arranged
- Authored
- Collaborated
- Convinced
- Corresponded
- Developed
- Directed
- Drafted
- Edited
- Enlisted
- Formulated
- Influenced
- Interpreted
- Lectured
- Mediated
- Moderated
- Negotiated
- Persuaded
- Promoted
- Publicized

- Reconciled
- Recruited
- Spoke
- Translated
- Wrote

Research Skills

- Clarified
- Collected
- Critiqued
- Diagnosed
- Evaluated
- Interpreted
- Interviewed
- Investigated
- Organized
- Reviewed
- Summarized
- Surveyed
- Systematized

Technical Skills

- Assembled
- Built
- Calculated
- Computed
- Designed
- Devised
- Engineered
- Fabricated
- Maintained
- Operated
- Overhauled
- Programmed
- Remodeled
- Repaired
- Solved
- Upgraded

Teaching Skills

- Adapted
- Advised
- Clarified
- Coached
- Communicated
- Coordinated
- Developed
- Enabled
- Encouraged
- Evaluated

Resume Action Verbs—cont'd

- Explained
- Facilitated
- Guided
- Informed
- Instructed
- Persuaded
- Set goals
- Stimulated
- Trained

Financial Skills

- Administered
- Allocated
- Analyzed
- Appraised
- Audited
- Balanced
- Budgeted
- Calculated
- Computed
- Developed
- Forecasted
- Managed
- Marketed
- Planned
- Projected
- Researched

Creative Skills

- Acted
- Conceptualized
- Created
- Customized
- Designed
- Developed
- Directed
- Established
- Fashioned
- Founded
- Illustrated
- Initiated
- Instituted
- Integrated
- Introduced
- Invented
- Originated
- Performed
- Planned
- Revitalized
- Shaped

Helping Skills

- Assessed
- Assisted
- Clarified
- Coached
- Counseled
- Demonstrated
- Diagnosed
- Educated
- Expedited
- Facilitated
- Familiarized
- Guided
- Motivated
- Referred
- Rehabilitated
- Represented

Clerical or Detail Skills

- Approved
- Arranged
- Catalogued
- Classified
- Collected
- Compiled
- Dispatched
- Executed
- Generated
- Implemented
- Inspected
- Monitored
- Operated
- Organized
- Prepared
- Processed
- Purchased
- Recorded
- Retrieved
- Screened
- Specified
- Systematized
- Tabulated
- Validated

Accomplishments

- Achieved
- Attained
- Convinced
- Expanded

Continued

Resume Action Verbs—cont'd

- Expedited
- Founded
- Improved
- Increased
- Initiated
- Introduced
- Invented
- Originated
- Overhauled

- Pioneered
- Reduced
- Resolved
- Restored
- Revitalized
- Spearheaded
- Strengthened
- Transformed
- Upgraded

Descriptive Resume Phrases

- Strong sense of responsibility
- Flexible and willing to take on a variety of tasks
- Neat, efficient, thorough
- Strong managerial skills
- Able to prioritize a heavy workload
- Cheerful outlook, positive attitude
- Strong motivation and dedication to the job
- Extensive artistic background
- Able to make important decisions on my own
- Take pride in a job well done
- Committed to completing a job
- Attentive to time schedules
- Self-motivated
- Goal-oriented
- Dedicated to the highest quality of work
- Resourceful problem solver
- Good organizational skills
- Willing to do extra work to gain valuable experience
- Ability to learn quickly
- Open-minded and imaginative
- Reliable and prompt
- Get along well with others
- Excellent communication skills
- Accurate in spelling and grammar
- Able to work well under pressure
- Able to work well unsupervised
- Outstanding leadership skills
- Good with numbers
- Enjoy a challenge
- Well-organized
- Able to meet deadlines
- Enthusiastic team member

employment. The first question may be, "Where do I look?" You can start the process by identifying various avenues that may lead to employment: newspaper advertisements, employment agencies, temporary agencies, professional networking, yellow pages, school placement, professional dental organizations, coworkers, family, and friends.

- **Newspaper advertisements** are one of the most common ways to look for a job. Employers place an advertisement describing the position available and inviting applicants to call for an appointment or send their resume.
- An **employment agency** offers placement services. It can be state run or may be a private business. State agencies usually provide their services free of charge, whereas private employment agencies charge the applicant or the employer. When you use a private agency, make sure you understand your liability and responsibilities.
- **Temporary agencies** place applicants in positions for a specified length of time. The agency charges a fee to the employer. The applicant works in a temporary position and is paid by the agency. When you work for a temporary agency, make sure you understand the details of your contract.
- **Educational institutes** often provide career placement services for their students. Depending on the institution, services can range from posting job opportunities to actually placing graduates in dental practices.
- **Professional networking** is a means of contacting other dental professionals and letting them know that you are seeking employment.

ANATOMY OF A COVER LETTER

1234 Valley Boulevard
Canyon View, CA 12345
Phone (123) 555-7890

April 12, 1999

(1) Family Dental Center
3841 Oak Drive
Canyon View, CA 91786

Dear Dr. Lamoure:

(2) I am interested in working as an administrative dental assistant for your organization. I am a knowledgeable administrative assistant with a year of experience to offer you. I enclose my resume as a first step in exploring the possibilities of employment with Family Dental Centers.

(3) My most recent experience was scheduling coordinator for Canyon View Dentistry. I was responsible for patient scheduling. I also coordinated revision of the practice policies and procedures manual. In addition, I initiated the conversion of patient scheduling from manual to computer.

As an administrative dental assistant with your organization, I would bring a focus on quality and enthusiasm to your dental team. Furthermore, I work well with others, and I am experienced in patient relations.

(4) I would appreciate your keeping this inquiry confidential. I will call you in a few days to arrange an interview at a convenient time for you. Thank you for your consideration.

Sincerely,

Ima Graduate

Ima Graduate

(1) INSIDE ADDRESS AND SALUTATION
Target the letter to a specific employer. Address the letter to a specific person, by name if possible.

(2) PARAGRAPH ONE
Tell why you are contacting the employer and identify the position in which you are interested.

(3) PARAGRAPHS TWO AND THREE
Express interest in the position and the dental practice or company. If applicable, tell how you became attracted to the particular dental practice (answering your ad in the Sunday paper, referred by John Evatt of the ABC Company). This demonstrates that you have done some research. Mention skills or qualifications that you possess that would be of particular interest to the dental practice. Identify at least one thing about you that is unique (must be relevant to the position).

(4) PARAGRAPH FOUR
Summarize specifically what you are asking and offering. Describe just what you will do to follow through.

- Your letter should be well organized, grammatically correct, and typed. If the letter accompanies a resume, use the same type of high-quality paper.

- Have someone proofread the letter before it is sent.

- Keep a copy in your personal career portfolio.

This is an informal job placement service and is one of the most effective means of seeking employment. The informal nature benefits the job seeker because people share more information about the job, personalities of the dental health-care team, working conditions, benefits, advantages, and disadvantages. Benefits to the employer are basically the same; they can let other professionals know that they have an open position and let them recommend possible applicants and get the word out. Professional networking includes:

- Attending local dental assistant society meetings, participating in study clubs, volunteering at local dental clinics

- Talking to supply house representatives who visit several dental offices in a local area (they may know when there is an open position and who may be looking for a position)

- **Professional organizations,** such as local chapters of the American Dental Association (ADA) and the American Dental Assistants Association (ADAA), may offer placement services for their members. A dental assistant can register with the local chapter by completing an informational survey. This survey will identify special skills, quantity of experience acquired, and type of employment sought, and will ask for your telephone number. Member dentists who have an opening can request a list of all applicants and will contact those who meet their qualifications. In addition to the ADA and the ADAA, other professional dental organizations may offer an employment placement service.

Other job search resources include the yellow pages (for a list of dentists; you may wish to send a cover letter and resume to attempt to schedule an interview). Former coworkers and employers may notify you when they learn of a job opening. Family and friends are also often willing to help you make a professional contact.

Organizing the Job Search

After you have identified sources and decided which direction you wish to pursue, take time to do some research on prospective employers. The primary reason for research is to help you gain information about a dental practice, including the type of practice—specialty, corporate, large group, or small solo practice. You can identify the type of dental insurance, if any, that they accept, the types of financial plans they offer, whether they use an active recall system, and whether they are members of a professional organization. This information can be gathered during informal networking or by checking the Web page of the organization. Such information will:

- Prepare you for the interview
- Demonstrate your initiative and ability to organize
- Help you feel more confident about your ability to respond to questions
- Assist you in deciding whether the dental practice meets your standards for employment

Job Search Log

The purpose of the **job search log** is to help you organize, plan, and follow through with employment leads. It tracks submitted applications and resumes and identifies the company name and telephone numbers of contact persons. Additionally, the log provides space in which you can keep track of important information for interviews and follow-up questions, such as directions, parking, date, time, name of interviewer, date of planned follow-up, and comments.

Personal Career Portfolios

A collection of documents that support your professional career is called a **personal career portfolio.**

Such portfolios are used as a source of information and a means of illustrating your skills, abilities, and strengths. Information contained in a portfolio is collected over time and is constantly changed and updated. Because they are personal collections, portfolios vary from person to person in content and appearance. They provide information for your use as you prepare applications and resumes and can serve as a study guide when you are preparing for a job interview. The portfolio is also a marketing tool; it presents your accomplishments, highlights your professional activities, and demonstrates to prospective employers your organizational abilities.

Components of a Personal Career Portfolio

- Resume
- Completed application
- Personal information

Write one or two paragraphs about yourself to be included in this section. To help you write a statement, see the Adjectives Describing Personal Qualities box for a list of adjectives that describe personal qualities. Complete the following statement: I am (select an adjective from the box). I have demonstrated this quality by ____. This quality is important in this field because ____.

Include a list of personal qualities that make you an excellent candidate for employment, personal references, volunteer experiences, areas of personal interest, and information on former employers along with salary history.

Have photocopies of report cards and transcripts, Social Security card, driver's license or picture ID, resident card (if not a US citizen), and passport.

Achievements are a good marketing tool. Keep a high-quality copy of certificates you have earned, and write a brief description that explains how you earned the award. Items that may be placed in this section of your portfolio include the following:

- Records of certificates earned
- Records of awards, honors, leadership shown
- Records of volunteer and extracurricular activities
- Records of published articles

Personal letters help you follow up on current leads and serve as models for future letters. These include:

- Cover letters
- Research letters

- Information interview letters
- Career information request letters

Reference letters are written by people who know you personally and are willing to speak on your behalf. Reference letters verify your abilities, skills, and positive attitude. Keep a quality letter in your portfolio, along with additional copies to give prospective employers when requested.

- **Thank you cards and letters** are letters that you have received from others.
- **Performance documentation** may include recent performance reviews, positively written comments regarding the quality of your work, and evidence of volunteer and nonpaid activities.
- **Work samples** may include actual completed works (samples of professional letters you have written) or pictures of completed work with a written statement that tells about the sample.

Going on an Interview

The purpose of the job interview is to share information; interviewers want to get to know the applicant better, and the applicant wants to tell why he or she is the best person for the job. During the interview, the interviewer asks questions designed to reveal information about the skills, abilities, and attitude of the applicant. The ways in which applicants respond to these questions helps the prospective employer to determine whether to offer the applicant the job. Sometimes, the person who is offered the job is not the best qualified but is the one who made the best impression.

Preparing for Interview Questions

During the interview, you will be asked several questions. These may range from "Tell me about yourself" to "Do you have any questions for me?" Following is a list of commonly asked questions. Take some time to answer each one of these questions. Write down your responses, and keep them in your personal career portfolio. Before you go on an interview, review these questions and your responses.

- *Please tell me about yourself.* This question is designed to reveal your level of self-confidence and your ability to handle yourself under pressure. The interviewer should be familiar with the

---

Adjectives Describing Personal Qualities

Accurate	Honest
Ambitious	Humorous
Articulate	Independent
Assertive	Insightful
Careful	Knowledgeable
Committed	Leader
Confident	Loyal
Conscientious	Motivated
Considerate	Neat
Consistent	Open-minded
Creative	Organized
Decisive	Outgoing
Dedicated	Patient
Dependable	Positive
Diligent	Productive
Disciplined	Professional
Efficient	Quick
Energetic	Responsible
Enterprising	Skillful
Enthusiastic	Strong
Flexible	Thorough
Friendly	Tolerant
Goal-oriented	

information you listed on the job application and your resume. Mention things that are easy for you to talk about, but keep them job related. For example, discuss your skills, abilities, personal qualities, work experience, or career technical training. Keep your response short.

- *What are your strengths and weaknesses?* Always answer this question in a positive tone. Be prepared to talk about your strengths. When asked to identify weaknesses, use this as an opportunity to list a weakness that may be a positive for the job for which you are applying. Becoming bored with simple tasks may be seen as positive in a job that requires complex tasks. When talking about a negative, give a positive solution: I have a tendency to procrastinate, but I work well under pressure.

- *Why do you want to work here?* On the basis of your research information, state reasons why you would like to work in this particular dental practice instead of another dental practice. Everyone wants to feel special, and this is a chance to show that you have done your homework and have considered other options.

- *How do you spend your spare time?* This question is designed to see if you spend your time constructively. Answer in a positive tone, and do not mention things that will appear negative or boring.

- *Where do you see yourself in 3 to 5 years?* This question is meant to reveal your goals. Be prepared to state your career goals. Goals can be stated in broad generic terms: "I see myself working in a profession that will provide room for growth and advancement." "I hope to complete advanced training in ••."

- *Why should I hire you? How are you qualified for this job?* This question allows the interviewer to see whether your skills, abilities, and personal qualities match the job description. You can answer the question by listing the qualifications of the job and explaining how your qualifications match.

- *What did you like/dislike about your last job/class?* Reference a similarity between your last job and the one you are applying for, and explain why you liked it. Use personal traits: "I enjoyed helping patients. I like to make them feel comfortable when they come to the dental office."

It is wise not to say negative things about a previous job because the interviewer may know your previous employer.

- *Do you have any questions for me?* The final question of the interview normally gives the applicant a chance to ask questions. Remember, you are also interviewing the prospective employer. Be prepared to ask one or two questions. Questions may relate to the future growth or expansion of the practice, a job description, or examples of a typical day, specific procedures, or opportunities for team development. Questions may also seek information on when the position will be filled and on whether you can answer any other questions about your qualifications.

During the interview, be prepared to think! Questions are designed to highlight your strengths and to assess your ability to respond when under pressure. These questions may identify personal work habits and philosophy, for example:

- Accomplishments that make you feel proud
- Who has had a positive influence on your life and why
- What rewards, other than money, motivate you
- Why you chose this career
- What you have learned from participation in extracurricular activities
- How a former employer or teacher would describe you
- A major problem you have encountered and how you dealt with it

For an interview to be successful, you must be prepared, make a good impression, and complete the interview process. Following are suggestions that will result in a successful interview.

Before the interview

- Research the company, salary range, and job qualifications.
- Prepare for questions by writing answers to questions that might be asked.
- Prepare questions for the interviewer.
- Review your resume and have a copy available.
- Organize your personal career portfolio to take with you.
- Review material in your portfolio and use as a study guide.
- Prepare your thank you letters.
- Locate the interview site, determine travel time, and check available parking.

- Practice good grooming and hygiene. Appropriate clothing for women includes suit, skirt and blouse, or dress with a jacket, medium-heeled shoes with closed toes and heels, and flesh-colored hosiery. Hair should be neatly groomed and jewelry kept to a minimum. Clothing for men includes suit or sport jacket, dress shirt, slacks, tie, belt, and dress shoes and dark socks. Hair should be neatly groomed and cut and facial hair shaved and trimmed. Jewelry for men should be limited to a watch and a ring. Color plays an important role, so choose solid colors or muted stripes for suits. The best colors are thought to be blue (believable) and gray (authoritative).
- Go alone, and prepare to arrive at least 15 minutes early.

REMEMBER

Dress conservatively. Clothing and accessories should not be trendy. Do not wear bright colors or extreme or excessive make-up and jewelry. This applies to both men and women.

During the interview
- Introduce yourself to the receptionist.
- Do not chew gum or smoke (before or during the interview).
- Introduce yourself to the interviewer, shake hands firmly (if the interviewer offers a hand), and be seated when directed.
- Maintain eye contact with the interviewer.
- Be enthusiastic.
- Keep a business-like attitude.
- Demonstrate good posture and mannerisms.
- Emphasize your qualities and skills.
- Ask questions (do not ask about salary until a position has been offered).

After the interview
- Thank the interviewer for his or her time, smile, and shake hands.
- Thank the receptionist, and ask for the interviewer's business card (which will provide information for the thank you letter).
- Send a thank you letter within 24 hours of the interview. The thank you can be a personal note or a typed letter.

- If you have not heard from the interviewer after 2 or 3 days, telephone the office, but keep the number of calls to a minimum.

Accepting a Job Offer

When a job is offered, you may or may not choose to accept it. Before you accept the position, it is necessary to know the particulars of the job: salary, benefits, vacation schedule, work schedule, and so forth. You should base your decision on conditions that you identified in your self-assessment. Do not feel that you are obligated to accept a position if it does not meet your needs. If a compromise cannot be reached, thank the employer for the offer and politely decline.

If you accept the offer, the employer should present an **employment agreement.** This agreement is an outline of conditions for employment. It may include a job title and description, work schedule, and salary and **benefits** (vacation days, sick days, insurance, and retirement plans). The agreement should clearly state when reviews are conducted and should describe termination procedures. The employer and the employee sign the agreement. A copy is given to the employee, and one is kept in the employee's personal employment file.

Leaving a Job

There are many reasons for leaving a job. It has been estimated that people have five to eight different careers during their lifetimes. This requires moving from job to job. A job change should be viewed as a chance to improve your employment status and achieve future success.

When it is time to leave a job, this must be done in a positive way and in accordance with the employment agreement. You will need to tell your supervisor that you are leaving. State the reason, and give a proposed date of exit (2 weeks' notice is average). Offer to train a new employee, and thank your employer for the opportunity to work for the organization.

A formal letter of resignation should be given to your employer when you speak to your supervisor. This letter is addressed to the personnel department. In the letter, state the position from which you are resigning, thank the company, and state the date of your resignation.

When employers initiate your termination, they should follow the procedure outlined in your employment agreement. If they ask you to leave without notice, they may offer severance pay. If you think that your termination is occurring without cause, you have rights under the law. For information concerning employment rights and a grievance process, consult the local labor board in your state.

KEY POINTS

- Career opportunities for administrative dental assistants include working in small and large dental practices, insurance companies, management and consulting firms, and educational institutions.
- Developing an employment strategy will prepare the administrative dental assistant for the job search process. The process includes completing a self-assessment, gathering information to be used in developing a master application form, creating a personal career portfolio, and writing a quality resume and cover letter.
- The interview process consists of three parts: preparing for the interview, responding to questions during the interview, and following up with a thank you note or letter.
- Before you accept a job offer, you should know what your salary requirements are and compare them with the salary offered by the employer. Employment agreements are outlines that highlight job descriptions, salary, benefits, and termination policy. When a job is terminated, this should be done in a professional and positive manner.

 Web Watch

Using Customer Reports: What Employers Need to Know

http://www.pueblo.gsa.gov/cictext/smbuss/credempl/credempl.htm

Reporting and Disclosure Guide for the Employee Benefit Plans

http://www.pueblo.gsa.gov/cictext/smbuss/employee-benefits/empbenef.txt

Small Business Handbook

http://www.pueblo.gsa.gov/cictext/smbuss/small-bus/smallbus.txt

Parting Ways: Effective Termination Techniques

http://www.sba.gov/test/wbc/docs/manage/terminations.html

 Log on to Evolve to access additional web links!

 Critical Thinking Activities

1. To help prepare yourself for employment, complete a self-assessment based on the questions listed earlier under "Assessing Yourself and Your Career Options."
2. Prepare for an interview by answering the following questions:
   - Would you tell me about yourself?
   - What are your strengths and weaknesses?
   - Why would you like to work here?
   - How do you spend your spare time?
   - Where do you see yourself in 3 to 5 years?
   - Why should I hire you?
   - In what ways are you qualified for this job?
   - What rewards, other than money, motivate you?
   - How would a former employer or teacher describe you?

Glossary

Abutment Tooth A tooth, a root, or an implant used for the retention of a fixed or removable prosthesis.

Account Aging Report Report that identifies the length of time that has elapsed since a charge was made.

Accounting Method used to verify and classify all transactions (accounts payable and receivable); this is usually the duty of an accountant.

Accounts Payable System that organizes, verifies, and categorizes all dental practice expenditures.

Accounts Receivable System that records all financial transactions between a patient and the dental practice.

Accounts Receivable Report Categorizes the amount of money patients and insurance companies owe the dental practice.

Administrative Dental Assistant Assistant assigned duties that pertain to the business side of dentistry.

Administrative Simplification Method designed to make the business of healthcare easier by providing standards for transaction code sets, privacy of patient information, security of patient information, and national provider identifiers.

Administrator Person or group of persons who represent dental benefit plans for the purpose of negotiating and managing contracts with dental service providers.

Aging Process that identifies how much of the money owed is 30, 60, 90, or 120 days past due.

Aging Labels Allow for quick and easy visual identification of when a patient was last seen in the dental practice.

Allowable Charges Maximum amount paid for each procedure by the insurance company.

Alphabetic Filing System that indexes names for filing purposes. Indexing rules have been standardized by the Association of Records Managers and Administrators (ARMA), which is recognized by the American National Standards Institute (ANSI) as an American National Standard.

Amalgam Alloy of various metals, silver in color, used as a dental restorative material.

American Dental Assistants Association (ADAA) Professional organization for dental assistants. The ADAA performs a variety of functions that promote professional growth, community involvement, and continuing education for its members.

Americans With Disabilities Act (ADA) Act signed into law on July 26, 1990, to prohibit discrimination on the basis of disability in employment, programs and services provided by state and local governments, and goods and services provided by private companies and commercial facilities.

AMS Administrative Management Society.

Amylase Enzyme found in saliva that is a function of the digestive process and serves as a source of minerals (fluorides, calcium, and phosphate) needed in the remineralization of tooth structure.

Anterior Toward the front.

Apex Anatomic area at the end of the tooth root.

Apical foramen Small opening at the apex of the root, where blood vessels and nerves enter.

Application Software Software designed for specific tasks, such as word processing, spreadsheet, database, and graphics.

Appointment Book A tool that, when used efficiently, helps one to organize the daily schedule of the dental practice. This book identifies who will be performing the work, on what date, and at what time.

Appointment Card Written reminder of the patient's next appointment.

Appointment Clerk Administrative personnel, within the business office of a dental practice, whose primary functions are to schedule and confirm appointments, maintain the recall system, and track patients who are in need of treatment.

Assignment of Benefits Authorization given by the subscriber or patient to a dental benefit plan, directing the company to make payment for dental benefits directly to the providing dentist.

Assistant (dental) Personnel who perform vital duties in the efficient operation of successful dental practices and who provide a link between the patient and the dentist. Several different types of dental assistants may be available to assist patients and dentists in a practice.

Attending Dentist Statement Form submitted by the dentist to the dental benefit plan that requests payment for services (dental claim form).

Attention Line (letter writing) Name of the person to whom a particular letter is being sent.

Audit Method used by third parties to check the accuracy of dental claim forms by comparing patient clinical records with information submitted on the dental claim form.

Avoiding Style (conflict resolution) Used when an issue is trivial, a cooling off period is needed, or the benefits do not go beyond the discord that a situation will cause between involved parties.

Back Order Items that were ordered but not shipped and will be sent at a later date.

Background Noise Noise that occurs as the result of activities that are going on outside of the immediate area; it can vary in intensity. Ambient sound level should not be higher than 55 decibels (dB).

Balance Billing Billing the patient for the difference between the amount paid by the dental benefits plan and the fee charged by the dentist (according to the specification of the dental benefits plan contract).

Bank Balance Balance of an account kept in a bank.

Bank Statements and Financial Reports Part of financial records that are filed according to subject and then subdivided chronologically.

Basic (practice management) System Method of organizing and creating a database and performing spreadsheet and word processing tasks.

Benefit Payment Amount paid by the dental benefits plan.

Benefit Services Services that are paid by the dental benefits plan.

Benefits (employee) Vacation days, sick days, insurance, and retirement plan.

Birthday Rule Method used to determine which parent is considered the primary provider of a child's dental coverage. This rule establishes that the parent whose birth date comes first during the year is the primary provider.

Blocked (letter writing) Letter format in which the margins are the same as those in the full-blocked style with the exception of dateline, complimentary close, company signature, and writer identification, all of which begin at the vertical center of the page.

Board of Dental Examiners Agency that has been assigned the task and authority to issue dental licenses.

Body of Letter Composed of the introduction, main body, and closing. The purpose of these paragraphs is to relay to the reader concise information that is organized in a logical sequence.

Bookkeeper Person who keeps records of the amount of money deposited into checking and savings accounts and uses a check paying system (manual check writing or electronic debt accounts) to pay vendors.

Bookkeeping Method of recording all financial transactions.

Bridge Fixed prosthetic.

Buccal Surface of posterior teeth that face the cheek.

Buccal Frenum Two buccal structures (right and left) that connect the cheek to the gingiva in the area of the maxillary first molar.

Buccal Vestibule Junction of the mucous membrane of the cheek and the gingiva.

Business Manager Person who manages the fiscal operation, develops marketing campaigns, negotiates contracts with managed care providers, and oversees the compliance of insurance, managed care, and government programs.

Business Office Area where most of the administrative assistant's duties are carried out.

Business Records Business documents that pertain to the operation of the dental practice. Business records are divided into several different types and require a variety of methods for retrieval and storage.

Business Reports Reports that focus on the fiscal operation of the dental practice, including profit and loss statements, practice production, and other specified reports that categorize a subject area. Reports are filed by subject and then are subdivided chronologically.

Call List Organized list that identifies patients who need to be scheduled for dental treatment, who can come in when there is a change in the schedule, or who wish to be notified when an opening in the schedule occurs.

Capitation Clause in a dental benefits plan that stipulates that payment will be made to the dentist per capita (per patient).

Card Files (Rolodex) Files designed for quick reference of telephone numbers and addresses and that can be used in a recall system.

Cast Crowns Cast restoration that covers the anatomic crown.

Cementum Thin, hard covering of the root surface of a tooth.

Central Incisors Anterior teeth (toward the front) characterized by thin, sharp incisal edges, which aid in cutting food.

Certified Dental Practice Management (CDPMA) Certification offered to administrative dental assistants who meet specified requirements and pass an examination administered by the National Dental Assisting Board.

Cervix Narrow portion of the tooth, where the root and the crown meet.

Chairside Dental Assistant Personnel who perform various duties, including scheduling appointments efficiently, communicating with the use of dental terminology, processing dental insurance claims, correctly coding procedures for posting, making entries in patients' clinical records, and doubling as assistant when additional help is needed in the clinical area.

Change Action that can be harmful or beneficial. When not accepted or understood, change places a barrier on communication. For some, change is seen as negative. Good communication provides a means for discussion of the need for change and how it will improve the organization.

Charge Slip Portion of a receipt, used in a pegboard system, that identifies treatment and charges.

Charting Methods Symbolic system used to identify teeth and current dental conditions.

Charting Symbols Series of symbols, numbers, and colors used to illustrate specific dental conditions.

Cheeks The sides of the face.

Chronological Filing System that allows one to locate documents according to date, month, or year.

Chronological Resumes Arrangement of information in the order of occurrence, with the most recent information provided first. The objective is presented, followed by work experience, education (order can be reversed, depending on the importance), skills and abilities, and miscellaneous information.

Circulating (roving) Assistant Assistants who perform a variety of duties, including assisting a dentist or chairside assistant as needed, taking dental x-rays, and maintaining responsibility for sterilization and infection control.

Claim (dental) Method used to request payment or authorization for treatment. Each claim provides necessary information about the patient, the treating dentist, and coded treatment.

Claims Payment Fraud Changing or manipulating of information (by a dental benefits plan) on a claim form that results in payment of a lower benefit to the treating dentist.

Claims Reporting Fraud Changing or manipulating of information (by the dentist) on a claims form that results in payment of a high benefit by the dental benefits plan. Intentionally falsifying information and services.

Clean Area Identifiable area of a sterilization center that is used for assembling and storing sterilized instruments and treatment trays.

Clinical Record (patient chart) Documents used to determine and record patient demographics, medical and dental health history, previous treatment, diagnosed treatment, radiographs, and treatment notes.

Closed Panel Groups of dental providers who are under contract with third parties to provide dental services.

Closing (letter writing) Describes the next step or expected outcomes of the letter.

Code on Dental Procedures and Nomenclature (the Code) National standard for codes used to report dental treatment.

Color Coding System used in filing that identifies various sections of the alphabet (or numbers) through specific colors or color combinations. Provides visual identification.

Columns Divisions of the pages of an appointment book. The functions of the columns are to organize the schedule and to indicate who is performing the dentistry, who the patient is, why the patient is being seen, and what is going to be done.

Combination Recall System Method of scheduling appointments according to patient preference. Some patients may be unwilling to schedule an appointment in advance but do not mind if you call them at work to schedule the appointment closer to the actual appointment date. Other patients may be very good at scheduling an appointment as soon as they receive the card in the mail.

Commissures Corners of the mouth at which the upper and lower lips meet.

Company Signature (letter writing) Identifies the company of the person who is sending a letter and is optional. It is used when the sender of the letter is representing the company.

Completeness A step in the organizational stage. When checking, make sure you have included all information, facts, and explanations needed by the reader. It is not uncommon to include a phrase that will appeal to the reader's emotions or understanding.

Complimentary Closing (letter writing) Final closing of a letter, such as "sincerely" and "truly yours."

Compromising Style (conflict resolution) A style that is best used when parties are equally powerful, consensus cannot be reached, integrating or dominating style is not successful, and a temporary solution to a complex problem is needed.

Computerized Letter Template A word processing software feature that allows you to save a letter in a file and reuse the letter as often as needed (making changes when needed).

Computerized Recall System Recall system that combines the elements of a manual system and is programmed to perform steps automatically. This type of system automatically schedules an appointment for a patient on the basis of stored information, prints a recall card, and places the patient's name on the recall list.

Concise Organized manner.

Conference Calls Several people are present on the telephone line at the same time.

Confidential Personnel Records Information about an employee's employment performance.

Consent Form Form used to receive authorization from a patient to continue treatment.

Consolidated Omnibus Budget Reconciliation Act (COBRA) Legislation that mandates guaranteed medical and dental coverage for a period of 18 months after the loss of group benefits coverage. Individuals are given the option of purchasing their own coverage at a group rate under special COBRA contracts.

Consultation Area Area used for meeting with patients when privacy is needed.

Consumable Supplies and Products Items that are used and that need to be replenished.

Contaminated Area Identifiable area of the sterilization center where instruments are processed before they are sterilized.

Coordination of Benefits (COB) System that coordinates the benefits of two or more insurance policies. The total benefits paid should not be more than 100% of the original service fee.

Copayment Portion of the service fee that remains after payment is made by the dental benefits plan.

Copy Notation (letter writing) The abbreviation "cc" for computer copy or carbon copy, used to notify the reader that a copy of the document is being forwarded to another party.

Corporate Dentistry Dental facilities that are owned and operated by companies for the purpose of providing dental care to their employees and dependents.

Correspondence Log Method used to document various types of correspondence that pertain to the patient. This form is kept in the patient's clinical record.

Cover Letter (letter of introduction or application) Introduces an applicant to a prospective employer. Cover letters should accompany all resumes sent by mail (including electronic transfer and fax).

Covered Charges Allowable services that are outlined in dental benefits plan contracts, fee schedules, or tables of allowance, as determined by the dental provider and paid for, in whole or in part, by the third party dental benefits plan.

CPU Central processing unit; the main operating component of a computer.

Cranium The eight bones that form a protective structure for the brain and the face.

Credibility The weight that is put on a message in accordance with the status or qualifications of the person sending the message.

Cross Referencing Method that identifies another name (or number) under which a record may be filed.

Current Dental Terminology (CDT) Terms and codes standardized by the ADA for the purpose of consistency in reporting dental services and procedures to dental benefits plans.

Current Procedural Terminology (CPT) Codes and procedures standardized by the American Medical Association (AMA) for the purpose of reporting medical treatment and services.

Cusp Pointed or rounded eminence on the surface of a tooth.

Cuspids Canines. Anterior teeth.

Customary Fee Fee, as determined by the third party administrator, from actual submitted fees, for specific dental services.

Daily Journal Form used to record business transactions.

Daily Schedule Sheets Posted schedules used in treatment rooms, dentists' private offices, laboratories, and other work areas.

Darkroom Place where dental x-ray film is processed.

Data Information.

Data Processor Person responsible for entering data into the computer system.

Dateline (letter writing) The date the letter is written.

DDS Doctor of Dental Surgery.

Deductible Service fee that the patient is responsible for paying before the third party will consider payment of additional services. The deductible may be payable annually, over a lifetime, or as a family.

Dental Arches (see Maxillary Arch and Mandibular Arch) Each dental arch contains the same number of teeth.

Dental Assisting National Board, Inc. National testing agency.

Dental Auxiliary Any person, other than the dentist, who provides a service in a dental practice.

Dental Healthcare Team All persons in the dental office. Someone who excels and becomes a vital member will have mastered multiple skills, will be flexible, and will work well in a team environment.

Dental History Information about previous treatment. It also alerts the dental healthcare team to fears and apprehensions that the patient may have concerning dental treatment.

Dental Hygienist Professionally educated and licensed member of the dental healthcare team who provides educational, clinical, and therapeutic dental services to patients.

Dental Insurance Method of financial assistance (provided by a dental benefit service) that helps pay for specified procedures and services concerning dental disease and accidental injuries to the oral structure.

Dental Practice Act Legislation that outlines the duties that can be performed by dental auxiliaries, the type of education required, and what licensure, if any, is necessary for these duties.

Dental Prophylaxis Removal of stains and hard deposits from teeth.

Dental Public Health Dentists who help organize and run dental programs that address the dental health of the general public.

Dental Radiographs X-rays of teeth.

Dental Service Corporation A legally formed, not-for-profit organization that contracts with dental providers for the sole purpose of providing dental care. Examples of dental service corporations are Delta Dental Plans and Blue Cross/Blue Shield.

Dentin Bulk of a tooth that consists of living cellular substance similar in structure to bone and softer than the hard outer shell of the crown (enamel) and the covering of the root surface (cementum).

Dependents Persons who are covered under another person's dental benefits policy.

DMD Doctor of Medical Dentistry.

Diagnostic Methods (study models) Casts of a patient's mouth used as a tool in treatment planning.

Direct Reimbursement Payment plan that allows an organization to be self-funded for the purpose of providing dental benefits.

Disposable (supplies) Items used only once and then thrown away.

Divided Payment Plan Payments are divided according to the length of treatment.

Dominating Style (conflict resolution) A style that is appropriate when speed is important in making a decision and the results are trivial, when an unpopular course of action is needed, when the decisions of others will be costly to you, or when one is handling an overly aggressive subordinate.

Downcoding Method of changing a reported benefits code by third-party payers so as to reflect a lower cost procedure.

Dual Addressing When a Post Office box and a street address are used in the same destination address. The address listed directly above the city, state, and ZIP code is where the mail will be delivered.

Electronic Protected Health Information (EPHI) Health information that is shared electronically; covered providers are required to protect the integrity, confidentiality, and availability of this information.

Emotions (communication) Feelings, such as being upset, angry, or even happy, that can keep listeners from hearing the message (barriers to effective communication).

Employment Agreement An outline of conditions for employment. May include job title and description, work schedule, salary, and benefits.

Enamel Hard, mineralized substance that covers the anatomic crown of a tooth. It consists of 99% inorganic matter and cannot regenerate.

Enclosure Reminder (letter writing) Notation stating that additional documents are enclosed with the letter.

Endodontics (root canal) Procedure that removes diseased pulpal tissue.

Ergonomics Science of fitting the job to the worker. When the job does not match the physical capacity of the worker, work-related musculoskeletal disorders may result.

Ethics Category of moral judgments.

Examination Form Form used in a clinical record to record examination information.

Exclusion The option in a dental benefits program to exclude dental services and procedures. These excluded services and procedures are outlined in the patient's contract (benefits book).

Expanded (extended) Function Assistants Assistants who have additional training and education in functions that enable more independent patient care. Functions are identified in each state's Dental Practice Act.

Expendable Supplies and products that can be reused for a specific length of time before they have to be replaced. Instruments, handpieces, and small equipment fall into this category.

Expiration Date Date that identifies when a product should no longer be used.

Express Mail The fastest service offered by the US Postal Service. Express mail is guaranteed for overnight delivery, 365 days a year.

Extended Payment Plan One of several methods that can be used when it is necessary to extend the schedule for payment of treatment.

Face The front of the head, consisting of 14 bones.

Federation Dentaire International Numbering System Tooth numbering system that is widely used in countries other than the United States. In this system, the quadrants and sextants are assigned numbers. Each configuration is a two-digit number that consists of a 0 and a number from 1 through 8.

Fee for Service Method of payment that compensates the dentist according to individual services and procedures. Reimbursement is determined by established fee schedules.

Fee Schedule List of charges for dental services and procedures. Fee schedules are established by the dentist or a dental benefits provider and are mutually agreed on.

Feedback Method for determining whether a message has been received and understood.

File Folders Used to store documents, patient record forms, and business reports.

File Labels Used to identify contents of files and indexing (filing procedure).

Filing Segment One or more filing units, such as the total name, subject, or number, that is being used for filing purposes.

Filing Unit A number, a letter, a word, or any combination of these used for filing.

Filtering by Level (organizational communications) Information sent is not received because it has been changed or stopped at one level. If, as an administrative assistant, you send a message or idea to the dentist and it is stopped or changed by the office manager, there is a breakdown in the upward flow of the message.

Financial Reports (filing procedure) Filed according to subject and then subdivided chronologically.

Financial Reports   Used to determine the financial health of a dental practice. Accountants use them to prepare business, income, and payroll tax reports.

First-Class Mail   Used for sending letters, postcards, and greeting cards that weigh less than 11 ounces. First-class mail will be delivered overnight to local areas, in 2 days to locally designated states, and in 3 days to all other areas.

Fluoride Treatments   Treatments provided to strengthen enamel and protect teeth from developing carious lesions.

Forensic Odontology   Method of identification based on dental conditions.

Formal Downward Channels (organizational communications)   Communication that originates at the top of the organizational structure and filters down to the lower levels of the organization.

Franchise Dentistry   Method of providing dental care under a common name. The purpose of franchised dentistry is to provide a common name, regional or national advertising, contract agreements with dental benefits providers, and financial and managerial support.

Frenum   Strip of tissue that connects two structures.

Full-Blocked (letter writing)   Format in which all letter sections begin at the left margin and proper spacing is applied between sections.

Full Denture   Prosthesis used to replace all teeth in an arch.

Full Gold and Metal Crowns   Replacements for tooth structures cast from gold alloy and other metals and categorized according to the amount of gold used: high noble, noble, low noble, and nongold (analogous to the carat classification for gold jewelry—18k, 14k, and 10k).

Functional Resumes   Resumes in which skills and abilities are placed first, according to importance, regardless of the time of occurrence. After the objective statement, skills and abilities are highlighted, followed by work experience, education, and miscellaneous information.

Gag Reflex   Contraction of the constrictor muscles of the pharynx in response to taste or touch on the posterior pharyngeal wall or nearby areas.

Geographic Filing   Means of categorizing records according to geographic location, such as city, ZIP code, area code, state, or country. Each document is coded and filed according to the selected geographic locator.

Geometric Chart   Method by which circles are used to represent teeth; the chart is divided into sections that represent the surfaces of the teeth.

Gingivae   Masticatory mucosa and the tissue that surrounds the teeth. Normal healthy gingiva is firm and attached tightly around the teeth; it is coral or salmon-pink in color (in races other than Caucasian, the color is commonly darker).

Guides   Used to divide filing systems into small sections.

Hard Palate   Hard plate or roof of the mouth, covered with masticatory mucosa. The soft palate is the posterior continuation of the hard palate.

Hardware   The physical part of the computer system. The hardware in a simple computer system includes the central processing unit (CPU), monitor, keyboard, mouse, and printer.

Hazardous Communication Program   Method of dealing with hazardous material. Consists of five parts: written program, chemical inventory, Material Safety Data Sheets, container labeling, and employee training.

Health Insurance Portability and Accountability Act of 1996   The *Portability* section of the Act simply guarantees that a person covered by health insurance provided by one employer can obtain health insurance through the second employer if he or she changes jobs. The *Accountability* section of the act answers the question of who and what should be accountable for specific healthcare activities.

Health Maintenance Organization (HMO)   Healthcare delivery system composed of providers who will accept payment for services on a per capita basis or a limited fee schedule.

Horizontal Channel (organizational communications)   Working across (horizontally) organizational structures, communication is transmitted between members. This type of communication occurs primarily between members at the same level.

HOSA (Health Occupations Students of America)   Student organization whose mission is to promote career opportunities in healthcare and to enhance the delivery of quality healthcare to all people.

Humanistic Theory   Based on the works of Maslow and Rogers. See under Maslow and Rogers.

Hybrid Resumes   Resumes that combine the best features of chronological and functional resumes in various arrangements while focusing only on information that is relevant to the current job objective.

Hyphenated Names (filing procedure)   Two surnames joined with a hyphen, treated as one unit.

Inappropriate Span of Control (organizational communications)   One person has control for too long a period. This leads to lack of trust and fuels resentment. It may be the result of poor communications, lack of direction, or poor or nonexistent policies and procedures.

Incentive Program   Payment schedule by which the copayment percentage changes when patients follow a preset standard of treatment.

Incisal Sharp cutting edge of anterior teeth (incisors and cuspids).

Incoming Mail Mail received by the dental office that requires sorting according to category and routing to the correct person or department.

Indemnity Plan Dental benefit plan that utilizes schedules of allowances, tables of allowances, or reasonable and customary fee schedules as the bases of payment calculations.

Indexing Method used to determine placement of files in an organized system.

Individual Patient File Folder Used to keep documents and forms (clinical record).

Individual Practice Association (IPA) Legally formed organization that enters into contracts with dental benefits plans to provide services to enrollees in the dental benefit plan.

Informal Channel (organizational communications) Communication that takes place in an informal setting and is not the official communication of the organization. Informal communications can be accurate or inaccurate and are often referred to as "the grapevine."

Information System Combination of equipment, software, data, personnel, and procedures that process information.

In-House Payment Plans (budget plans) Financial arrangements between the dental practice and the patient.

Initial Oral Examination Performed during the patient's first visit to the dental practice. Consists of diagnostic aids that will help the dentist determine existing conditions and restorations, as well as the dental needs of the patient.

Inlay Partial coverage of a tooth, usually on the same surfaces as amalgam restorations. Cast from gold or composite materials.

Input Devices Peripherals that transfer data into a computer system. Common input devices include keyboard, mouse, and scanner.

Inside Address (letter writing) Address of the person or company to whom a letter is being sent.

Inspecting (filing procedure) Checking the document to make sure it is ready to file.

Insurance Billing Process of billing a benefits provider for services rendered a patient.

Insurance Clerk Administrative dental assistant responsible for insurance billing.

Insurance Information Information needed for insurance billing.

Insurance Records Records that include contracts with third party carriers (insurance companies).

Insured A person who has enrolled with an insurer (third party) to arrange for payment for dental services and procedures.

Insurer Third party who assumes responsibility for payment for dental services and procedures on behalf of enrollees in the program.

Integrating Style (conflict resolution) Style that works best when time is available to address the problem. Usually, problems are complex, and solving them requires the expertise of more than one person. The problem must be identified, and then input from all members is needed to develop a solution.

Intergroup Conflict Conflict between two or more groups because members of one group disagree with members of another group.

Intermediate (practice management) System Intermediate level of software used in computerized practice management systems.

International Standards Organization See Federation Dentaire International Numbering System.

Interorganizational Conflict Conflict between two or more organizations.

Interpersonal Communication Communication in which the sender and the receiver exchange information in real time. This includes face-to-face, telephone, and video conferencing.

Interpersonal Conflict Conflict (between two team members) that occurs when members of the team at the same level (assistant and assistant) or at different levels (hygienist and assistant) disagree about a given matter.

Intragroup Conflict Conflict (within the group) that occurs when members at the same level (assistant and assistant, dentist and dentist) disagree. This conflict normally occurs when differences in goals, tasks, and procedures are discussed.

Intraorganizational Conflict Conflict within the organization.

Intrapersonal Conflict Conflict within oneself when one is expected to perform a task that does not meet personal goals, values, beliefs, or expertise.

Introduction (letter writing) The first paragraph in the body of a letter. It should contain a brief list of the important points discussed in the main body of the letter.

Invoice Document that indicates charges or products sent.

Jargon Specialized words, acronyms (groups of initials), and other terms that are unique to a given group.

Job Search Log Method used to organize, plan, and follow through with employment leads. Tracks submitted resumes and identifies company names and telephone numbers of contact persons.

Keyboard Common type of computer input device that is similar in configuration to a typewriter. The keyboard may include a variety of function keys.

Labial The surface of anterior teeth that faces or touches the lips.

Labial Frenum Connects the tissue of the lips (labia) to the gingival tissue.

Labial Vestibule   Junction of the lips and the gingiva.

Laboratory (dental)   Area of the dental office where nonpatient procedures can be performed.

Laboratory Form   Prescription used to communicate instructions to a laboratory technician.

Lack of Trust and Openness (organizational communications)   Situation that can occur at all levels of the organization, possibly leading to conflict.

Lateral File Folders   Folders used for clinical records. Tabs are located on the side of the folder.

Lateral Files   Open file cabinets used to store lateral file folders.

Lateral Incisors   Anterior teeth characterized by thin, sharp incisal edges that aid in cutting food.

Lead Time   The time it takes for supplies to arrive at the office once an order has been placed.

Least Expensive Alternative Treatment (LEAT)   A provision in dental benefits plans that allows payment for dental services and procedures according to the least expensive treatment.

Legal Standards   Legislation regulated by boards and commissions.

Letterhead   Name, address, and telephone number of the sender.

Licensure   Identifies members of a profession who meet minimal standards and are qualified to perform set duties outlined in regulations and standards (Dental Practice Act).

Lighting   Critical factor for a comfortable and productive workstation. The correct type and optimal level depend on the task at hand.

Line Spacing   The number of lines between the elements of a letter.

Lingual   Surface of teeth that faces the tongue or inside of the mouth.

Lingual Frenum   Connects the tongue to the floor of the mouth.

Lining Mucosa   Covers the cheeks, lips, vestibule, ventral (under side) surface of the tongue, and soft palate. This tissue is very thin and can be injured easily.

Lips   Tissue that surrounds the opening to the oral cavity.

Locker Room   Place to change from street clothes into uniforms.

Loose Leaf Appointment Books   Book whose pages can be removed and placed in permanent storage as they are used, providing for a less bulky appointment book. It is easy to insert new pages as needed, and at the end of the year, pages for the new year can be added to provide for a smooth transition from year to year.

Loudness (speech)   Volume of a voice.

Mail Recall System   System that requires the mailing of recall cards to patients to remind them that they are due in the dental office for an appointment.

Main Body (letter writing)   Details of the points stated in the introduction. One or two paragraphs in length.

Major Equipment   Equipment that can be depreciated, such as dental chairs, radiology units, computers, office equipment, and laboratory equipment.

Malocclusion   Teeth that are out of alignment or occlusion.

Managed Care   Method employed by some benefits plans that is designed to contain the cost of healthcare. These methods involve limiting access to care (enrollees are assigned healthcare providers), services and procedures covered, and reimbursement amounts.

Mandibular Arch   Lower teeth or jaw.

Mandibular Left   One of the dental arches that are divided into four sections or quadrants. Each quadrant has the same number and type of teeth as the opposite quadrant. Quadrants consist of maxillary right, maxillary left, mandibular left, and mandibular right.

Mandibular Right   See Mandibular Left.

Maslow, Abraham H. (1908–1970)   Psychologist who believed that individuals have to satisfy a level of physiologic need before they are motivated to seek the next level. These levels range from the basic needs of life (food, shelter, and safety) to the higher needs of love, belonging, and self-esteem, and the highest—self-actualization.

Mastication   Chewing and grinding of food with the teeth.

Masticatory Mucosa   Thick, dense mucosa attached tightly to bone (with the exception of the tongue). It is designed to resist the pressure of chewing food and is not easily injured. This tissue type forms the gingiva (gums), the hard palate, and the dorsum (top) of the tongue.

Material Safety Data Sheets (MSDS)   Components of a Hazardous Communication Program that contain information about a product.

Matrixing   Outlining.

Maxillary Arch   Upper teeth or jaw.

Maxillary Left   See Mandibular Left.

Maxillary Right   See Mandibular Left.

Maximum Allowance   The total amount of dental benefits (dollars) that will be paid toward dental services and procedures. Maximums are determined by the provisions of individual group contracts.

Maximum Benefit   The total amount of dental benefits that will be paid for an individual or family for dental services and procedures. This amount is determined by the individual group contract and may involve a yearly maximum or a lifetime maximum.

Maximum Fee Schedule   The total acceptable fee for a dental service or procedure that will be charged by a dental provider under a specific dental benefits plan.

Medical History (clinical record) Comprehensive medical information that alerts the dentist to drug allergies and medical conditions that may be affected by certain dental procedures.

Medium (communication) Method of transferring information. Can be verbal, nonverbal, or a combination of the two.

Mesial Proximal surface of a tooth that is facing toward the midline.

Message Idea to be shared with another person or group.

Mixed Dentition Primary and permanent teeth are both present.

Modem Unit that electronically transfers information from the CPU through a transmission line (commonly a telephone line) to another location.

Modified Blocked (letter writing) A blocked format with one change: paragraphs are indented 5 spaces.

Molars Posterior teeth that have flat surfaces with rounded projections and are used for chewing.

Mouse Computer input device.

Mucous Membrane Moist membrane that covers the inside of the cheeks.

National Provider Identifier Standard (NPI) A distinctive standard identification number issued by the US government that can replace the Social Security Number, Individual Tax ID, or other identifiers on standard electronic healthcare transactions such as dental insurance claim forms.

Necessary Treatment Dental services and procedures that have been established by the dental professional as necessary for the purpose of restoring or maintaining a patient's oral health. Treatment is based on established standards of the dental profession.

Networking (employment strategy) A means of contacting other dental professionals and letting them know that you are seeking employment. This is an informal job placement service and is one of the most effective means of seeking employment.

Noise (communication) Something that alters the message because the sender and the receiver cannot hear the message. When conversations take place around machinery, large groups of people, and other noisy areas, the message that is being sent may not be completely received.

Nonconsumable Products Items that can be used for only 1 or 2 years before they must be replaced because of wear.

Nonparticipating Dentist A dental professional who is not under contract with a dental benefits plan to provide dental services and procedures to enrollees.

Nonverbal Communication Method of communication in which the message is sent through facial expressions and body gestures.

NSF "No significant findings"; also, "nonsufficient funds."

Numeric Filing Records are filed according to an assigned number.

Objective (resume) Important component of your resume that identifies the position for which you are applying and is supported by the information listed in the body of your resume.

Obliging Style (conflict resolution) Style used when the issue is unimportant and you are willing to give in to the other party to preserve a relationship.

Occlusal The broad, flat chewing surface of posterior teeth (premolars and molars).

Occlusion Relationship between the maxillary arch and the mandibular arch and the way they meet or touch.

Occupational Safety and Health Administration (OSHA) Federal government agency that was enacted to protect the worker from workplace injury. OSHA regulates all areas of employment. In addition to OSHA, most states have their own versions, which in some cases, are stricter than the federal agency.

Office Letter Portfolio Collection of samples of letters that can be used for different occasions. The portfolio is similar to computerized templates, with the exception that a hard copy of the letter is placed in a notebook.

Office Manager Person who organizes and oversees the daily operations of the office staff.

Onlay Partial coverage of a tooth; the same as an inlay, except that it includes more tooth structure and replaces a cusp. Cast in gold or composite.

Online Resume Resume that is posted on Web sites for prospective employers to review.

Open Enrollment Period of time (occurs annually) when a member of a dental benefits program has the option of selecting the type of coverage and the provider of dental services.

Open Panel Dental benefits plan in which any licensed dentist can participate. The enrollee (insured) can seek treatment from any licensed dentist with payment of benefits provided to the enrollee or the dentist.

Open Punctuation (letter writing) Format in which no punctuation is used in the salutation and complimentary closing (punctuation is, however, used in the body of the letter).

Operating Systems Software Information needed to operate and run a computer.

Oral and Maxillofacial Radiology Specialty that produces and interprets images and data generated by all modalities of radiant energy (x-rays and other types of imaging) that are used for the diagnosis and management of diseases, disorders, and conditions of the oral and maxillofacial region.

Oral Cavity Anatomic area in which dentistry is performed. It is also the beginning of the digestive system, contains sensory receptors and is used to form speech patterns; it is a source of human pleasure and a weapon for defense (verbal and physical).

Oral and Maxillofacial Pathology Area of dentistry in which diseases of the mouth or oral structures are diagnosed and treated.

Oral and Maxillofacial Surgery Surgical procedures of the head and neck, ranging from simple tasks such as extraction of teeth to complex surgical procedures designed to reconstruct facial structures.

Oral Mucosa Tissue that lines the oral cavity.

Orthodontics and Dentofacial Orthopaedics Area of dentistry in which conditions of malocclusion (the way teeth meet) are diagnosed and treated. An orthodontist is a member of a complex team of medical and dental doctors who restore facial features and oral functions of patients.

Outgoing Mail Mail sent from the dental practice.

Out-Guides Used to replace a file that has been removed from the system.

Output Devices Devices used to transfer data out of the computer, such as monitors, printers, and peripheral storage devices.

Outside Payment Plans Financial arrangements made by the dental office and administered by an outside agency.

Overbilling Fraudulent practice of not disclosing to benefit plan organizations the waiver of patient copayment.

Overcoding Billing of dental benefits plans for procedures that results in higher payments than are justified by the service or procedure that was actually performed.

Panographic X-ray Unit Machine that takes extraoral (outside the mouth) radiographic films.

Parotid Glands Salivary glands.

Participating Dentist Dentist who has a contract with a dental benefits organization to provide dental care to specific enrollees.

Patient Education Room Area designated for activities prepared to educate and motivate patients.

Patient Information (clinical record) Information within the record that strictly pertains to the treatment of the patient. Does not include financial accounting or insurance forms.

Payer Dental fees made on behalf of patients by insurance companies, dental benefits plans, or dental plan sponsors (direct reimbursement, unions).

Payment in Full Plan Office policy that requires the patient to pay in full after each visit. Payment may be made in the form of cash, check or credit card.

Payroll Records Documents that contain payroll information pertaining to employees.

Pediatric Dentistry Area of dentistry in which dentists (pedodontists) treat patients from newborn to about the age of 15 years in all phases of dentistry. They may work in a hospital setting to provide treatment to patients under general anesthesia, work with patients with special needs, and provide treatment for children who are in need of preventive and restorative dental treatment.

Pegboard System Also referred to as a "one-write system." Components of this system consist of ledger board, day sheet, patient ledger, and receipt. Forms are arranged one on top of the other to facilitate entry of data one time only. Pegboard checkwriting system components include ledger board, check register, and checks.

Periodic Method (filing procedure) System by which all financial reports, payroll records, and other monthly reports are transferred to an inactive file, making room for the new year's reports and records.

Periodontal Ligament Connective fibers that helps to hold teeth in the alveolar socket; provides protection and nourishment for the tooth.

Periodontics Area of dentistry in which dentists (periodontists) treat patients who have diseases of the soft tissue surrounding the teeth (periodontal disease). Periodontal disease occurs in several different stages, which vary in severity. The treatment performed by a periodontist focuses on correcting and preventing the progression of disease.

Permanent Dentition The second set of teeth (32 in number) that are intended to remain in the mouth for a lifetime.

Perpetual Method (filing procedure) Method that identifies files and records that have been inactive for a predetermined length of time or that are no longer required for quick reference.

Personal Career Portfolio A collection of samples from your professional career. These are used as a source of information and an illustration of your skills, abilities, and strengths.

Personal Names (filing procedure) Indexing method by personal names or business or organizational names, in accordance with the ARMA Simplified Filing Standard Rules.

Personnel Records Nonpayroll information about employees.

Phenomenological Viewing a situation from the other person's point of view.

Pitch (voice) A quality of the sound of your voice.

Pontic Artificial replacement of a missing tooth or teeth.

Porcelain Fused to Metal Gold-cast crown with a porcelain cover (tooth colored).

Postage Amount of money that is required to mail an item.

Postal Cards One-sheet items used to send short messages through the mail.

Posterior Toward the back.

Posting Transactions Placing the correct patient information on the ledger, receipt, and day sheet (manual system), or keying the information into a computerized system.

Preauthorization Certification by a dental benefit plan that a pretreatment plan has been authorized for payment in accordance with the patient's group policy.

Precertification Confirmation by a dental benefit plan that a patient is eligible to receive treatment according to the provisions of the contract.

Predetermination See Preauthorization.

Preexisting Condition A clause, in most dental benefit plans, that limits coverage of dental benefits to conditions that existed before the patient was enrolled in the benefit plan.

Preferred Provider Organization (PPO) A contract between a dental benefit plan organization and a provider of dental care that states that, in return for the referral of dental patients, the dentist will provide dental services and procedures at a reduced fee, or will adhere to a pre-established fee schedule.

Prefiling of Fees A procedure in which a dental professional files a fee schedule with the dental benefit plan organization for the purpose of gaining preauthorization of the fee schedule.

Premolars (bicuspids) Posterior teeth, smaller than molars, with 2 cusps, used for tearing and grinding.

Prescheduled Recall System Scheduling of patients in advance of their recall.

Primary Dentition A set of 20 teeth, including central, lateral, cuspid, 1st primary molar, and 2nd primary molar. Often referred to as "baby teeth."

Priority Mail A faster delivery service than first-class at a reasonable rate.

Privacy Officer Person who is appointed to oversee the written policy and procedure manual for handling PHI (protected health information).

Private Office A personal office.

Production Reports Reports that identify what types of procedures have been performed and by whom.

Productivity Fees charged for dental treatment, or monies collected.

Products Materials used in direct patient care, including dental materials and dental therapeutics.

Profit and Loss Statements Statements that identify overhead (the cost of operating a business) and determine whether the dental practice is making or losing money.

Progress Notes (clinical record) Notations kept in a patient's clinical record, including those related to diagnosis, treatment, amount and type of anesthetic, and brand name of materials used.

Proof of Posting Method used to check posting transactions.

Prosthodontics Area of dentistry for which dentists (prosthodontists) receive advanced training in performing procedures that replace lost and damaged teeth and tooth structures with partial dentures (fixed and removable), full dentures, or crowns over implants.

Protected Health Information (PHI) Health information that is required to be protected in all formats and in all locations; this is necessary during the transfer of information in oral, written, and electronic formats and when information is stored (paper and electronic copies).

Proximal Surfaces that are adjacent or next to another surface of a tooth.

Pulp Chamber Center of the crown.

Pulpal Tissue Connective tissue, blood vessels, and nerves.

Quadrants The four sections of the dental arches. Each quadrant has the same number and type of teeth as the opposite quadrant.

Radiology Room Place where dental radiographs are obtained.

Rank and Status (organizational communications) Factors that may interfere with communication in several ways. Some people use position (rank) as a means of power over others, which closes channels of communication.

Rate of Use Length of time between purchase and use of a product.

Reasonable Fee A determination by the third-party administrator that a specific service has been modified to take into consideration unusual complications.

Recall Appointment Scheduled appointment for preventive treatment or reevaluation of dental conditions.

Recall System Method used to ensure timely scheduling of patients for preventive treatment.

Receipt Document given to a patient that shows charges and payments.

Reception Area The first office area to be viewed by the patient; the place where patients wait.

Receptionist Administrative dental assistant responsible for answering the telephone, greeting patients, and scheduling appointments.

Records Manager Person who organizes and maintains all aspects of patients' clinical charts according to preset standards. Establishes and maintains an efficient filing system to ensure the precise location of all clinical records.

Record and Supply Storage Areas where storage shelves and large file cabinets are stored.

Reference Initials (letter writing) Initials of the sender of the letter (in upper case) and initials of the typist (in lower case).

Referral Letters Method for sending information about patients to other professionals. The purposes of the referral letter are to introduce the patient and to state the purpose of the referral.

Registration Form of licensure that has been established by some states as a method of protecting the public. Requirements for registration are outlined in each state's Dental Practice Act.

Registration Form (clinical record) Introduces the patient to the dental practice and provides demographic and financial information for insurance forms and patient billing.

Removable Partial Removable prosthesis.

Resin Tooth-colored restorative material.

Resin-Based Composite Type of restorative material that is tooth colored and used primarily on anterior teeth.

Resumes Personal marketing tools prepared with one goal—to get a job interview. A good resume will give a competitive advantage, help organize thoughts, and make a good impression.

Retention (filing procedure) Keeping records. The retention of patient records varies according to the extent of treatment provided, whether radiographs have been taken, and regulations established by third party insurance carriers. Business record retention is determined by office policy and government regulations.

Return Address Identifies the sender of a piece of mail. Placed in the upper left-hand corner of an envelope.

Risk Management Process that identifies conditions that may lead to alleged malpractice or procedures that are not in compliance with mandated regulations.

Rogers, Carl (1902–1987) Psychologist who theorized that each healthy individual believes in an ideal self and is constantly trying to achieve the ideal self as much as possible.

Root Anatomic portion of a tooth located in the alveolar process.

Root Canal (endodontics) Procedure that replaces diseased pulp.

Routing Slips Used to communicate details of patient treatment between the business office and the treatment area.

Royal and Religious Titles (filing procedure) Convention that states that when titles are followed by one name, they are filed as written.

Rugae Ridges located within the hard palate.

Saliva Substance produced by the salivary glands to moisturize mucous membranes, lubricate food, clean the teeth, and supply an enzyme (amylase) that begins the digestive process.

Salutation (letter writing) A greeting, such as "Dear—" and "To Whom it May Concern."

Scanner Computer input device that digitizes images.

Sealant Substance that covers the chewing surfaces of teeth with a thin coat of resin. The purpose of this coating treatment is to seal and protect the tooth from the effects of acid attacks, which cause demineralization of enamel and lead to carious lesions.

Semantics Meanings of words and language.

Semi-Blocked (letter writing) Format that is the same as blocked with one change: Paragraphs are indented 5 spaces.

Sender (communication) Person who has the responsibility to ensure that the proper message is sent and that the receiver understands the content of the message.

Sextants The six sections into which the dental arches are sometimes divided. This method of division is most commonly used in periodontal evaluations. Sextants consist of maxillary right posterior, maxillary anterior, maxillary left posterior, mandibular left posterior, mandibular anterior, and mandibular right posterior.

Signer's Identification (letter writing) Identifies the sender of the letter.

Simple Extraction Removal of one or more teeth without the need to remove bone or cut tissue.

Simplified or AMS (letter writing) Format similar to full-blocked, except that open punctuation is used, no salutation or complimentary closing is included, a subject line in all capital letters must be used, the word "subject" is omitted, the signer's identification appears in all capital letters, and lists are indented 5 spaces. If a numbered list is used, the period is omitted and the list is not indented.

Sincerity (communications) An emotion that patients can perceive from members of the dental healthcare team when barriers are removed. Barriers can take the form of desks and other objects that come between the team members and the patient.

Skip Tracing Process for locating a person who has moved and not left a forwarding address.

Skull Bones in the head made up of two sections. The cranium consists of 8 bones that form a protective structure for the brain, and the face consists of 14 bones.

Smile (communication) Facial expression that communicates a positive thought. Smiles can be used to ease a patient's apprehension, send a warm greeting to a child, or acknowledge the arrival of a patient.

Soft Palate Posterior tissue region of the roof of the mouth. This region is soft and flexible.

Software Instructions in a computer for performing functions specific to dental-related procedures.

Sorting (filing procedure)   Phase of the filing process during which records and documents are separated into categories according to the filing method used and the locations of files.

Speed of Speech   The quickness with which a message is spoken.

Square-Blocked (letter writing)   The same format as full-blocked with minor changes. The date line is on the same line as the first line of the inside address and is right justified. Reference initials and enclosure reminders are typed on the same line as the signature and the signer's identification and are right justified. This style allows for squaring of the letter and is used when space is needed.

Staff Room   Area set aside for the exclusive use of staff for activities such as eating lunch and holding meetings.

Standard Mail (A)   Used by retailers, cataloguers, and other advertisers to send out mass mailings.

Standard Mail (B)   Used for sending parcels that weigh less than 70 pounds. Parcels are delivered in 2 to 9 days.

Standard Punctuation (letter writing)   The salutation is followed by a colon (:), and the complimentary closing is followed by a comma (,).

Standards for Privacy of Individually Identifiable Health Information (The Privacy Rule)   The intent of the rule is to protect health information; the rule applies to three types of covered entities: health plans, healthcare clearinghouses, and healthcare providers who use an electronic mode to transfer information.

Standards for Security of Individually Identifiable Health Information (The Security Rule)   Covered providers must run a risk analysis to protect the integrity, confidentiality, and availability of electronic health information.

Statement   Summary of individual invoices and requests for payment.

Stationery   Collection of paper products that are used in correspondence. Effective professional communication combines selected stationery with messages.

Sterilization Area   Room in which contaminated instruments are cleaned, packaged, sterilized, and prepared for reuse. The room is separated into two areas—contaminated and clean.

Stereotyping (communication)   Attitude that blocks effective communication because assumptions are made about nonfactual information or preconceived ideas about a person, an idea, or a procedure.

Subject Filing   Method of storing information according to subject. In this system, files are labeled according to the subject of the contents and then are filed alphabetically.

Subject Lines (letter writing)   Words that draw attention to the nature of the correspondence.

Sublingual Gland   Salivary gland.

Submandibular Gland   Salivary gland.

Subscriber   A term used to describe the holder of a dental benefit (insurance).

Supplies   Consumable goods that are used in support of dental treatment.

Surfaces of the Tooth   Sections into which each tooth is divided. Each surface has a name that is used by the dental professional to describe the exact location of tooth decay, restorations, and other conditions.

Surgical Extractions   Procedures that include the cutting of tissue and the removal of bone to facilitate removal of a tooth.

Symbolic Numbering System   Method in which each tooth in a quadrant is assigned a number and the quadrant is assigned a symbol.

Table of Allowances   A list of the services and procedures that a dental benefits plan will pay for, with a dollar amount assigned to each procedure. Also referred to as a "schedule of allowances" and an "indemnity schedule."

Tax Records (filing procedure)   Payroll, business, and corporate tax reports that are filed by subject and then subdivided into the type of report or record. These records normally cover a specified period of time and therefore are subfiled chronologically.

Telecommunications   The use of equipment to transfer information or to communicate with someone over a distance. In a dental practice, telecommunication methods include the telephone system and intraoffice memoranda.

Telephone Recall System   Method by which an assistant personally calls all patients before the month they are due for recall and scheduling of their appointment.

Third Party   A group or organization that has the capacity to collect premiums, accept financial risk, and pay dental claims. In addition, the third party performs other administrative services. Also known as an administrative agent, carrier, insurer, or underwriter. (First party, patient; second party, healthcare provider.)

Titles and Suffixes (filing procedure)   Titles and suffixes are not used as a filing unit, except when they are needed to distinguish between two or more identical names. If used, they are placed in the last filing unit, and they are filed as written but without punctuation (specific filing guidelines specify that suffixes are filed in numeric sequence when needed for identification).

Tone (communication)   A quality in the sound of your voice.

Tone (letter writing)   The way that words and phrases are used to convey a message.

Tongue A strong muscle in the mouth that is covered with taste buds, aids in the digestive process, and contributes to speech formation.

Touch (communication) Conveys a message of warmth, reassurance, understanding and caring.

Transactions and Code Sets HIPAA states that any practice that electronically sends or receives certain transactions must send or receive them in a standard format. This means that all transactions and codes must be available in the same format.

Transfer Methods Methods of relocating files. A filing system works best when the location is accessible and the files are not overcrowded. Therefore, this space should be used only for active files. Those that are not active are transferred to a more remote area.

Treatment Plan Outline of proposed dental treatment.

Treatment Rooms Areas where patients are treated by the dentist, dental hygienist, and dental assistant. Also referred to as "operatories" (although this term is fading from use because patients associate it with "surgical operating room"; some dental personnel may still use it).

Unconditional Positive Regard (communication) Total love and respect, no matter what.

Units (scheduling) Each column of an appointment book is divided into time segments. Each segment represents a unit (units consist of 10- or 15-minute intervals).

Universal Numbering System Tooth numbering system developed in the United States to ensure consistency in identifying individual teeth. Each tooth is assigned a number, with the maxillary right third molar as tooth number 1; maxillary left third molar, tooth number 16; mandibular left third molar, tooth number 17; and mandibular right third molar, tooth number 32.

Upward Channel (organizational communications) Flow of information from one level to a higher level.

Usual, Customary, and Reasonable (UCR) Plan A dental plan that uses the following criteria to establish a fee schedule: usual fee, the fee the dentist uses most often for a given dental service; custom-ary fee, the fee determined by the third party administrator from actual submitted fees for specific dental services; and reasonable fee, a determination by the third party administrator that a particular service for a given procedure has been modified to take into consideration unusual complications. This fee may vary from the dentist's usual fee and the administrator's customary fee.

Usual Fee Fee that the dentist uses most often for a given dental service.

Uvula A projection of tissue located on the posterior of the soft palate that hangs down into the center of the throat.

Veneer Crown Thin coverage on the facial surface that is made with only a cast composite or resin material.

Verbal Messages Messages communicated with words, which can be divided into two categories: spoken and written. Spoken verbal messages can be delivered face to face or transferred electronically (via telephone, voice mail, or video conferencing). Written communication may consist of letters, memos, faxes, e-mails, and newsletters.

Vermilion Border The junction of the tissue of the face and the mucous membrane of the lips.

Vertical File Folders Those folders used with vertical filing systems with tabs located at the top of the file.

Vertical Files Filing cabinets that consist of one to five drawers that, when pulled out, present files from the side rather than the front. When these are used for storage of business records, a frame can be inserted into each drawer that provides a means of hanging files. Hanging files can be labeled, and then individual files can be organized within each hanging file.

Voice Mail Recorded messages accessed by telephone.

White Space (letter writing) Space that surrounds the text of the letter. It should be uniform and balanced.

WNL Abbreviation for "within normal limits."

Work Overload Any amount or type of work that adds to daily stress.

Bibliography

Adler NJ: International Dimensions of Organizational Behavior. 4th edition. Mason, Ohio, South-Western College Publishing, 2001.

American Dental Association. ADA Principles of Ethics and Code of Professional Conduct. Available at: http://www.ada.org/prof/prac/law/code/index.asp.

American Dental Association: Current Dental Terminology: CDT 2005. Chicago, Ill, American Dental Association, 2005.

American Dental Association: Efficient Appointment Scheduling: Training and Management. Chicago, Ill, American Dental Association, 1995.

American Dental Association: Principles of Ethics and Code of Professional Conduct. Chicago, Ill, American Dental Association, 1999.

Applegate EJ: The Anatomy and Physiology Learning System: Instructor's Manual. 3rd edition. Philadelphia, Pa, WB Saunders, 2006.

Applegate EJ: The Anatomy and Physiology Learning System: Textbook. 3rd edition. Philadelphia, Pa, WB Saunders, 2006.

Applegate EJ: The Anatomy and Physiology Learning System: Workbook. 3rd edition. Philadelphia, Pa, WB Saunders, 2006.

ARMA International: Establishing Alphabetic, Numeric, and Subject Filing Systems. Prairie Village, Kansas, Association of Records Managers and Administrators, Inc., 2005.

ARMA International: Professional Resource Catalog: Guides for Effective Information Management. Prairie Village, Kansas, Association of Records Managers and Administrators, Inc., 1996–1997.

Baker SK: Creating positive relationships with dental patients. Paper presented at the Loma Linda University School of Dentistry, October 30, 1997.

Bird D, Robinson D: Modern Dental Assisting. 8th edition. St. Louis, Elsevier Saunders, 2006.

Blunk D: Perfecting the new-patient experience. Dental Practice & Finance 1997;5:47–48.

Bobrow DA: Total recall and reactivation. Dentistry 1997;17:21–23.

Boswell S: Understanding behavioral styles: the art of communicating with patients, peers. Dental Teamwork 1996;9:22–25.

California Dental Association: CDA dental patient bill of rights. Available at: http://www.cda.org/public/rights.html.

California Dental Association: Practice Promotion Seminar: Private and Public Relations: A Wet-Fingered Primer for Dental Office Communications. Sacramento, Calif, California Dental Association.

Caplan CM: The Handbook of Letters and Verbal Responses to Patients for the Dentist and Staff. 3rd edition. Champaign, IL, Colwell Systems Incorporated, 1980.

Carr-Ruffino N: The Promotable Woman: Advancing Through Leadership Skills. 4th edition. Franklin Lakes, NJ, Career Press, 2004.

Christensen GJ: Developing a great dental team. Journal of the American Dental Association 1997; 12:1703–1704.

Cooper TM, DiBiaggio JA: Training dental office personnel. Preview 1995;4:11–20.

Denhardt RB. Public Administration: An Action Orientation. 5th edition. Belmont, Calif, Wadsworth Publishing Company, 2005.

Ehrlich A: Business Administration for the Dental Assistant. 4th edition. Champaign, Ill, Colwell Systems, 1991.

Finkbeiner BL, Finkbeiner CA: Practice Management for the Dental Team. 6th edition. St. Louis, Elsevier Mosby, 2006.

Furlong A: Electronic claims filing made easy. Available at: http://www.ada.org/prof/resources/pubs/adanews/adanewsarticle.asp?articleid=1240.

Furlong A: HIPAA security required April 2005. Available at: http://www.ada.org/prof/resources/pubs/adanews/adanewsarticle.asp?articleid=490.

Furlong A: Inform patients with new HIPAA posters, brochure. Available online at: http://www.ada.org/prof/resources/pubs/adanews/adanewsarticle.asp?articleid=260.

Hartley C, Jones E: American Medical Association: HIPAA plain and simple: a compliance guide for health care professionals. Chicago, AMA Press, 2004.

Internal Revenue Service: Employer's Tax Guide. Publication 15, Circular E. Available at http://www.irs.gov/publications/p15/index.html. Accessed January 2006.

Internal Revenue Service: Starting a Business and Keeping Records. Publication 583. Available at www:http://www.irs.gov/publications/p583/index.html. Accessed January 2006.

International Organization for Standardization: New ISO standard for managing business records. Available at: http://www.iso.org/iso/en/commcentre/pressreleases/archives/2002/Ref814.html.

Jameson C: Don't let patients fall through the cracks. Dental Practice & Finance 1998;6:21–25.

Jones DG: Evolving business: keeping up with the profession is the challenge. CDA Journal 1998;26:29–36.

Kehoe B, Blunk D: The new "gold standard" in patient service. Dental Practice & Finance 1998;6:15–19.

Limoli TM, Limoli TM Jr: Insurance reimbursement. Compendium 1997;18:604–612.

Los Angeles County Office of Education: Job Finders Guide: How to Obtain and Advance in the Job of Your Choice. 4th edition. Downey, Calif, Los Angeles County Office of Education, 2001.

Manji I: Beyond the bells and whistles: what high technology really delivers. Dental Teamwork 1996;9:13–17.

Manji I, Snyder T, Freydberg B: Taking Care of Business: Selecting a Dental Computer: A Step-by-Step Workbook, vol 3. Cherry Hill, NJ, ExperDent Consultants Inc., 1994.

Mann L: Payment cards: a practical rx for dental office collections. The Dental Assistant Journal 1993;62:13–15.

McKenzie S: 4 key elements of a successful recall system. The Dental Assistant 1995;64:13–16.

Occupational Safety and Health Administration: Ergonomics. Available at http://www.osha.gov/SLTC/ergonomics/.

Price Waterhouse LLP: Cover Letters and Other Correspondence. Available at http://www.career.virginia.edu/students/resources/handouts/coverletters.pdf. Accessed 2005.

Rahim MA: Managing Conflict in Organizations. 3rd edition. Westport, Conn, Quorom Books, 2000.

Reiter C: Taking charge of your career. The Dental Assistant 1995;64:5–9.

Robinson D, Bird D: Essentials of Dental Assisting. 4th edition. St. Louis, Elsevier Saunders, 2006.

Schwab D: Today's impatient patient. Journal of the American Dental Association 1997;128:1646–1649.

Sweeney C: Leadership vs. management: can you define the difference? The Dental Assistant Journal 1993;62:4–5.

Trombly RM: Taming the paper tiger: recordkeeping and documentation in the dental office. Dental Teamwork 1996;9:18–21.

Troyka LQ, Hesse D: Simon & Schuster Handbook for Writers. 8th edition. Englewood Cliffs, NJ, Prentice Hall, 2006.

United States Department of Justice: Americans with Disabilities Act: ADA Home Page. Available at www:http://www.usdoj.gov/crt/ada/adahom1.htm. Accessed June 5, 2006.

United States Postal Service: Consumer's Guide to Postal Services and Products. Washington, DC, United States Postal Service, 1996.

United States Postal Service: Get More From Your Post Office. Washington, DC, United States Postal Service, 1997.

University of Wisconsin-Madison: Tips for enhancing the office environment. Available at http://www.uwm.edu/Dept/EHSRM/EHS/ERGO/genergotips.html. Accessed February 8, 2006.

US Department of Health & Human Services: HHS patient privacy protection press release. Available at: http://www.hhs.gov/news/press/2002pres/20020809a.html.

US Department of Health & Human Services: HIPAA overview. Available at: http://www.cms.hhs.gov/HIPAAGenInfo/.

US Department of Health & Human Services: Protecting the privacy of patient's health information. Available at: http://www.hhs.gov/news/facts/privacy.html.

Vale GL: California Law and You: A Continuing Education Program. Self-published.

Washington T: Resume Power: Selling Yourself on Paper in the New Millennium. 7th edition. Bellevue, Wash, Mount Vernon Press, 2003.

Wiles CB: The Complete Dental Letter Handbook: Your Fingertip Resource for Practice Communications. Phoenix, Ariz, Semantodontics, 1989.

Wisconsin Dental Association, Inc.: The Dental Record by Dentists, for Dentists: The Dentist's Manual on Record Keeping. Milwaukee, Wis, Wisconsin Dental Association Professional Services, Inc., 1995.

Index

Page numbers followed by f indicate figure; t, table.